Plastic Surgery

FACTS

Christopher Stone

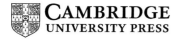

CAMBRIDGE
UNIVERSITY PRESS

CAMBRIDGE UNIVERSITY PRESS
Cambridge, New York, Melbourne, Madrid, Cape Town, Singapore, São Paulo

CAMBRIDGE UNIVERSITY PRESS
The Edinburgh Building, Cambridge CB2 2RU, UK

Published in the United States of America by Cambridge University Press, New York

www.cambridge.org
Information on this title: www.cambridge.org/9780521674492

First published 2001 by Greenwich Medical Media Limited
Second edition 2006

Printed in the United Kingdom at the University Press, Cambridge

A catalogue record for this publication is available from the British Library

ISBN-13 978-0-521-67449-2 paperback
ISBN-10 0-521-67449-2 paperback

Plastic Surgery: Facts (Second Edition)

This text has been designed specifically to help senior plastic surgery trainees to prepare for and pass their postgraduate examinations in plastic surgery. It will also appeal to trainees with less experience who may use it as a core text during their training. The first edition of this text was written by the author in preparation for the FRCS(Plast) examination. It is a collection of notes that addresses the whole curriculum of plastic surgery providing information on clinical anatomy, points of technique and the fundamental principles relevant to each subject area. There are self-assessment sections and hundreds of reviews of published articles. This text has become essential reading for all trainees and the second edition has sought to update the text, mainly with regard to material published over the past 5 years. There is no other textbook of plastic surgery of this kind available to trainees in plastic surgery.

Contents

Abbreviations

A

AA	amyloid A
ABGs	arterial blood gases
ACE	angiotensin converting enzyme
ACTH	adrenocorticotrophic hormone
AD	autosomal dominant
ADH	anti-diuretic hormone
ADM	abductor digiti minimi
AER	apical ectodermal ridge
AIDS	acquired immunodeficiency syndrome
AKA	above knee amputation
AK	actinic keratosis
AL	amyloid L
ALM	acral lentinginous melanoma
Ab	antibody
AP	antero-posterior, abductor pollicis
APB	abductor pollicis brevis
APL	abductor pollicis longus
AR	autosomal recessive
ARDS	adult respiratory distress syndrome
ASA	American Society of Anesthesiologists
ASD	arterial septal defect
ASIS	anterior superior iliac spine
ATLS	advanced trauma life support
AV	arteriovenous
AVM	arteriovenous malformation
AVN	avascular necrosis

B

BAPS	British Association of Plastic Surgeons
BBA	British Burn Association
BBR	bilateral breast reduction
BCC	basal cell carcinoma
BEAM	bulbar elongation and anastomotic meatoplasty
bFGF	basic fibroblast growth factor

BJPS	British Journal of Plastic and Reconstructive Surgery
BKA	below knee amputation
BMP	bone morphogenetic protein
BOA	British Orthopaedic Association
BP	blood pressure
BPB	brachial plexus block
BSA	body surface area
BXO	balanitis xerotica obliterans

C

CAH	congenital adrenal hyperplasia
CCF	congestive cardiac failure
CEA	cultured epithelial autografts
CF	craniofacial
CGRP	calcitonin gene related peptide
CJD	Creutzfeldt-Jakob disease
CL/P	cleft lip/palate
CMC	carpo-metacarpal
CMF	cisplatin, melphalan, 5-fluorouracil
CNS	central nervous system
CO	carbon monoxide
COHb	carboxyhaemoglobin
CPAP	continuous positive airways pressure
CP	cleft palate
CRP	C reactive protein
CRPS	complex regional pain syndromes
CSAG	Clinical Standards Advisory Group
CSF	cerebrospinal fluid
CT	computed tomography
CTR	carpal tunnel release
CTS	carpal tunnel syndrome
CURA	comprehensive urgent reconstruction alternative
CVA	cardiovascular accident
CXR	chest X-ray

D

DCIA	Deep circumflex iliac artery
DCIS	ductal carcinoma in situ
DD	Dupuytren's disease
DIC	disseminated intravascular coagulation
DIEA	deep inferior epigastric artery
DIEP	deep inferior epigastric perforator (flap)
DIPJ	distal interphalangeal joint
DISI	dorsal intercalated segment instability
DMCA	dorsal metacarpal artery (flap)
DNA	deoxyribonucleic acid

DoH	Department of Health
DP	distal phalanx
DPA	deep peroneal artery
DPT	dental panoramic tomogram
DRUJ	distal radioulnar joint
DSA	digital subtraction angiogram
DTIC	dimethyltriaxeno imidazole carboxamide
DVT	deep venous thrombosis

E

EC	extensor communis
ECG	electrocardiograph
ECMO	extracorporeal membrane oxygenation
ECRB	extensor carpi radialis brevis
ECRL	extensor carpi radialis longus
ECU	extensor carpi ulnaris
EDC	extensor digitorum communis
EDL	extensor digitorum longus
EDM	extensor digiti minimi
EGF	epidermal growth factor
EGFR	epidermal growth factor receptor
EHL	extensor hallucis longus
EI	estensor indicis
ELND	elective lymph node dissection
EM	electron microscopy
EMG	electromyograph
ENT	ear, nose and throat
EPB	extensor pollicis brevis
EPL	extensor pollicis longus
ESR	erythrocyte sedimentation rate
ET	endotracheal
EUA	examination under anaesthetic

F

FBC	full blood count
FC	fasciocutaneous (flap)
FCR	flexor carpi radialis
FCU	flexor carpi ulnaris
FDA	Food and Drug Administration
FDL	flexor digitorum longus
FDM	flexor digiti minimi
FDP	flexor digitorum profundus
FDS	flexor digitorum superficialis
FGF	fibroblast growth factor
FGFR	fibroblast growth factor receptor
FHL	flexor hallucis longus

FNA	final needle aspiration
FPL	flexor pollicis longus
FT	full thickness
FTSG	full thickness skin graft

G

GA	general anaesthesia
GAG	glycosaminoglycan
GFR	glomerular filtration rate
GGF	glial growth factor
GI	gastrointestinal
GM-CSF	granulocyte-macrophage colony stimulating factor
Gp&S	(blood) group and save
GRAP	glanular reconstruction and prepucioplasty
GRH	gonadotrophin releasing hormone
GRO	growth related gene
GTN	glyceryl trinitrate
GU	genitourinary

H

Hb	haemoglobin
HBV	hepatitis B virus
HCG	human chorionic gonadotrophin
HCL	hydrogen chloride
HCV	hepatitis C virus
HF	hydrofluoric acid
HIV	human immunodeficiency virus
HLA	human leukocyte antigen
HPV	human papilloma virus
HR	heart rate
HSV	herpes simplex virus

I

ICD	idiopathic cervical dystonia
ICP	intracranial pressure
IDDM	insulin-dependent diabetes mellitus
IEA	inferior epigastric artery
IF	interferon
IGF	insulin-like growth factor
IL	interleukin
ILP	isolated limb perfusion
IM	intramuscular
IM	intramedullary
IMF	intermaxillary fixation
IP	interphalangeal (joint)
ITU	intensive therapy unit
IV	intravenous

K

KCI	Kinetic Concepts Inc.
KTP	Potassium, Titanyl, Phosphate (laser)

L

La	Latin
LA	local anaesthetic
LAK	lymphokine-activated killer
LASER	light amplification by stimulated emission of radiation
LB	leukotriene (B)
LCIS	lobular carcinoma in situ
LC	Langerhans cell
LD50	lethal dose (50%)
LD	latissimus dorsi
LFTs	liver function tests
LH	luteinising hormone
LHRH	luteinising hormone releasing hormone
LIMA	left internal mammary artery
LM	lentigo maligna
LMM	lentigo maligna melanoma
LND	lymph node dissection

M

MAGPI	meatal advancement and glanulopasty incorporated
MASER	microwave amplification by stimulation emission of radiation
MGSA	melanocyte growth-stimulating activity
MM	malignant melanoma
MND	motor neurone disease
MP	metacarpophalangeal (joint)
MRI	magnetic resonance imaging
mRNA	messenger RNA
MRSA	methicillin-resistant Staphylococcus aureus
MSG	Melanoma Study Group
MTP	metatarsophalangeal (joint)
MUA	manipulation under anaesthetic

N

NAI	non-accidental injury
NCS	nerve conduction studies
Nd: YAG	neodymium:yttrium aluminium garnet
NF-2	neurofibromatosis-2
NGF	nerve growth factor
NGT	nasogastric tube
NK	natural killer (cell)
NL	nasolabial
NMDA	N-methyl-D-aspartate

NO	nitrous oxide
NSAID	non-steroidal anti-inflammatory drug
NV	neurovascular

O

OA	osteoarthritis
OI	osteogenesis imperfecta
OM	occipitomental
OPT	orthopantomogram
ORIF	open reduction and internal fixation
OT	occupational therapist

P

PA	postero-anterior
PAWG	posterior auricular Wolff graft
PB	peroneus brevis
PBCM	particulate bone and cancellous marrow
PBS	phosphate buffered saline
PCR	polymerase chain reaction
PD	proximo-distal
PDA	patent ductus arteriosus
PDG	(glucose-6-) phosphate dehydrogenase
PDGF	platelet derived growth factor
PDS	polydioxanone
PE	pulmonary embolus
PG	prostaglandin
PIPJ	proximal interphalangeal joint
PL	peroneus longus
PMA	pectoralis major advancement (flap)
PMSH	past medical and surgical history
PNS	peripheral nervous system
POP	plaster of Paris
PP	proximal phalanx
PRCA	posterior radial collateral artery
PRS	*Plastic and Reconstructive Surgery* (journal)
PSA	pleomorphic salivary adenoma
PSIS	posterior superior iliac spine
PT	peroneus tertius
PTFE	polytetrafluoroethylene
PWS	plagiocephaly without synostosis
PWS	port wine stain
PZ	progress zone

Q

| QDS | four times daily |

R

RA	radial artery
RA	retinoic acid
RA	rheumatoid arthritis
RAFF	radial artery forearm flap
RBBB	right bundle branch block
RCL	radial collateral ligament
RF	rheumatoid factor
RFF	radial forearm flap
RhPDGF	recombinant human PDGF
ROM	range of movement
RSD	reflex sympathetic dystrophy
RSS	rotatory subluxation of the scaphoid
RTA	road traffic accident

S

S-GAP	superior gluteal perforator (flap)
S-QUATTRO	Stockport serpentine spring system
SC	subcutaneous, subcuticular
SCC	squamous cell carcinoma
SCI	superficial circumflex iliac
SCIA	superficial circumflex iliac artery
SCM	sternocleidomastoid
SDD	selective digestive tract decontamination
SL	scapholunate
SLAC	scapholunate advanced collapse
SLE	systemic lupus erythematosus
SMAS	superficial musculo-aponeurotic system
SMR	submucous resection
SNS	sympathetic nervous system
SSD	silver sulfadiazine
SSG	split skin graft
SSM	superficial spreading melanoma
SSM	skin sparing mastectomy
SVR	systemic vascular resistance

T

TAP	tunica albuginea plication
TBSA	total body surface area
Tc	cytotoxic T cell
TC	Treacher Collins (syndrome)
TCA	trichloroacetic acid
TCC	transitional cell carcinoma
TENS	Transcutaneous Electric Nerve Stimulation
TE	tissue expansion
TFCC	triangular fibrocartilaginous complex

TFL	tensor fascia lata
TGF	transforming growth factor
TICAS	trauma-induced cold-associated symptoms
TLND	therapeutic lymph node dissection
TMJ	temporomandibular joint
TMN	tumour, metastases, nodes (classification)
TMT	tarsometatarsal (joint)
TNF	tumour necrosis factor
TPN	total parenteral nutrition
TRAM	transverse rectus abdominis muscle (flap)
TXA2	thromboxane A2

U

U&Es	urea & electrolytes
UAL	ultrasonic assisted liposuction
UCL	ulnar collateral ligament
UC	ulcerative colitis
UMN	upper motor neurone
URTI	upper respiratory tract infection
USS	ultrasound scan
UTI	urinary tract infection
UV	ultraviolet

V

VAC	vacuum assisted closure
VCF	velocardiofacial
VCs	venae commitantes
VEGF	vascular endothelial growth factor
VF	ventricular fibrillation
VISI	volar intercalated segment instability
VPI	velopharyngeal incompetence
VRAM	vertical rectus abdominis muscle (flap)
VSD	ventricular septal defect

W

| WLE | wide local excision |

X

| XFNG | cross facial nerve graft |
| XP | xeroderma pigmentosa |

Z

| ZPA | zone of polarizing activity |

Preface

Five years have elapsed since the publication of the first edition of *Plastic Surgery: Facts*, a text that essentially consolidated my preparation for the FRCS(Plast) examination in 1999. Since then I have been gratified and encouraged by the feedback that I have received from many trainees in plastic surgery who have found the book useful as part of their own structured revision for examinations or simply as a source of information in their training.

The second edition of *Plastic Surgery: Facts* updates much of the plastic surgery and related literature over the past 5 years. Some areas have developed rapidly, while others have changed little. Plastic surgery encompasses many different disciplines under one umbrella and at times it would seem that future disintegration into a number of factions allied to other surgical specialties is inevitable. However, it is precisely this broad spectrum of principles and techniques that is fundamental to our cohesion and versatility as plastic surgeons and this remains our greatest strength.

In each chapter there are new citations that have been selected either for their educational value or scientific importance but, perhaps predictably, my own sub-specialty interests have received particular attention. Consequently, the sections on malignant melanoma and soft tissue sarcoma have expanded to reflect my own greater understanding of these areas.

Future editions of the book are likely to increasingly rely upon contributions from other authors and my intention is that *Plastic Surgery: Facts* will propagate as a text written by trainees for trainees. This transition begins with the second edition and I am enormously indebted to my friend and colleague David Oliver, who, despite busy family and clinical commitments in Australia over the past year, has managed to make significant contributions to the manuscript, co-editing chapters on cleft surgery, hypospadias, hand and breast surgery.

I hope that this text continues to provide a useful overview of the plastic surgery curriculum for all aspiring plastic surgeons, as well as for those of us charged with the responsibility for educating them.

Cutaneous neoplasia and hamartomas (BCC, SCC, melanoma, vascular malformations, sarcomas)

1

Overview of aetiology of neoplasms

Clin Plastic Surg 1997; 24(4)
A neoplasm is an abnormal mass of tissue, the growth of which exceeds, and is uncoordinated with that of the normal tissues and which persists in the same excessive manner after cessation of the stimulus which evoked the change
A malignant neoplasm is one that invades surrounding tissues and has a propensity to metastasize
Initiation, promotion and progression lead to unrestrained growth and proliferation:
Initiation: a change in the genome of a cell
Promotion: the change made permanent by cellular division (initiators and promoters include UV and ionizing radiation, chemical carcinogens, viruses)

Progression: further cell division to form an invasive tumour

Inappropriate activation of normal cellular proto-oncogenes to become oncogenes – these proto-oncogenes encode growth factors, growth factor receptors or transcription factors

Inactivation of other cellular genes called tumour suppresser genes

p53 tumour suppresser gene is mutated in the majority of human cancers

UV radiation is the most important factor

First, mutations in cellular DNA and a failure of DNA repair

Second, production of immunosuppressive cytokines, depletion and alteration of antigen-presenting LCs and systemic induction of Ts-cells by altered LCs, inflammatory macrophages and cytokines

Sunburn, suntanning, local and systemic immunosuppression, photo-ageing, skin cancer and precancer are attributed to **UVB radiation (290–320 nm)**

UVA radiation (320–400 nm) generates oxygen-free radicals that damage cell membranes and nuclear DNA, contributing to erythema, photo-ageing and carcinogenesis

Interruption of intercellular and intracellular signalling cascades regulating transcription and function of viral oncoproteins in human keratinocytes

Interaction between a physical carcinogen (UV part of the sunlight) and a 'low risk' (non-mutagenic) papillomavirus infection

Benign epithelial tumours

Seborrhoeic keratosis (seborrheic wart, senile wart, basal cell papilloma)

Incidence
Males = females, fifth decade onwards

White races

Stucco keratosis – non-pigmented seborrhoeic keratosis on the limbs

Dermatosis papulosa nigra – multiple facial lesions, dark skinned races, early onset

Aetiology
Familial – autosomal dominant

Inflammatory dermatosis

Manifestation of visceral malignancy

Oestrogen administration

Pathology
Accumulation of immature keratinocytes between basal and keratinizing layers

Acanthosis – thickening of the epidermis

Elongation of dermal papillae

Malignant transformation reported but rare (squamous type)

Clinical
Verrucous plaque

Face, hands and upper trunk

May be heavily pigmented

Multiple lesions aligned in direction of skin folds

May bleed, become inflamed and itch

May shed but then reform

Treatment

Curettage or excision

Cryotherapy

Topical trichloroacetic acid

Digital fibrokeratoma

Papillary or keratotic outgrowth in the region of a finger joint

Adults, males > females

Follows trauma

Hyperkeratosis and acanthosis (thickening of the epidermis, specifically the stratum spinosum)

Distinguish from supernumerary digit

Treat by excision

Keratoacanthoma (*Molluscum sebaceum*)

Rapidly evolving tumour which resolves untreated

Keratinizing squamous cells originating in pilosebaceous follicles

Incidence

White races

Males > females (×3)

One-third frequency of SCC

Middle age onwards

Aetiology

Sun exposure

Coal, tar and carcinogenic hydrocarbons (multiple lesions)

Injury and infection including skin graft donor sites

Association with carcinoma of the larynx, internal malignancies and leukaemia

Association with deficient cell-mediated immunity (multiple lesions)

Pathology

Keratin-filled crypt

Rapidly dividing squamous cells deriving from skin appendages

Atypical mitoses and loss of polarity

Clinical

Globular tumour

Keratin plug or horn

Radial symmetry

Resolution begins after 6 weeks, takes 3 months
Face, dorsum of hand
Torre's syndrome: multiple internal malignancies, KAS and sebaceous adenomas
Distinguish from SCC

Treatment

Excise to provide good histological specimen
Spontaneous resolution leaves unsightly scar
5-FU and radiotherapy shorten time to resolution

Hair follicle tumours

Trichilemmal cyst

Sebaceous cyst of hairy skin
Wall resembles hair follicle
Situated on the scalp
Women > men
Middle age
Familial (AD)
Rupture causes cell proliferation and occasionally malignant change
Ruptured cell wall may fuse with surrounding skin (marsupialization)
Treat by excision

Trichofolliculoma

Multiple malformed hair roots arising from an enlarged follicle canal
Keratin-filled crater
Hairs may emerge from a central punctum
Mainly on the face

Tricholemmoma

Hair follicle tumour usually diagnosed clinically as BCC
Plaques of squamous cells containing glycogen
Occurs on the face
Middle-aged/elderly men

Tricho-epithelioma

Epithelial tumour differentiating towards hair follicle cells

Incidence
Rare, onset at puberty

Aetiology
Familial (AD)

Pathology

Resembles BCC

Rounded masses of fusiform cells

Lacunae filled with keratin

Tumour islands may connect with hair follicles

Malignant change (BCC)

Clinical

Pinkish nodules

Cheeks, eyelids and nasolabial folds

Often diagnosed as BCC, pigmented lesions mistaken for MM

Treatment

Excision

Pilomatrixoma (benign calcifying epithelioma of Malherbe)

Hamartoma composed of dead, calcified cells, which resemble those of hair matrix

Incidence

Uncommon

Mainly <20 years

Females > males

Association with myotonia atrophica

Pathology

Well-circumscribed dermal tumour

Cells mature from outer to inner layers

Similar to hair matrix cells maturing from cortex to root sheath

Central calcification and ghost cells, lacking basophilic granules

Clinical

Dermal/subcutaneous tumour

Head, neck, upper extremity

Stony hard consistency

Treatment

Excision

Tumours of sebaceous glands

Sebaceous adenoma

Benign tumour composed of incompletely differentiated sebaceous cells

Incidence

Rare tumour

Either sex
Mainly in the elderly

Pathology
Multilobular tumour of the upper dermis
Small basophilic sebaceous matrix cells
Larger cells containing fat globules

Clinical
Ulcers/plaques/sessile or pedunculated lesions
Yellowish hue
Face (including eyelid) or scalp
Sudden increase in growth rate

Treatment
Excision
Recur if incompletely excised
Radiosensitive

Sebaceous carcinoma

Malignant growth of cells differentiating towards sebaceous epithelium

Incidence and aetiology
Rare – 0.2% of skin cancers
May follow radiodermatitis

Pathology
Deeply set in dermis, epidermis usually uninvolved
Outer basophilic undifferentiated cells
Central differentiating cells with cytological atypia
Cytoplasmic vacuolation and fat droplets
Invasion

Clinical
Yellowish nodules on face and scalp
Slow or rapid growth
Metastasis uncommon

Treatment
Excision

Epidermoid cyst (sebaceous cyst)

Incidence and aetiology
Young and middle-aged adults
Inflammation and obstruction of a pilosebaceous follicle

Pathology

Epidermal lining

Birefringent keratin and breakdown products

Cholesterol clefts

Clinical

Spherical cyst in the dermis

Tethered to epidermis

Enlarge and suppurate through punctum

Treatment

Excision

Sweat gland tumours

Apocrine glands release lipid secretions in membrane-bound vesicles (e.g. breasts)

Eccrine glands release secretions by exostosis into ducts

Holocrine glands discharge whole cells which then disintegrate to release secretions

Sweat glands: mainly eccrine secretion, some apocrine

Sebaceous glands: holocrine secretion of sebum

Three benign eccrine sweat gland tumours: syringoma, acrospiroma, cylindroma

Syringoma (papillary eccrine adenoma)

Benign tumour of eccrine sweat gland origin

Incidence

Uncommon

Females > males

Onset during adolescence

Multiple tumours associated with Down's syndrome

Pathology

Collections of convoluted sweat ducts in the upper dermis

Tail-like projection of cells – characteristic tadpole appearance

Clinical

Small, yellowish dermal papules, usually <3 mm

May appear cystic – injury may cause release of a small amount of clear fluid

Chest, face, neck

May resemble tricho-epithelioma or xanthelasma

Treatment

Excision

Intralesional electrodesiccation

Laser

Eccrine acrospiroma

Tumour derived from eccrine sweat duct epithelium
Epidermal, juxta-epidermal or dermal
Eccrine poroma commonest subtype: juxta-epidermal

Incidence
Male = female
Middle age
Usually acral – palms and soles

Pathology
Sweat gland duct cell proliferation
Cells contain glycogen and glycolytic enzymes
Overlying hyperkeratosis
Malignant change (malignant eccrine poroma) reported

Clinical
Hyperkeratotic plaque on sole or palm
May ulcerate

Treatment
Excision

Dermal cylindroma (dermal eccrine cylindroma, turban tumour, Spiegler's tumour)

Derived from the coiled part of sweat glands (part secretory, part duct)

Incidence
Uncommon
Females > males ($\times 2$)
Often familial (AD)
Early adult life

Pathology
Columns of cells interspersed with hyaline material
Large and small (peripheral) cell types

Clinical
Scalp and adjacent skin
Pinkish fleshy tumours
Usually multiple and hairless
May be painful
Malignant change very rare
Distinguish from trichilemmal cyst

Treatment
Excision

Adenoid cystic carcinoma of the scalp

Malignant tumour of eccrine glands
Usually arises in salivary glands
Lacrimal glands and mucous glands of upper respiratory tract
Rarely arises primarily in the skin, mainly eccrine sweat glands of the scalp
Slow growing
Invades fascial planes, nerves and bone
Characteristic lattice-type appearance microscopically
Rarely completely excised
Not radiosensitive
Treat by excision with histological control of margins

Sweat gland carcinoma

Malignant epithelial tumour of the sweat glands

Incidence
Rare
Males = females
Middle age onwards

Pathology
Adenocarcinoma within the dermis
Eccrine or apocrine varieties
Eccrine commonest, frequently metastasizes

Clinical
Painful, reddish nodules within the dermis
Firm/hard
Irregular border
Occur anywhere, mainly scalp and face
Slow growth but may metastasize

Treatment
Wide excision
Monitor lymph nodes

Basal cell carcinoma (basal cell epithelioma, rodent ulcer)

Malignant tumour composed of cells derived from the basal layer of the skin

Incidence
Commonest malignant tumour of the skin in white races
Increased prevalence in locations of high sunlight exposure
Males > females except lower extremity lesions (female:male ratio = 3:1)

Uncommon in non-Caucasians

75% of patients > 40 years old

Aetiology

UV and ionizing irradiation

Burn and vaccination scars

Arsenicals

Immunosuppression

Occasionally has a familial inheritance

Malignant change in sebaceous naevi and other adnexal hamartomas

Face at much greater risk than other sun-exposed areas (may be related to density of pilosebaceous follicles)

Pathology

Tumour cells arranged in palisades

Cell–cell desmosomes preserved

Well-organized surrounding stroma

Varying degrees of atypia

Small buds of tumour off the main mass

Occasionally harbour a melanocytic proliferation

Mucin accumulation and central necrosis characteristic of cystic lesions

Clinical

Pinkish, pearly nodules

Telangiectasia

May be ulcerated, encrusted or pigmented

Nodular, ulcerated, superficial, sclerosing, cystic, morphoeic, desmoplastic

Usually slow growing

Very rarely metastasize via lymphatics

Long-standing tumours may invade deep into subcutaneous tissues

Distinguish from sebaceous hyperplasia

Gorlin's syndrome (basal cell naevus syndrome): AD inheritance, multiple BCCs, palmar pits, jaw cysts, sebaceous cysts, abnormalities of ribs and vertebrae, dural calcification

Bazek's syndrome: association of multiple BCCs with follicular atrophoderma

Treatment

Excisional biopsy: 2–5 mm margins, antibiotic cover if ulcerated

35% of incompletely excised tumours recur; re-excision of incompletely excised tumours shows residual tumour in only 30% of cases

5-FU or photodynamic therapy for superficial lesions

Radiotherapy

Guidelines for the management of basal cell carcinoma

Telfer. *Br J Dermatol* 1999

- Review of surgical and non-surgical modalities used in the treatment of BCCs including
  - Mohs' micrographic surgery
  - Radiotherapy

- Topical chemotherapy
- Intralesional interferon
- Photodynamic therapy

Audit of incompletely excised basal cell carcinoma

Griffiths. *Br J Plastic Surg* 1999
- Retrospective review of 99 BCCs incompletely excised in one surgeon's practice over a 10-year period
- Incompletely excised BCCs accounted for 7% of all lesions removed
- 13% of periorbital lesions and 12% of BCCs on the nose were incompletely excised
- lateral margin involvement most common (55%), deep margin involved in 36% and both lateral and deep margins involved in 9%
- 74 out of 99 incompletely excised lesions were re-excised: residual tumour present in 40 specimens (54%)
  - but only 25% of periorbital re-excision specimens contained residual tumour and none of five patients with incompletely excised tumours developed recurrence after a mean follow-up period of 2 years without further treatment

Incomplete excision of basal cell carcinoma

Kumar. *Br J Plastic Surg* 2002
- Prospective audit of completeness of BCC excision in a plastic surgery department, supra-regional cancer unit and a district general hospital
- Overall incidence of incomplete excision 4.5%
- Similar rates in plastic surgery and DGH settings, slightly higher rate in the cancer unit (syndromal lesions)
- Trunk and extremity BCCs less frequently incompletely excised than facial BCCs
- Lowest incomplete excision rates were amongst non-consultant career grade surgeons (associate specialist and clinical assistant)
- Recurrent and multifocal lesions most prone to incomplete excision, superfical BCC least prone
- Incidence of incomplete excision inversely proportional to excision margin (lowest rates with margins 5 mm or more)
- 50% of patients with incompletely excised BCC underwent early additional treatment, remaining 50% opted for observation (higher average age group)

Premalignant conditions

Solar keratosis

Premalignant keratosis in sun-damaged skin

Pathology

Epidermal hyperplasia, hyperkeratosis (thickening of the keratin layer which is otherwise normal), acanthosis
Basaloid cells adjacent to basement membrane
Elastotic degeneration

Clinical

Keratosis, telangiectasia

Face and dorsum of hands

Clinical conversion into SCC after 10 years (minority)

Resultant SCC slow growing and unlikely to metastasize

Treatment

5-FU

Excision

Photodynamic therapy

Bowen's disease

Intra-epidermal carcinoma

Aetiology

Sun damage

Exposure to arsenicals

Pathology

Squamous proliferation, acanthosis and atypia (nuclear and cellular pleomorphism, hyper-chromatism and frequent mitoses)

Loss of intercellular connections

Basement membrane intact

Clinical

Red hyperkeratotic plaque

Ulceration an indication of invasion

Association with internal malignancy

Erythroplasia of Queyrat: Bowen's disease of the glans penis

Potential for malignant transformation into an invasive SCC (fairly aggressive)

Treatment

5-FU

Photodynamic therapy

Excision

Xeroderma pigmentosum

First described by Kaposi in 1874

Familial disorder (AR) in which a deficiency in DNA repair processes leads to photosensitivity and a predisposition to cutaneous malignancy

Incidence and aetiology

Incidence: 2 per million

All races, male = female

XP (group A) protein (an endonuclease) involved in the process of nucleotide excision and repair: defends cells against the deleterious effects of UVB

Carcinogenesis due to defective DNA repair pathways following UV irradiation (80%)

XP variants (20%) have a defect of DNA replication during the S-phase of the cell cycle following UV irradiation

XPA-deficient transgenic mouse now available

Pathology

Cutaneous atrophy similar to that seen in photo-ageing

Atypical melanocytes

Keratosis

Clinical

>2000-fold increased risk to develop skin cancer at sun-exposed areas

Onset within the first 3 years of life (75%), pursuing a relentless course thereafter

Often small stature, occasionally mentally retarded

Pigmentation/hypopigmentation

Keratoses and susceptibility to infections

Photophobia and conjunctivitis in 80%

Development of cutaneous malignancy (basal and squamous carcinoma, malignant melanoma)

Often fatal before the age of 10 years, 60% die by 20 years of age

Treatment

Protect against sunlight exposure

Excise lesions early

Leukoplakia

Oral or genital mucosa

Oral lesions associated with smoking, intra-oral sepsis (caries), drinking spirits

White–grey verrucoid plaques

Classical histological features of hyperkeratosis, parakeratosis (thickened keratin layer containing nuclear remnants) and acanthosis

15–20% malignant transformation into aggressive SCCs

Treat by avoiding precipitating factors

CO_2 laser or surgery

Poikiloderma

Diffuse atrophy

Leukomelanodermia

Telangiectasia

Predisposition to SCC

Rothmund–Thomson syndrome

Rare inherited disorder

Poikilodermatous skin changes that appear in infancy

Autosomal recessive

Skeletal abnormalities

Bone tumours

Juvenile cataracts

Higher-than-expected incidence of malignancy

Diminished capacity of DNA repair in the fibroblasts following exposure to oncogenic stimuli

Kindler syndrome

Rare inherited skin disease

Acral bullae formation and generalized progressive poikiloderma

Fusion of fingers and toes

Squamous cell carcinoma (squamous epithelioma)

Malignant epidermal tumour whose cells show maturation towards keratin formation

Incidence

Uncommon in dark skinned races

Late middle age onwards

Male:female ratio + 2:1

Aetiology

UV irradiation

Burn scar (Marjolin)

Osteomyelitis sinuses

Granulomatous infections

Hidradenitis superativa

Dermatoses such as poikiloderma

Venous ulcers

Industrial carcinogens and oils

Immunosuppression

Actinic keratoses and Bowen's disease

Xeroderma pigmentosum

Leukoplakia

Pathology

Dermal invasion of atypical Malpighian (spindle) cells

Variable degrees of cellular atypia and differentiation

Well-differentiated tumours exhibit parakeratosis and keratin pearls

Clinical

Firm skin tumour of dorsum of hands, scalp, face

May have everted edges with a keratotic crust

Well-differentiated tumours have a keratin horn

Less well-differentiated lesions flat and ulcerated

Surrounding hyperaemia

Lymph node metastases

Treatment

Excision, antibiotic cover if ulcerated

Radiotherapy

Therapeutic lymph node dissection

Guidelines on the management of squamous cell carcinoma

Motley. *Br J Plastic Surg* 2003

- Review of the overall management of SCC including surgical and adjuvant treatment modalities
- Metastatic potential determied by:
  - Location of tumour
    - Highest in sun-exposed areas including lip
  - Diameter of tumour
    - Tumours >2 cm twice as likely to recur locally and three times more likely to metastasize than smaller tumours
  - Depth of invasion
    - Tumours >4 mm thick most likely to metastasize (>45% incidence)
  - Histological differentiation
    - Poor differentiation and perineural involvement correlate with local and distant recurrence
  - Host immunosuppression

Prognostic indicators in SCC

Griffiths. *Br J Plastic Surg* 2002

- Retrospective review of one surgeon's experience in the management of 171 patients with cutaneous SCC
- 8 of 93 patients available for follow-up died of their disease within 5 years
  - in these patients tumour thickness and tumour diameter were greater compared with surviving patients
  - all eight patients developed nodal disease as their first presentation of metastatic disease, none developed local recurrence
  - mean interval from primary surgery to first metastasis was 9 months (range 1–34 months)
- lateral excision margins similar in surviving and non-surviving patients (7 and 6 mm, respectively)

Epidermal naevi

Naevus: maternal impression (La)

Definition: best defined as a **cutaneous hamartoma**, usually incorporating a proliferation of melanocytes (melanocytic naevus), vascular tissue (vascular naevus) or sebaceous glands (sebaceous naevus)

Sebaceous naevus (Jadassohn)

Hamartomatous lesion comprised predominantly of sebaceous glands

Pathology
Accumulation of mature sebaceous glands with overlying epidermal hyperplasia

Clinical
Pinkish plaques

Mainly scalp/head and neck

Present at birth in 0.3% of neonates but enlarge at adolescence

Malignant transformation in <5%

Mainly BCC, also SCC, sebaceous and apocrine carcinomas

Epidermal naevus syndrome: association of sebaceous naevi with developmental anomalies, especially of the CNS, eye and skeleton

Treatment
Excision to prevent malignant transformation

Vascular birthmarks

Haemangiomas: increased turnover of endothelial cells, proliferate and involute (e.g. strawberry naevus)

Vascular malformations: inborn errors of vascular morphogenesis, permanent and progressive: capillary, lymphatic, venous, arterial, combined

Salmon patch

Pinkish patch, mostly on the nape of the neck, in 50% of infants

Usually disappears within 1 year

Ectatic superficial dermal capillaries

Thought to reflect persistence of fetal-type dermal circulation

Transient flushing during crying and exertion, etc.

Strawberry naevus (capillary haemangioma)

Benign neoplasm of vasoformative tissue

Well-defined life cycle of proliferation and involution

Immature vasoformative cells fill the dermis

Progressive maturation towards capillary or cavernous channels

bFGF and VEGF over-expression?

90% appear at birth or within the first month of life

White races > dark races

?Low birth weight

Female:male = 3:1

Twenty times more common than PWS

May be deeply located, i.e. subcutaneous, and appear bluish

Most common birthmark, mostly head and neck

- by 1 year of age 10% of white children have a haemangioma
- 80% single, 20% multiple

Grow rapidly in the first 5–8 months of life

Intravascular thrombosis and fibrosis result in regression

Also corresponds with mast cell infiltration

(50% aged 5 years, 60% aged 6, 70% aged 7, etc.)

Pale pink scar, wrinkled scar

Multiple haemangiomas may be associated with internal haemangiomas of CNS, liver, lungs, gut

Non-operative treatments:

- observation only
- dressings for minor bleeding
- corticosteroids:
  - high dose short course (4 mg/kg/day for 2 weeks followed by a gradual tailing off) used for the treatment of rapidly growing haemangiomas but must be under close supervision of a paediatric endocrinologist. Of lesions in the active phase, 100% respond but rebound growth can occur as steroids are gradually withdrawn
  - administration of intralesional steroids (triamcinolone) has been reported when treating peri-orbital haemangiomas but complications include:
    - globe perforation
    - infection
    - fat atrophy
    - dyspigmentation
    - bleeding
    - blindness
    - eyelid necrosis
    - adrenal suppression
    - retinal artery embolization
  - compression
  - pulsed-dye laser (or argon laser for deeper tissues)
  - radiation
  - cryotherapy
  - interferon – used for life-threatening lesions only, e.g. systemic haemangiomatosis, 10–25% of children develop permanent spasticity as a result of interferon treatment

Complications

Ulceration, recurrent bleeding and infection

Skeletal distortion

High output cardiac failure

Late: scarring, residual colour, residual mass, redundant skin

Indications for surgery

Obstruction of lumina (oral cavity, airways) – neonates are obligate nasal breathers

Impingement on visual axis causing amblyopia. Upper lid haemangiomas → deformation of the growing cornea → astigmatism

Severe bleeding or ulceration unresponsive to conservative treatments

Kasabach–Merritt syndrome: sequestration of platelets leading to thrombocytopenia, consumption coagulopathy and DIC → 30–40% mortality rate

Very small lesion, with psychological morbidity, easily excised and directly closed. Nasal tip (Cyrano de Bergerac nose) and vermilion lesions very slow to resolve

Late scar revision

Uncomplicated haemangiomas should, in general, be left alone until complete involution

If a surgical route is taken and the haemangioma is big, consider tissue expansion

Management of haemangioma of infancy

Achauer. *PRS* 1995

Review of treatment vs. outcome in strawberry naevi

Laser therapy proved to be most efficacious in terms of volume reduction, colour and texture compared with observation, steroids, surgery or combined modalities

Recommended for consideration for early use in complicated haemangiomas and to avoid psychological morbidity

Haemangiomas of the lip

Zide. *PRS* 1997

Difficulty in eating and drinking

Psychosocial morbidity

Early intervention advocated to avoid teasing and childhood depression (2–3 years of age)

Debulking procedures – horizontal and vertical elliptical/wedge excisions

Mucosal advancement to reconstruct vermilion

Bulk reconstruction with free scalp–fascial grafts

Steroids → control of endothelial cell proliferation

- 30–90% response rate during the proliferative phase
- but → growth retardation

Waiting for involution and scar revision is psychologically debilitating

Reduction of haemangioma bulk should be conservative

Over-reduction results from excision of muscle

Surgery itself may expedite involutional changes

Avoid lip denervation by central or paracentral reduction

Intralesional photocoagulation of peri-orbital haemangioma

Achauer. *PRS* 1999

Bare tip laser introduced **into** the haemangioma

More effective in reducing bulky tumours without affecting the overlying skin

KTP and Nd:YAG lasers used

Avoids amblyopia secondary to a mechanical ptosis

23 patients treated

Two-thirds had a >50% reduction in haemangioma bulk at 3 months

Ulceration provoked in four patients

Vascular anomalies: hemangiomas

Gampper. *Plastic Reconstruc Surg* 2001

Haemangiomas:

- vascular lesion, increased endothelial cell turnover
- grow rapidly then involute
- most common tumour of infancy
- typically appear after 3 months of life
- 2–5x more common in girls
- 60% in cervicofacial region
- 20% multiple
- may have autosomal dominant inheritance pattern in some patients
- may be associated with other congenital abnormalities
  - PHACES syndrome
    - Posterior cranial fossa malformations
    - Haemagiomas
    - Arterial anomalies
    - Cardiac anomalies
    - Eye anomalies
    - Sternal cleft
  - Dandy–Walker malformation
    - Absence of carotid or vertebral vessels
    - Bifid or cleft sternum
    - Supraumbilical raphe
    - Haemangiomas
    - Female:male 9:1
- superfical or deep location
  - deep lesions may have a bluish colour and be confused with a venous vascular malformation
  - visceral lesions can occur without cutaneous lesions
- early onset of resolution leads to opitmal cosmetic outcome
  - rate of resolution unaffected by ulceration, size or depth of lesion
  - VEGF expression decreases with resolution but bFGF remains high
  - Mast cell population dramatically increases in involuting lesions

Vascular malformations

Mullikan and Glowacki classification 1982

Low flow	High flow
Capillary (PWS)	Arterial
Venous	Arteriovenous
Lymphatic	

Port-wine stain

Pathology
Combined capillary **vascular malformation**

Progressive ectatic dilatation of mature superficial dermal vessels

Developmental weakness of vessel wall

In distribution of fifth cranial nerve suggesting a neurogenic pathogenesis

Relative or absolute deficiency of sympathetic innervation

Relative deficiency – slow growing

Absolute deficiency – rapidly growing

Incidence

Male:female + 1:1

Almost always present at birth

Clinical

Deep red–purple colour

Mostly face, also upper trunk

Growth in proportion to the child

Flat but may progress to become nodular (cobblestoning) and hypertrophic over time (related to density of SNS innervation – absolute deficiency causes an aggressive lesion)

Some fade, others deepen in colour

May be associated with congenital glaucoma or ipsilateral leptomeningeal angiomatosis (**Sturge–Weber syndrome**)

- affects trigeminal nerve distribution
- may have intractable epilepsy
- V2 and V3 malformation only → low risk of brain involvement

Limbs – **Klippel–Trenauney syndrome**: associated with limb bone and soft tissue hypertrophy and **lateral** varicose veins; if AV malformations are present this is **Parkes–Weber syndrome**

Differential diagnoses

Flat haemangioma

Naevus flammeus neonatorum

- affects supratrochlear or supra-orbital nerve territories, one-half resolve spontaneously, remainder persist but never progress
- fading macular stain, affects 50% of neonates

Treatment

Cosmetic camouflage

Argon/pulsed-dye laser

Laser treatment: 10% completely ablated, 60–70% improved, 20% no benefit

Up to 50% may recur after 4 years

Port-wine machrochelia

Zide. *PRS* 1997

Lasers effective in treating colour but do little to reduce bulk

PWS does not involute therefore no rationale for delayed surgery

Lip reduction surgery to debulk the malformation

Laser depigmentation post-operatively

Low flow lesion so bleeding is not excessive but expect oozing

Aim for slight over-reduction

Venous malformation

May be hereditary

Usually multiple

No involution

Superficial or deep venous lakes

May form phleboliths – pathognomonic – as young as 2 years of age

Thrombophlebitis

Lips are site of predilection, usually laterally, also tongue

Soft blue skin and subcutaneous swellings

Empty with compression and elevation

No pulsation

Drains under gravity

Cosmetic deformity, possibly some functional sequelae

Increased activity with trauma, infection

Also crying, straining in an infant

Also responds to hormonal environment

Deep involvement of masseter and parotid

Bony involvement is rare – but mandible is commonest

Orbital venous malformation can → enophthalmos or exorbitism (depending upon filling) and may communicate with the infratemporal fossa via the inferior orbital fissure

May have a coagulopathy due to decreased fibrinogen

MRI:

- T_1-weighted image – iso-intense with muscle
- T_2-weighted image – hyperintense, phleboliths appear as dark holes

Treatment

Conservative – compression garments

Pre-operative sclerotherapy – 95% ethanol or sodium tetradecyl sulphate 3% (maximum 30 ml), staged injections every 3 months

Then surgical – carefully define the extent of involvement of the soft tissues

Evaluation and treatment of head and neck venous malformations

Pappas. *Ear, Nose Throat J* 1998

Low flow, non-proliferative lesions

Percutaneous puncture and injection of contrast defines the lesion using digital subtraction angiography

Head and neck venous malformations become engorged during Valsalva manoeuvre

Sclerotherapy effective in reducing the size of the lesion

- 95% ethanol
- immediate coagulation
- intense inflammatory response
- late fibrosis
- extravasation → soft tissue necrosis

Assess at 4 months following sclerotherapy

Surgery reserved for residual disease

Sclerotherapy contraindicated where the venous malformation communicated with the ophthalmic veins to avoid cavernous sinus thrombosis

Some patients underwent laser treatment as an adjunct to sclerotherapy (argon and Nd:YAG)

AV malformations

Warm, pulsating, thrill, bruit

High flow

Present at birth at a microscopic level

Enlarge at puberty or following puberty

Localized or diffuse

Midline upper lip common

High output cardiac failure

Need MRI and DSA before operating

Intracranial > limbs > trunk > viscera

May → ulceration, bleeding, pain

Schobinger classification

(International Workshop for the Study of Vascular Anomalies 1990)

- Stage 1 – AV shunting – **quiescence**
- Stage 2 – thrill, pulsation, bruit – **expansion**
- Stage 3 – ulceration, bleeding, pain – **destruction**
- Stage 4 – high output cardiac failure – **decompensation**

Treatment

Directed predominantly at stages 3 and 4

Embolization → recruitment of other feeding vessels so inadequate treatment alone

Pre-operative angiography and embolization followed by surgery within 24–48 h

High-grade lesions may involve skin making skin excision mandatory

- skin involvement can be the source of recurrence
- may need free flap skin replacement

Excise early in life

Arteriovenous malformations of the head and neck

Kohout. *PRS* 1998

AV malformations are due to errors of angiogenesis during the fourth-to-sixth weeks

81 patients retrospectively reviewed

Most patients had a cutaneous blush during infancy or at birth, resembled a PWS

Bleeding episodes in one-third of patients – either spontaneously or after trauma, e.g. dental extraction. Loose tooth in a bleeding socket → treat with caution – occult AVM

Bony involvement in 22 patients – cranium, maxilla or mandible

Most patients treated by embolization combined with resection

Outcome adversely affected by increasing Schobinger stage

Bony resection and reconstruction secondary to soft tissue procedures

Most soft tissue defects closed with local tissues or skin grafts, free flaps in 11 patients

Intervention at stage I to prevent progression may be indicated in children with discrete scalp and lip lesions

Puberty and pregnancy may provoke progression from stages I to II or III

Treatment with laser and steroids has not been shown to be effective

Arteriovenous malformations of the face

Bradley. *PRS* 1999

Grotesque disfigurement and life-threatening haemorrhage

Highly selective embolization and resection used to treat 300 facial AVMs

Hypovascularity develops in neighbouring tissues → dubious reliability of local tissues for expansion, etc.

'Cure is elusive and recurrence can be rapid'

Resection of scalp AVMs must include the periosteum to avoid recurrence

Acquired vascular malformations

Campbell de Morgan spots

- sun-exposed skin in older patients
- AV fistula at the dermal capillary level

Spider naevus

- angioma appearing at puberty and disappearing spontaneously
- also affects two-thirds of pregnant women → disappear in the puerperium

Lymphatic malformations

Microcystic (previously known as lymphangioma)

- diffuse
- violate tissue planes
- facial or cervicofacial

Macrocystic (previously known as cystic hygroma)

- localized
- respect tissue planes
- shell out easily

Never involute – fill and empty

- sudden enlargement due to intralesional bleeding
- enlarge in response to infection

Most are present at birth, others arise during late childhood or adolescence

May have a significant venous component – lymphovenous malformation

Fluid levels on MRI scan diagnostic

Head and neck lymphatic malformations are often a combination of macro- and microcystic

- cause of macroglossia
- involve face and orbits
- secondary bony (including mandibular) hypertrophy → class III malocclusion and anterior open bite
- may cause airway obstruction

Thoracic lymphatic malformations → involve mediastinum → pleural and pericardial effusion

Intralesional bleeding → enlargement and confusion with vascular malformation or lymphovenous malformation

Lymphatic malformation in the groin → lymphoedema and limb hypertrophy

- management:
  - antibiotics and NSAID if inflamed

- sclerotherapy with 95% ethanol or sodium tetradecyl sulphate 3%. Used before surgery
- surgical excision
  - define extent of involvement
  - define acceptable blood loss
  - recurs following incomplete excision – lymphatics regenerate
- laser (Nd:YAG) for cutaneous lesions

Management of giant cervicofacial lymphatic malformations

Lille. *J Paediatr Surg* 1996

Most lymphatic malformations occur in the head and neck, mostly in the posterior triangle

Abnormal development of lymphatics

Grows in proportion with growth of the child

Rapid enlargement may follow URTI

Regression or involution is uncommon

Compression → **airway obstruction**, difficulty feeding

Excessive mandibular growth, abnormal speech and dentition

Inadequate excision → high rate of recurrence but surgical excision is the definitive management of lymphatic malformation

Infiltration along tissue planes → extensive involvement of intra-oral structures and nerves

Skin involvement → need to excise skin and reconstruct (free VRAM in this case)

Mandibular osteotomy to improve intra-oral access

Cervicofacial lymphatic malformations

Padwa. *PRS* 1995

Up to 95% occur in the neck and axilla

Massive cervicofacial lesions account for ~3%

Priorities are:

- airway problems → tracheostomy frequently required (two-thirds in this series)
- establish a feeding line

Episodic bleeding, recurrent cellulitis, dental caries, abnormal facial growth

Cellulitis secondary to minor trauma or URTI

Dental caries secondary to difficulty in access for cleaning

Speech problems due to infiltration of the tongue

Phleboliths were seen in some patients – secondary to intralesional bleeding

Surgery

- soft tissues
  - staged debulking surgery limited to a defined anatomical region at each stage
  - tongue reduction
- mandible
  - correction of class III malocclusion and anterior open bite after completion of skeletal growth
  - segmental mandibulectomy
  - inferior border resection
  - le Fort I osteotomy

Surgery complicated by injury to facial and hypoglossal nerves

Lymphatic malformation present within medullary bone

Cystic hygroma of the chest wall

Ardenghy. *Ann Plast Surg* 1996

75% of macrocystic lymphatic malformations (cystic hygromas) occurs in the neck

Predilection for the left side, mainly in the posterior triangle

20% occurs in the axilla

Transillumination test

Lack of a communication between the cystic sac and the venous system *in utero*

USS shows multiloculated cyst

CT or MRI used to define relationship with surrounding tissues

75% diagnosed at birth

Treat by conservative excision

Melanocytic naevi

Junctional naevus

Flat (macular) deeply pigmented lesion

Any site, but benign acral or mucosal lesions are usually junctional naevi

Childhood or adolescence

Melanocytic proliferation at the dermo-epidermal junction

Progresses to compound or intradermal naevus with age

Compound naevus

Maculopapular pigmented lesion in adolescence

Junctional proliferation of melanocytes

Nests and columns of dermal melanocytes

Intradermal naevus

Papular faintly pigmented lesion in adults

Cessation of junctional proliferation

Clusters of dermal melanocytes

Congenital naevus (giant pigmented naevus)

Histologically similar to a compound naevus

Tendency towards dermatomal distribution

Large, pigmented, hairy, verrucose

1–2% malignant transformation, mainly within first 5 years of life

Lesions overlying sacrum may be associated with meningocoele or spina bifida

Treat by excision, often serial

Also dermabrasion, laser, curettage

Spitz naevus (juvenile melanoma)

Benign melanocytic tumour with cellular atypia occurring predominantly in childhood

Incidence

Usually in childhood

Has been reported as congenital and also occurring > 70 years of age

<1% of melanocytic naevi in children

Pathology

Resembles a compound naevus

Spindle-shaped or epithelioid cells at dermo-epidermal junction

Multinucleated giant cells

Acanthosis and atypia – may be difficult to differentiate from MM

Abundant melanin

Clinical

Reddish-brown nodule, occasionally deeply pigmented

Bleeding after minor trauma

Initial rapid growth then remains static

Face and legs most commonly

Treatment

Excision to obviate malignant change

Dysplastic naevus

Pathology

Irregular proliferation of atypical melanocytes around the basal layer

Clinical

Variegated pigmentation

Irregular border

>5 mm in diameter

Sun-exposed areas

Often multiple: dysplastic naevus syndrome

Familial inheritance

5–10% risk of malignant change to SSM type

Found in 2–5% of the population

Spindle cell naevus

Dense black lesion most commonly on the thigh

Females > males

Spindle cell aggregates and atypical melanocytes at the dermo-epidermal junction

Malignant potential unclear

Dermal melanocytosis

Mongolian spot

Macular pigmentation present at birth on the sacral area of >90% of Mongoloid and ~1% of Caucasian neonates

Pathology

Ribbon-like melanocytes around the neurovascular bundles of the dermis

Lack of melanophages

Clinical

Blue–grey patch

Up to 10 cm diameter

Pigmentation increases after birth but regresses by the age of 7 years

No treatment required

Blue naevus

Benign blue–black pigmentation due to a collection of dermal melanocytes

Pathology

Arrested migration of melanocytes bound for the dermo-epidermal junction

Melanocytes gathered around dermal appendages

Presence of melanophages distinguishes from Mongolian spot

Clinical

Nodular blue–black lesion

Extremities, buttocks and face

Change to malignant melanoma very rare

80% occurs in females

60% present during infancy

Treatment

Excision

Naevus of Ota

Dermal melanocytosis of the sclera or skin adjacent to the eye

Pathology

Features are those of Mongolian spot

Clinical

Presents in the distribution of the ophthalmic and maxillary divisions of fifth cranial nerve

Blue–brown pigmentation

Commonest in the Japanese

Not usually present at birth

Darkens during childhood, persists in adult life

Development of malignant melanoma very rare

Malignant melanoma

Malignant tumour of epidermal melanocytes

First described by John Hunter in 1799 as a 'cancerous fungous excrescence' behind the jaw in a 35-year-old man

Accounts for <5% of all skin cancers but >75% of deaths from skin cancer

Abbreviations

Malignant melanoma – MM

Lentigo maligna – LM

Lentigo maligna melanoma – LMM

Superficial spreading melanoma – SSM

Acral lentiginous melanoma – ALM

Incidence

Six per 100 000 per year in the UK

33 per 100 000 per year in Australia

Commonest cancer in young adults (20–39 years)

Accounts for most deaths from cutaneous malignancy

Uncommon in black populations

Increasing rapidly, especially in men

Celtic and Caledonian races

Female:male ratio = 2:1

Possible familial tendency

Rare before puberty

Transplacental spread to foetus reported

Estimated that people born in 2000 will have a 1:75 risk of developing melanoma sometime during their lifetime

Aetiology

Short, intense episodes of sun exposure (UVB)

Sunburn

Lentigo maligna

Significance of a pre-existing naevus

Only ~10% of melanomas arise in a pre-existing naevus

Vast majority of melanocytic naevi are benign – each adult has 30 naevi on average

Congenital and dysplastic naevi at greatest risk

Lifetime risk of congenital naevus ~4% (2–42%)

Clinical

Characteristic features which should alert suspicion:

- variegated pigmentation
- irregular border
- irregular surface
- asymmetry

History of increased size, darkening, itching

Bleeding and ulceration are suggestive of well-established malignancy

Colour

Typically a haphazard array of brown–black pigmentation

Red lesions indicative of host inflammatory response

Nodular MM often blue-black

Depigmentation indicates either an amelanotic area or a focus of regression

Asymmetric halo around an asymmetrical lesion is strongly indicative of a MM

Amelanotic lesions stain positively for tyrosinase: tyrosinase is the rate-limiting enzyme critically associated with melanin synthesis

Border

Irregularity most commonly with SSM and LMM

Nodular MM often symmetrical, well-defined border

Differential diagnoses

Acquired melanocytic naevi, especially dysplastic naevus

Dermal melanocytoses

Pigmented BCC

Pigmented actinic keratosis

Pigmented seborrhoeic keratosis

Pyogenic granuloma (amelanotic MM)

Histological types

Radial growth phase

- proliferation of neoplastic melanocytes within the epidermis
- focal/single cell invasion of papillary dermis
- SSM, LM
- acral lentiginous MM
- atypical *in situ* lesions may present as reddish macules

Vertical growth phase

- invasion of malignant melanocytes into papillary and reticular dermis
- LMM
- nodular MM

Lentigo maligna melanoma (Hutchinson's melanotic freckle)

Sun-exposed skin, especially face, of older patients

5–10% of all MM

Women > men

Invasive counterpart of LM – 30–50% of LM will become invasive

May take up to 30 years before vertical growth phase

Nodules and foci of darkened pigmentation (LMM) within areas of LM

Melanocytes typically large and pleomorphic (fusiform/dendritic)

Invasive melanocytes are spindle-shaped and infiltrate along neurovascular structures

Superficial spreading melanoma (pagetoid melanoma)

Commonest type of MM

50–70% of all melanomas

Backs and legs in women

Trunk on men

Radial growth phase may be as short as 6 months or as long as 6 years

Flat, irregular border, pigmentation and surface

Invasion heralded by ulceration

Dense lymphocytic and fibroblast aggregations indicate regression

Difficult to distinguish histologically from Paget's disease when located at the nipple

Nodular melanoma

10–20% of all MM

Concurrent radial and vertical growth

Acral lentiginous melanoma

Palms, soles, mucocutaneous junctions, subungal

2–8% of MM in Caucasians but up to 60% of MM in dark-skinned races

Radial growth followed by vertical growth after ~2 years

Usually affects the elderly (>60 years)

Histologically similar to LMM but more aggressive locally and more likely to metastasize

Subungal melanoma

Accounts for 1–3% of MM

Great toe affected in ~50% of cases, thumb next most common

Splitting of the nail, paronychia, nail dystrophy; distinguish from pigmented naevus of the nail matrix

Treat by amputation of the affected digit

Level of amputation does not affect local recurrence or survival

ILP reduces local recurrence but not survival; Balch, *Ann Surg* 1994

Subungal melanoma of the hand

Quinn. *J Hand Surg* 1996

Series of 38 patients, mean tumour thickness 3 mm

Mean duration of symptoms before diagnosis ~12 months

- commonly treated for 'fungal' infection
- often an associated history of trauma
- high incidence of amelanotic subungal MM (~30%; 7% of cutaneous MM overall are amelanotic)

Male > female (even though upper limb MM is more common in females)

Mean age at presentation 58 years (older than cutaneous MM)

Distal (or functional) amputation recommended:

- through the neck of the PP of the thumb
- through the PIP joint of the fingers

Poorer survival rates than for non-ALM

Secondary melanoma (no identifiable primary)

Accounts for ~5% of melanomas

Usually presents as lymph node disease, primary lesion having undergone regression

Non-lymph node metastatic sites:
- skin
- brain
- lung
- bone
- spinal cord
- adrenals

Radiotherapy may offer effective palliation of brain metastases

Surgery may be indicated for a solitary brain metastasis

Abdominal presentation of MM:
- usually metastatic
- obstruction or **intersusseption**
- usually amelanotic

Desmoplastic melanoma

Most commonly in the head and neck

Desmoplastic spindling stroma

Melanocytic dysplasia

May be non-pigmented

Predilection for local recurrence due to perineural infiltration

May need special stains for diagnosis

Tumour markers

Gene encoding melanoma associated antigen (ME941) may be an anti-invasion gene: reduced expression in invasive and metastatic melanoma compared with LM and SSM

p53 tumour suppresser gene

HLA-DQB1*0301 is a genomic marker that independently identifies melanoma patients in whom recurrence is more likely, and is potentially useful in selecting those most likely to benefit from adjuvant therapy

Polymerase chain reaction assay of tyrosinase activity assesses occult (micrometastasis) tumour burden

Prognosis and prognostic indicators

Clinical variables

Better prognosis in women and in the <50 years of age group (but the elderly tend to have thicker lesions and more ALM)

Better prognosis if MM develops in a pre-existing naevus (20% of cases)

BANS lesions – significance disputed

Pathological variables

Tumour thickness (**Breslow**) measured from the stratum granulosum to the deepest part of the tumour

Level of invasion (Clark and McGovern)
- I – confined to the epidermis
- II – invasion of papillary dermis

- III – filling of papillary dermis
- IV – invasion of reticular dermis
- V – invasion of subcutaneous fat

Ulceration

Mitotic activity

Neurovascular invasion

Microscopic satellites

Two-year survival of patients undergoing positive radical neck dissection approaches zero

See AJCC staging

Outpatient follow-up

Moloney. *BJPS* 1996

602 patients followed for a minimum of 5 years following excision of primary lesions <0.76 mm (Frenchay)

All primaries excised with at least 1 cm margins

Recurrence in 14/602 within 5 years

Mean time to recurrence ~4.5 years

Only 5/14 were treatable (1% of all patients) including a need for TLND

- in four of these five, treatment resulted in survival beyond 5 years
- these four patients all presented within 2 years of primary excision

9/14 returned with disseminated disease

After 5 years there were a further four treatable recurrences and six non-treatable, but none survived >10 years

Hence, total recurrence = 24/602 (4%)

Conclusion: treatable recurrences after excision of thin melanomas were all detected within 2 years, questioning the need for continued follow-up beyond this point

Multiple primaries (Yale Melanoma Unit, 423 patients in 10 years)

Ariyan. *PRS* 1995

5% of patients with primary cutaneous MM will develop a second primary

27 patients examined with multiple primaries

Histologically confirmed not to be in-transit metastases or satellite lesions

Mean age 52 years, 16 male, 11 female

22/27 developed two primaries

5/27 developed three primaries

In eight patients the second primary arose within 1 month of the first

17% arose within the first year

29% within the second year

54% beyond the second year

Anatomical site:

- 14/27 totally different
- 4/27 same anatomical region but widely spaced
- 9/27 same anatomical region but closely spaced
- first primaries were between 0.2 and 6.0 mm thick but all subsequent primaries were *in situ* or <1 mm (?earlier diagnosis, host immune response)
- patient's prognosis is related to the thickness of the thickest lesion

Adjuvant therapy

Radiotherapy

Is adjuvant radiotherapy necessary after positive neck dissection?

Shen, Wanek, Morton. *Ann Surg Oncol* 2000

- Retrospective review of 217 patients undergoing positive neck dissection
  - 80% TLND, 20% positive ELND
- 196 patients did not receive radiotherapy
  - 27/196 (14%) developed recurrence in the dissected nodal basin (predictor: extracapsular spread)
- 21 received post-operative radiotherapy (insufficient number for statistical analysis)
  - 3/21 (14%) developed recurrence in the dissected nodal basin
- No role for adjuvant radiotherapy unless there is widespread extracapsular spread

Survival and prognostic factors in patients with brain metastases from malignant melanoma

Meier. *Onkologie* 2004

A retrospective review of the factors influencing survival in patients with melanoma brain

- 100 patients treated between 1966 and 2002
- overall median survival time was 4.8 months
  - 6-month, 1-year and 2-year survival: 36%, 14% and 5%, respectively
- Survival correlated significantly with
  - radiotherapy (partial and whole brain)
  - surgery (stereotactic radiosurgery)
  - chemotherapy
  - Clark level and Breslow thickness
- Treatment with temozolomide ($P = 0.052$) and number of brain metastases ($P = 0.07$) failed to be statistically significant.

Conclusion

- Radiotherapy, chemotherapy and especially surgery and stereotactic radiosurgery significantly prolong survival, as shown by multivariate analysis

A multi-institutional retrospective analysis of external radiotherapy for mucosal melanoma of the head and neck in Northern Japan

Wada. *Int J Radiat Oncol Biol Phys* 2004

- A multi-institutional retrospective study of external radiotherapy as the definitive treatment modality for localized mucosal melanoma of the head and neck in 31 patients
  - Radiotherapy alone was performed in 21 patients
  - Ten patients received adjuvant radiotherapy for gross post-resectional disease
  - fraction size 1.5–13.8 Gy
  - total dose 32–64 Gy (median 50 Gy).
- Complete response in 9/31 patients
- Partial response in 18/31 patients
- Most incidences of local recurrence and distant metastasis developed within 2 years

- Age the only significant prognostic factor by multivariate analysis
- No significant locoregional control or survival benefit in patients with gross post-resectional disease

Conclusion

- Local control achievable using radiotherapy at a dose of 3 Gy or more per fraction in patients with localised mucosal melanoma of the head and neck

Immunotherapy

Antibody to melanoma ganglioside antigen GM2

High-dose interferon-α

Interferon-γ

Non-specific lymphokine-activated killer (LAK) cells

IL-2

Vaccines currently experimental

Eastern Cooperative Oncology Group Trial (E1684): Interferon alfa-2b in the management of melanoma

Kirkwood. *J Clin Oncol* 1996

Maximum-dose interferon alfa-2b trialled in patients with T4 primary melanoma or regional nodal disease (N1 – 1 node either microscopically or macroscopically involved)

Compared with observation only in a total patient group of 287

Median follow-up 6.9 years

Conclusion: high dose IFN alpha-2b prolongs the relapse-free interval and overall survival in high-risk resected melanoma patients

High and low dose interferon alfa-2b trial (E1690)

Kirkwood. *J Clin Oncol* 2001

642 patients enrolled in to 3 treatment arms following resection of high-risk melanoma

- High dose IFN alpha-2b for 1 year
- Low dose IFN alpha 2-b for 2 years
- Observation

5-year relapse-free survival:

- HDI 44% (significant advantage)
- LDI 40%
- Obs 35%

No overall survival benefit from high dose or low dose IFN alpha-2b compared with observation

High dose IFN-alpha 2b compared with ganglioside vaccine (E1694)

Kirkwood. *J Clin Oncol* 2001

888 patients randomized to two treatment groups:

- high dose IFN for 1 year
- GM2 ganglioside for 96 weeks

Conclusion: Significant relapse-free survival and overall survival in the IFN-treated group

Role of SLNB in adjuvant therapy trials

Kretschmer. *J Clin Oncol* 2002

Microscopic nodal staging is necessary in order to compare treatment outcomes in adjuvant therapy trials

In patients with clinically negative nodes, some patients may have N1a or N2a disease while others may have true N0 disease

- Patients with N1a or N2a disease have a worse prognosis compared with patients with true N0 disease

Unequal distribution of these patients into cohorts comparing treatment vs. observation will therefore affect results

This criticism levelled at the E1684 trial

Adjuvant interferon in high-risk melanoma: the AIM HIGH Study – United Kingdom Coordinating Committee on Cancer Research randomized study of adjuvant low-dose extended-duration interferon alfa-2a in high-risk resected malignant melanoma

Hancock. *J Clin Oncol* 2004

To evaluate low-dose extended duration interferon alfa-2a as adjuvant therapy in patients

- Thick (> or = 4 mm) primary cutaneous melanoma and/or
- locoregional metastases
- Radically resected stage IIB and stage III disease
- Randomized controlled trial involving 674 patients
- Effect of interferon alfa-2a (3 megaunits three times per week for 2 years or until recurrence) on overall survival and recurrence-free survival was compared with an observation group
  - OS and RFS rates at 5 years were 44% and 32%, respectively
  - no significant difference in OS or RFS between the interferon-treated and control
  - Subgroup analysis by disease stage, age, and sex did not show any clear differences between interferon-treated and control groups in either OS or RFS
- Interferon-related toxicities were modest:
  - fatigue or mood disturbance in 7% and 4%, respectively
  - 50 withdrawals (15%) from interferon treatment group due to toxicity

Conclusion

- extended-duration low-dose interferon is no better than observation alone in the initial treatment of completely resected high-risk malignant melanoma

Systemic chemotherapy

Single agent or combination chemotherapy

Little evidence for survival benefit in patients with dissemniated disease

Dacarbazine used for advanced disease

Temozolomide for the treatment of brain metastases associated with metastatic melanoma: a phase II study

Agarwala. *J Clin Oncol* 2004

Temozolomide is a well-tolerated oral alkylating agent with activity in the CNS

Study design:

- A phase II study to assess the safety and efficacy of temozolomide in patients with melanoma brain metastases who did not require immediate radiotherapy
- Treatment continued for 1 year or until disease progression or unacceptable toxicity
  - 151 patients enrolled
  - 117 had received no prior systemic chemotherapy
    - 25% had more than four brain lesions
  - 34 had received prior chemotherapy
- Median overall survival was 3.5 months
  - median overall survival was 2.2 months in previously untreated patients
- Temozolomide was generally well tolerated
  - haematologic toxicities included:
    - thrombocytopenia (3%)
    - neutropenia (2%)
    - leukopenia (1%)
  - Headache (9%) and vomiting (8%)

Conclusion

Temozolomide was well tolerated and demonstrated activity in the treatment of melanoma brain metastases

The role of SLNB and staging of malignant melanoma

Node management in melanoma

Stone and Goodacre. *Br J Surg* 1995

ELND acts as an independent prognostic variable for lesions 0.76–3.99 mm thick:

Collaborative study of 1786 patients in Alabama (Balch) and Sydney (Milton)

Series of ELND indicate that 40% of node metastases are subclinical

Occult disease increases with depth (38% > 1.5 mm) and level of invasion (58% > level V)

Survival advantage of ELND over TLND only if <10% of the node basin harbours occult disease

70% of lesions are drained by a single 'sentinel' node

10% of lesions drain to contralateral nodes

Overall discordancy between predicted and actual drainage patterns averages 40%, especially for head and neck lesions

Node-positive ELND for head and neck lesions may contribute to locoregional control but not survival in comparison with TLND

Complications of groin dissection: marginal wound necrosis (20%), seroma (35%), infection (30%), lymphoedema (noticeable 10%, severe 3%)

Argument against ELND mainly based on Veronesi (WHO) study which had a gender bias (women > men) and lesion bias (mostly lower limb – better prognosis in women).

Potential survival advantage to ELND in ulcerated intermediate thickness melanoma

Long term results of the Intergroup Melanoma Surgical Trial

Balch. *Ann Surg Oncol* 2000

- Intergroup Melanoma Surgical Trial established in 1983 to determine the role of ELND for patients with intermediate thickness melanoma (1–4mm)

- Trial recruitment closed in 1989, median of 10 years follow-up
- 740 patients prospectively randomized to ELND or observation groups
- Lymphoscintigraphy undertaken for all truncal lesions to identify draining nodal basin
- Calculation of survival advantage in subgroups of patients stratified for ulceration, tumour thickness and age
- Survival at 10 years, compared with observation:
  - non-ulcerated melanoma + ELND → survival advantage (84% vs. 77%, $P = 0.03$)
  - tumours 1–2 mm + ELND → survival advantage (86% vs. 80%, $P = 0.03$)
  - limb primary + ELND → survival advantage (84% vs. 78%, $P = 0.05$)
  - age 60 or younger + non-ulcerated primary + ELND → significant survival advantage at 10 years (89% vs. 79%, $P = 0.004$)
- No analysis of survival difference between positive ELND patients vs [observation + TLND] patients
- Risk of distant metastatic disease in patients with ulcerated melanomas and tumours >4mm offsets benefit of ELND

Immediate vs. delayed node dissection in truncal melanoma

Cascinelli. *Lancet* 1998
- Multicentre trial on behalf of the WHO
- 240 patients <65 yrs with truncal melanoma >1.5 mm randomised to:
  - ELND (median Breslow thickness 3.4 mm, M:F 2:1, $n = 122$)
  - Observation and TLND (median tumour thickness 3.2 mm, M:F 2:1, $n = 118$)
- 5 year survival in *positive* ELND patients ($n = 27$, 22%) was 48.2%
- 5 year survival in patients undergoing TLND ($n = 36$, 30%) was 26%

Efficacy of SLND vs ELND for early stage melanoma

Essner. *Ann Surg Onol* 1999
- Comparison of outcome in 267 pairs of patients undergoing either SLNB/completion or ELND, matched for gender and age, and site and thickness of the primary tumour
- No overall significant difference in survival or number of tumour positive dissections
  - a significant increase in number of tumour positive dissections was seen in the SLN group for intermediate thickness primaries (related to immunohistochemical diagnosis of occult microscopic disease)
- similar incidence of same-basin recurrence (4.8% in SLNB group) and in-transit disease (3%) after tumour negative dissection

ELND vs observation/TLND for head and neck melanoma

Fisher. *Laryngoscope* 2002 (Carolina)
- retrospective analysis of database of 1444 patients with head and neck melanoma grouped by:
  - ELND at time of diagnosis, $n = 219$, (27+ ve, 11%)
  - No initial LND but (delayed) TLND for regional recurrence >3 months of diagnosis, $n = 1045$, TLND in 106
  - LND for palpable lymphadenopathy within 30 days of diagnosis, $n = 112$ (99 +ve)
- 5-year survival from date of diagnosis:
  - + ve ELND 24%
  - + ve TLND <3 m 36%

- + ve delayed TLND 56%
- BUT small number of patients in the + ve ELND group (only 27)
- Postulate that micrometastatic disease may stimulate T-cell activation, removal by ELND may adversely affect survival

Lymphatic mapping and lymphadenectomy for early stage melanoma

Morton. *Ann Surgery* 2003 (John Wayne Cancer Institute)

Patterns of metastatic spread:

- in some patients, the SLN harbours cells that, after and latent period of growth, are responsible for later haematogenous spread (incubator hypothesis)
  - a critical mass of cells must be achieved in order to allow passage of cells along the lymphatic chain (generation of immunosuppressive factors)
  - Incubator hypothesis of spread supported by observation of 15-year survival in up to 32% of patients undergoing therapeutic LND, i.e. node removal before progression to distant metastases
- in other patients, SLN positivity is simply a marker for metastatic disease that has bypassed the node (marker hypothesis)
- afferent lymphatics drain in a compartmentalized fashion in to the node: specific areas of skin map to specific compartments within the node
- PCR facilitates detection of micrometastases that are missed by serial sectioning

Analysis of data:

- Data on 6189 patients since 1971
- 1599 underwent SLNB
  - mean age 51 yrs, median tumour thickness 1.43 mm
  - positive in 322 (20%)
- 4590 underwent wide local excision and observation of regional nodes (dissection when clinically positive)
- Analysis of overall survival in 287 pairs of patients matched for clinical/pathological stage showed improved survival in the SLNB/completion lymph node dissection group compared with delayed LND (73% and 51% survival at 5 years, respectively)

Five years' experience of SLNB at St Georges

Topping *et al* (B Powell). *Br J Plastic Surg* 2004

- Prospective data on 347 patients undergoing SLNB between 1996 and 2001
  - Largest UK series to date
- Breslow thickness >1 mm or <1 mm if > Clark III
- Technique
  - pre-operative lymphoscintigraphy (Nanocoll) and surface marking of the node (and depth estimation)
  - intra-operative patent V dye injected around the biopsy scar for visual localization of the SLN
  - hand-held gamma probe for detection of the 'hot' node
  - WLE with 1 cm margin (if primary <1 mm) or 2 cm (primary >1 mm)
  - Patients discharged the following day
- Results
  - Mean tumour thickness 2.04 mm
  - 17.6% positive

- positive SLNB followed by completion LND within 3 weeks in all patients
  - 87% had no further disease in the node basin
- 11 patients have subsequently died of disseminated disease
  - 2 of these had further disease in the nodal basin at completion lymphadenectomy
  - 9 had no further disease in the node basin at completion lymphadenectomy
- lower limb most common positive primary site in males and females
- mean number of SLNs 2.1 (range 0–7)
- mean positive thickness 3.13 mm
  - ratio of negative:positive SLNB for primary tumours
    - <1 mm was 29:1
    - 1–2 mm was 5:1
    - >2 mm was 2:1
- mean negative thickness 1.81 mm
- false-negative rate 2%
- Patients with a positive SLNB were six times more likely to die from their disease than patients with a negative SLNB during the follow-up period
- SLN positivity was an independent prognostic indicator for survival but was not as significant as tumour thickness

Microanatomy of sentinel node metastases as a predictor of non-sentinel node involvement

Dewar. *J Clin Oncol* 2004

Positive SLNs from 146 nodal basins examined for intra-nodal location of metastases

Anatomical site of metastases and depth of involvement of the SLN corellated with non-sentinel node (NSN) involvement at completion lymphadenectomy

- Subcapsular involvement ($n = 38$) → no NSN involved
- Combined subcapsular and parenchymal metastases ($n = 54$) → 11% NSN involvement
- Parenchymal deposits ($n = 16$) → 19% NSN involvement
- Multifocal metastases ($n = 19$) → 37% NSN involvement
- Extensive disease ($n = 19$) → 42% NSN involvement

Final update of the AJCC staging system for melanoma

Balch *et al. J Clin Oncol* 2001

- database on 30 450 patients
- full data on 17 600 available for production of survival data

T classification	Thickness	Ulceration/level
T1	<1 mm	a: without ulceration/level II–III
		b: with ulceration/level IV–V
T2	1.01–2.0 mm	a: without ulceration
		b: with ulceration
T3	2.01–4.0 mm	a: without ulceration
		b: with ulceration
T4	>4 mm	a: without ulceration
		b: with ulceration

N classification	Number involved regional nodes	Nodal metastatic mass
N1	1	a: micrometastases
		b: macrometastases
N2	2–3	a: micrometastases
		b: macrometastases
		c: in transit/satellite *without* nodal disease
N3	4 + or in-transit/ satellite *plus* nodal disease (inc microscopic)	

M classification	Site	Serum lactate dehydrogenase
M1a	Distant skin metastsis	Normal
	Distant node involvement	
M1b	Lung	Normal
M1c	Other visceral	Normal
	Any	Elevated

Micrometastases detected by SLNB

Macrometastases = palpable positive nodes or gross extracapsular spread

Survival in node positive patients depends upon stage of disease taking into account ulceration of the primary lesion

Clinical staging

Stage I: Localized disease, T stage T2a or less

Stage II: Localized disease, T2b or more

Stage III: Nodal disease

Stage IV: Metastatic disease

Pathological staging

- Based upon further information about the regional nodes following SLNB and completion LND
- Subdivides stage 3 disease by N stage
- positive SLNB upstages the patient to stage III, irrespective of tumour thickness
- but survival in a patient with a *non-ulcerated* melanoma and micrometastases in the sentinel node only (stage IIIa) is likely to exceed survival in a patient with stage IIc disease, i.e. a thick, *ulcerated* primary (69% and 45% survival at 5 years, respectively)
- pathological staging of nodes (by SLNB) recommended before entry of patients into melanoma trials

Stage	T	N	M	5y survival%
IA	1a	0	0	95
IB	1b or 2a	0	0	90
IIA	2b or 3a	0	0	78
IIB	3b or 4a	0	0	65
IIC	4b	0	0	45
IIIA	Any (no ulceration)	1a or 2a	0	60
IIIB	Any (ulcerated)	1a or 1b	0	51
	Any (no ulceration)	1b or 2b	0	53
	Any	2c	0	
IIIC	Any (ulcerated)	1b or 2b	0	27
	Any	3	0	
IV	Any	Any	1a	19
			1b	7
			1c	10

Patterns of recurrence after SLNB

Gershenwald. Recurrence after negative SLNB
J Clin Oncol 1998
Follow-up study of 243 patients following negative SLNB to determine pattern of relapse
- 11% of patients overall developed recurrent disease
  - 10 patient (4.1%) developed in transit disease
  - 18 patients (7.4%) developed distant disease
  - 14 patients (5.8%) developed nodal disease in the biopsied node basin

SLNB in melanoma – WHO experience
Cascinelli. *Ann Surg Oncol* 2000
- 829 patients participating in WHO SLNB programme
- 18% positive SLNB
- of the SLNB-negative patients
  - 6% developed regional nodal recurrence (but these sentinel nodes were identified by blue dye only)
  - 3% developed in transit disease
  - 7% developed distant metastases
- SLN positivity, tumour thickness and ulceration were independent prognostic variables by multivariate analysis

Recurrence after SLNB
Clary. *Ann Surg* 2001
- Review of 332 sentinel node biopsy procedures over a 7-year period
- Positive rate 17%
- Mean Breslow thickness 2.7 mm, ulceration in 29%

- Disease-free survival at 3 years:
  - SLNB negative 75%
  - SLNB positive 58%
- Overall recurrences:
  - SLNB negative 14%
  - SLNB positive 40%
- Re-evaluation of negative SLN status by PCR in patients developing recurrent disease showed 7/11 patients actually had metastatic disease

Recurrence after SLNB for melanoma

Chao. *Am J Surg* 2002

- Data from the Sunbelt Melanoma Trial group
- 1183 patients within the study group
  - 13% had T4 disease
  - 233 patients (19.7%) positive
  - completion LND $+/-$ adjuvant interferon alpha-2b
- predictors of tumour recurrence
  - Breslow thickness
  - Clark level
  - Ulceration
  - Positive SLNB
  - Number of positive nodes at SLNB
- After negative SLNB
  - Biopsied nodal basin recurrence 1.2%
  - In-transit recurrence 1%
  - Distant recurrence 2.7%
- After positive SLNB
  - Dissected nodal basin recurrence 0.4%
  - In-transit recurrence 2%
  - Distant recurrence 10.3%

SLNB in 200 patients

Doting. *Eur J Surg Oncol* 2002

200 patients underwent SLNB for stage I/II melanoma

24% of patients had positive nodes

- Completion lymphadenectomy results:
  - 1–2 mm thick tumour → 23% had at least one positive node at completion
  - 2–4 mm primary → 23%
  - >4 mm primary → 33%
- causes of recurrence in the biopsied nodal basin
  - biological failure (in transit cells yet to reach nodal basin)
    - advocate introducing time delay between diagnosis and SLNB
  - technical failure (SLN not correctly identified, wrong node harvested)
  - pathological failure (metastatic cells not identified within the SLN)

Long term follow-up after SLNB

Vuylsteke. *J Clin Oncol* 2003

5-year follow-up undertaken on 209 patients following SLNB $\pm$ completion LND

40/209 patients had a positive sentinel node (19%)

Recurrence after positive SLNB:

- 13/40 patients developed in-transit recurrence (32%)
- 9/40 patients developed systemic disease (22.5%)
- no regional node recurrence

Recurrence after negative SLNB:

- in-transit disease 6.5%
- nodal recurrence 2.4%
- distant disease 4.8%

Overall survival at 5 years:

- SLN negative 92%
- SLN positive 67%

Patterns of recurrence and prognosis after SLNB

Wagner *et al. Plastic Reconstruc Surg* 2003 (Indianapolis)

- 408 patients with melanomas >1 mm staged by SLNB
- mean thickness 2.8 mm
- 84 patients (20.8%) positive
- completion lymphadenectomy positive in 18/84 patients (21.4%)
- of SLN negative patients
  - 3% subsequently developed nodal disease in the SLN basin
  - 4% developed in-transit disease
  - 4.6% developed metastatic disease
- SLN positive patients more likely to experience distant recurrence
- SLN negative patients may develop isolated distant recurrence due to haematogenous spread

6 year follow-up of 250 sentinel node procedures

Estourgie, Nieweg *et al. Ann Surg Oncol* 2003

52% female/48% male

Mean Breslow thickness 2.7 mm

Ulceration in 32%

24% of patients had a positive SLNB

- high compared with previous studies
- three patients had metastatic disease in more than one nodal basin

Minor local wound complications occurred in 9.2%

Mild limb oedema occurred in 23 patients (all lower limb except one patient)

12 patients developed nodal disease in the biopsied basin

- of these, five patients developed in-transit metastases first

Positive SLNB patients ($n = 60$) were at high risk of in-transit metastases (23%) or distant disease (42%) within the follow-up period

Sentinel node positivity confirmed as a poor prognostic indicator:

Disease-free survival at 3 and 5 years:

- SLNB negative 85%, 80%
- SLNB positive 62%, 53%

Summary of recurrence rates after SLNB

Negative SLNB	Biopsied nodal basin	In-transit	Distant
Gershenwald, 1998	4.1%	5.8%	7.4%
Essner, 1999	4.8%	2.6%	4.0%
Clary, 2001	4.4%	2.8%	5.6%
Chao, 2002	0.4%	1%	2.7%
Wagner, 2003	2%	5%	5.9%
Doting, 2002		4%	
Estourgie, 2003	6%	7%	12%
Vuylsteke, 2003	2.4%	6.5%	4.8%
Topping, 2004	2%	0.7%	2.8%

Positive SLNB	Positive rate	Number of +ve	Biopsied nodal basin	In-transit	Distant
Essner, 1999	15.7%	42	12%	10%	16.7%
Clary, 2001	17%	56	5.4%	12.5%	17.9%
Chao, 2002	20%	233	0.4%	2%	10.3%
Doting, 2002	24%			8%	
Estourgie, 2003	24%	60	8%	23%	42%
Vuylsteke, 2003	19%	40	0%	32%	22.5%
Wagner, 2003	20.8%	84	4.7%	9.4%	16.5%

Non-nodal metastases of cutaneous melanoma

Cascinelli. *Eur J Surg Oncol* 1986

Review of 1503 patients treated in Milan

- 380 patients underwent ELND at the same time as excision of the primary lesion
- 577 patients underwent delayed ELND or TLND
- 546 patients had no nodal surgery

In-transit recurrence rates:

- 8.9% in patients who had no nodal surgery (546 patients)
- 12.5% in patients who had positive nodal disease (519 patients)
- no significant difference in incidence of post-lymphadenectomy in-transit disease in patients subjected to in-continuity vs. discontinuity dissection

Distant disease:

- diagnosed in 22% of patients at the time of appearance of in-transit disease (usually distant skin or subcutaneous disease)
- median survival following the diagnosis of in-transit disease was 30 months

Metastatic pathways and time courses in the orderly progression of melanoma

Meier. *Br J Dermatol* 2002

- 182 patients presented with metastases
- 75 patients presented with metastases but an unknown primary

- 3001 patients with stage I/II disease followed for 20 years
  - 466 patients developed metastases
    - satellite or in-transit metastases 21% (3.4% of all patients as first recurrence)
    - regional node metastases 50.2% (7.8% of all patients)
    - distant metastases as first recurrence 28.1% (4.4% of all patients)
  - 51.5% of patients with in-transit disease were subsequently diagnosed with systemic disease
  - 20.8% of patients with in-transit disease subsequently developed nodal disease
  - 59% of patients with nodal disease subsequently developed distant disease
- most first recurrences were to the lymph nodes
- lower limb primaries are most at risk of develoiping in-transit disease (31.8%)
- upper limb and trunk primaries most at risk of developing distant disease as first recurrence (35%)
- in-transit pathway for first metastasis significantly more common in women compared with men
- median time interval to development of in-transit metsatases 17 months
- median time interval to development of regional node metastases as first recurrence 14 months
- development of distant metastases occurred after around 25 months, irrespective of whether or not this occurred as a first recurrence or was preceded by either in-transit or nodal disease

In-transit metastases following therapeutic lymph node dissection for melanoma

Kretschmer. *Melanoma Rese* 2002

Overall incidence of in-transit disease after excision of a primary melanoma may be as high as 19% (Cascinelli, *Eur J Surg Oncol* 1986)

- review of 224 patients subjected to therapeutic axillary or inguinal lymphadenectomy for metastatic melanoma with histological confirmation of disease
- 65 (29%) of these patients developed in-transit metastases during the course of their disease
  - of these 65 patients 24 (11% of the total TLND group) developed in-transit disease before the development of palpable disease
    - 5-year survival in this group 27%
  - 11 patients presented with simultaneous in-transit disease and palpable lymph nodes
  - 15 patients developed in-transit disease as the first recurrence after TLND
    - 5-year survival 28%
  - 26 patients developed in-transit disease after nodal basin recurrence following TLND or distant recurrence following TLND
    - 5-year survival 0%
- thicker primaries and lower limb primaries were predictive of the development of in-transit disease

Management of in transit cutaneous metastases from melanoma

Hayes. *Br J Surg* 2004

Patients with in-transit metastases are staged either IIIB or IIIC disease

- Survival 18%–60% at 5 years

Non-nodal cutaneous or subcutaneous deposits between the primary site and draining nodal basin

Rapid acceleration in development of in-transit metastases often coincides with development of distant disease

Satellite lesions occur within 5 cm of the primary lesion site (probably biologically the same entity as in-transit disease)

Local recurrence is growth of persistent disease at the biopsy site due to incomplete excision

Treatment of in-transit disease

- Palliation of disease
- Complete excision (narrow margins acceptable)
- Carbon dioxide laser therapy
- Isolated limb perfusion
  - Melphalan
  - Dacarbazine
  - Good response rates reported
- Radiotherapy
  - 52% response rate reported by Feng, *Am J Clin Oncol* 1999
- Chemotherapy
  - Widespread truncal or head and neck in-transit disease
- Amputation only considered for palliation of fungating disease or exsanguinating haemorrhage

PET scanning for staging of melanoma

Positron emission tomography and sentinel lymph node biopsy in staging primary cutaneous melanoma

Havenga, *Eur J Surg Oncol* 2003

- fluorodeoxyglucose–positron emission tomography (FDG–PET) compared with SLN biopsy in staging primary cutaneous melanoma
- 55 patients with melanomas >1.0 mm Breslow thickness and no palpable regional lymph nodes underwent a FDG–PET scan before SLNB
- SLNs were retrieved in 53 patients
  - Melanoma metastases were found in the SLN of 13 patients.
- FDG–PET detected the lymph node metastases in 2 of the 13 patients with positive sentinel nodes
- In five patients FDG accumulation was recorded in a regional lymph node basin where the SLNB was negative
- In eight patients FDG–PET showed increased activity at a site of possible distant metastasis
  - Metastatic disease was confirmed in one patient
  - No explanation for the positive FDG–PET result could be found in five cases
- SLN biopsy reveals regional metastases that are too small to be detected by FDG–PET

The role of positron emission tomography in patients with metastatic melanoma

Gulec. *Nucl Med* 2003

- Study evaluates the accuracy of fluorine-18 deoxyglucose (FDG) whole-body positron emission tomography (PET) in determination of extent of disease (EOD) in patients with metastatic melanoma and its impact on surgical and medical management decisions

- 49 patients with known or suspected metastatic melanoma underwent EOD evaluation using computerized tomography (CT) of the chest, abdomen, and pelvis, and magnetic resonance imaging (MRI) of the brain
- After formulation of an initial treatment plan, patients underwent FDG–PET imaging
  - PET scan identified more metastatic sites in 27 of 49 patients (55%) compared with conventional imaging
    - in 6 of those 27 patients, PET detected disease outside the fields of CT and MRI
- 51 lesions were resected surgically
  - 44 confirmed to be melanoma on histology
  - all lesions larger than 1 cm were positive on PET
  - 2 of 15 lesions smaller than 1 cm were detected by PET
- The results of PET-led treatment changes in 24/49 patients (49%)
  - In 6 of these 24 patients, chemotherapy, radiation therapy, or an experimental immunotherapy protocol was prompted by identification of new foci of disease

Excision margins in high risk melanoma

Thomas. *N Engl J Med* 2004

Outcome data from the UK Melanoma Study Group trial

- 1 cm vs. 3 cm margins ($n = 900$)
- All tumours Breslow thickness 2 mm or thicker
- 60-month follow-up

Results

- 1 cm margin of excision associated with a significantly increased risk of local recurrence
- 168 locoregional recurrences (as first events) in 1 cm margin group ($n = 453$)
  - 128 deaths
- 142 locoregional recurrences in 3 cm margin group ($n = 447$)
  - 105 deaths
- overall survival was similar in the two groups

Conclusion

- a 1 cm margin of excision for melanomas 2 mm thick or greater is associated with a significantly greater risk of locoregional recurrence than a 3 cm margin, but with a similar overall survival rate

Axillary lymphadenectomy

Anatomy

Floor: axillary fascia

Anterior wall: pectoralis major, pectoralis minor, subclavius and clavipectoral fascia

Posterior wall: subscapularis, teres major, tendon of latissimus dorsi

Medial wall: serratus anterior

Apex: bounded by outer edge of first rib medially, clavicle anteriorly and scapula posteriorly

Contents: axillary artery, axillary vein, lymph nodes, brachial plexus

Margins data

Trial	Design	Number of patients	Follow-up	Local control	Overall survival
Veronesi (WHO) *N Eng J Med* 1988	1 vs. 3 cm WLE for MM <2 mm	612	5 yrs	No difference	No difference
Cohn-Cedermark (Swedish Melanoma Study Group) *Cancer* 2000	2 vs. 5 cm WLE for primary MM 0.8–2.0 mm trunk or extremeities	989	11 yrs	No difference	No difference
Balch (Intergroup Melanoma Surgical Trial) *Ann Surg Oncol* 2001	2 vs. 4 cm WLE for primary MM 1–4 mm trunk/ upper limb	468	10 yrs	No difference	No difference
Khayat (French Co-operative Study) *Cancer* 2003	2 vs. 5 cm WLE for primary MM <2.1 mm	337	16 yrs	No difference	No difference
Thomas (MSG study) *New Engl J Med* 2004	1 vs. 3 cm WLE for MM >2 mm	900	5 yrs	Increased local recurrence in 1 cm group	No difference

Axillary artery

Three parts, second part lies behind pectoralis minor

Superior thoracic A branches from first part

Second part: thoraco-acromial A and lateral thoracic A (follows inferior border of pectoralis minor lying on the fascia investing serratus anterior)

Third part: subscapular A (largest branch) which runs down the posterior axillary wall and divides into the circumflex scapular A and the thoracodorsal A, and the medial and lateral circumflex humeral As

In its second part the axillary A is clasped by the medial, lateral and posterior cords of the brachial plexus

Invested by fascia projected off the paravertebral fascia – the axillary sheath

Axillary vein

Lies on the medial side of the axillary A in the apex of the axilla

Not invested by fascia hence free to expand

Receives the cephalic vein in its first part (above pectoralis minor)

Long thoracic nerve

C5,6,7 – emerging from posterior aspect of nerve **roots**

Lies posterior to the mid-axillary line

Lies upon and supplies serratus anterior

Thoracodorsal nerve

C6,7,8 – from **posterior cord**

Runs down the posterior axillary wall

Closely related to the subscapular A

Enters latissimus dorsi on its deep surface

Intercostobrachial nerve

Lateral cutaneous branch of the second (occasionally third) intercostal N

Supplies an area on the medial aspect of the upper arm

Lateral pectoral nerve

Arises from the **lateral cord**

Crosses the axillary V

Enters the deep surface of pectoralis minor

Penetrates this to enter pectoralis major

Pectoralis minor

Arises from third, fourth and fifth ribs

Inserts into the coracoid process

Supplied by medial and lateral pectoral Ns (C6,7,8)

Assists serratus in protraction of the scapula

No great functional significance

Lymph nodes

Between 35 and 50 in number

Surgical groups

Level I – lateral to pectoralis minor

Level II – beneath pectoralis minor

Level III – medial to pectoralis minor

Anatomical groups

Anterior (pectoral) – medial wall of axilla, along the lateral thoracic A at the lower border of pectoralis minor, drain the majority of the breast (level I)

Posterior (subscapular) – medial wall of axilla in its posterior part, along the subscapular A, drain the posterior trunk and tail of the breast (level I)

Lateral – along the medial side of the axillary V, drain the upper limb (level II)

Central – within the fat of the axilla, receive lymph from all the above groups (level II)

Apical – at the apex of the axilla, receive lymph from all the above groups (level III)

Technique

Arm position:

- abduction initially to raise skin flaps and dissection of fat off the medial wall
- flexion to 90° allows relaxation of pectoralis major and dissection of improves access to the apex

Steps:

- raise skin flaps – inverted U-shaped incision – with arm in abduction
- sweep fat off pectoralis major, continuing on its deep surface and identifying, and preserving, the lateral pectoral N as it emerges from pectoralis minor
- flex the arm to relax pectoralis major and allow access to pectoralis minor
- divide the insertion of pectoralis minor on the coracoid process and dissect fat off the axillary vein, following this from medial to lateral, tying off tributaries
- sweep the specimen downwards and off the medial wall of the axilla, preserving the long thoracic N anteriorly and the thoracodorsal N and subscapular A posteriorly

Inguinal lymphadenectomy

Anatomy

Femoral triangle

Boundaries include the **medial** border of sartorius laterally, the **medial** border of adductor longus medially and the inguinal ligament superiorly

Further medially are adductor magnus and gracilis

Further laterally is rectus femoris

Gutter-shaped floor is formed by pectineus, psoas and iliacus (medial to lateral)

Femoral sheath containing the femoral V and A lies in the gutter of the femoral triangle with the femoral N most lateral and **outside** the femoral sheath

Just medial to the femoral vein, but within the femoral sheath, is the femoral canal which serves two functions:

- allows dilatation of the femoral vein
- transmits lymphatics from the deep inguinal nodes to the iliac nodes

Lymph node of Cloquet lies in the femoral canal, draining lymph for the clitoris/glans penis

Opening of the femoral canal in the thigh is the femoral ring – site of femoral hernia

Femoral artery, vein and nerve

Femoral artery

Four branches in the thigh, just below the inguinal ligament:

- superficial circumflex iliac
- superficial epigastric
- superficial external pudendal
- deep external pudendal

Profunda femoris A given off just beneath the distal edge of the femoral sheath, passing medially deep to adductor longus

Femoral A passes into subsartorial (adductor, Hunter's) canal to emerge as the popliteal A in the popliteal fossa

Adductor canal contains the femoral artery and vein and the saphenous nerve and distally communicates with the popliteal fossa at the adductor hiatus – hamstring and adductor heads of adductor magnus

Femoral vein

Femoral vein lies medial to the artery at the level of the inguinal ligament and deep to the artery at the inferior apex of the femoral triangle

Vein receives four tributaries corresponding to the arterial branches as above plus the long saphenous vein

Femoral nerve

Femoral nerve gives off:

- muscular branches to the extensor compartment of the thigh
- sensory branches: intermediate and medial cutaneous nerves of the thigh
- saphenous nerve

Other nerves include:

- lateral cutaneous nerve of the thigh which passes deep to the inguinal ligament at the origin of sartorius at the lateral apex of the femoral triangle
- femoral branch of the genitofemoral nerve (L1) pierces the femoral sheath to supply the skin overlying the femoral triangle

Lymph nodes and vessels

Lymphatics accompany the long saphenous vein

Superficial inguinal nodes:

- vertical group – lie along the termination of the long saphenous vein (lower limb)
- lateral group – below the lateral part of the inguinal ligament (buttocks, flank, etc.)
- medial group – below the medial part of the inguinal ligament (anterior abdominal wall below the umbilicus and the perineum)
- deep inguinal nodes lie medial to the femoral vein and communicate with superficial nodes via the cribriform fascia at the saphenous opening

Technique

Superficial circumflex iliac A and the deep external pudendal A are usually preserved during groin dissection as they lie deep, applied to the floor of the femoral triangle, and may help reduce skin necrosis

Other superficial vessels are usually scarified

Position: hip extended, slightly abducted and externally rotated

Begin 5 cm above the inguinal ligament, two-thirds along its length from the pubic tubercle and curve down to the inferior apex of the femoral triangle

Raise flaps to include fascia – all nodes are deep to fascia and skin flaps less prone to necrosis/wound breakdown

Clear fat to the margins of the femoral triangle working from above infer-laterally

Sartorius switch to cover the femoral vessels

Closure and drain

Complications of lymphadenectomy

Intra-operative – accidental damage to vessels and nerves

Early postoperative – skin necrosis, dehiscence, infection, seroma

Late postoperative – numbness and dysaesthesia, lymphoedema, hernia (groin dissection)

Superficial vs. radical inguinal node dissection

Kretschmer. *Acta Oncol* 2001

- Patients with deep inguinal (iliac) nodes have a poor prognosis with a high likelihood of distant disease
- Iliac node dissection significantly increases morbidity (limb oedema)
- Data conflicting on survival benefit following radical clearance of deep nodes
- Inguinal node clearance = femoral triangle up to inguinal ligament
- Iliac clearance = iliac and obturator nodes up to bifurcation of common iliac artery (or if nodes clinically enlarged up to aortic bifurcation)
- 69 patients underwent extended clearance, 35 underwent inguinal clearance only
  - 24/69 (35%) patients had positive iliac nodes
  - positive iliac nodes corellated with a significant increase in mortality (5-year survival 6% compared with 37% in iliac node – negative patients)
- no difference in overall survival between extended and superficial dissection groups
- unless there is evidence for pelvic nodal disease, a superficial (inguinal) node clearance should be undertaken

Superficial vs. combined superficial and pelvic node dissection

Hughes, A'Hern, Thomas. *Br J Surg* 2002

- Retrospective analysis of 132 patients (60 inguinal dissections, 72 extended dissections)
- Presence of pelvic lymph node metastases reduced survival from 47% (iliac node negative) to 19% (iliac node positive) at 5 years
- Other prognostic factors were extracapsular spread and number of positive superficial nodes
- Authors observed no significant increase in morbidity following extended dissections in comparison with superficial lymphadenectomy

Isolated limb perfusion

Isolated limb perfusion

Ariyan, *PRS* 1997

ILP in 67 limbs (16 upper, 51 lower) in 60 patients >21 years (Yale Melanoma Unit)

Pump oxygenator for 1 h, non-melphalan drugs including DTIC, cisplatin, carboplatin

Median leak up to 1.6% (upper) and 7.5% (lower) – ^{131}I-labelled serum albumin

4/60 → two perfusions, 2/60 → three perfusions

21% complication rate: oedema, seroma, dehiscence, infection, PE

Permanent oedema in 11 patients – all lower limb

No systemic toxicity

43 patients underwent therapeutic ILP:

- 11/43 patients alive and disease free at ~5 years (median figure)
- 5/43 patients alive with disease at ~4 years
- 27 patients died, 14 without local recurrence
- 17/60 patients treated prophylactically (six upper, 11 lower)
- 12/17 alive and disease-free at ~6.5 years
- five patients died, one without local recurrence

Conclusion: non-toxic drug alternatives to melphalan enable safe palliation and achieve good locoregional control

Used for locally advanced disease

Main agent used is melphalan, also cisplatin and recombinant TNF-α

General anaesthesia

Mild hyperthermia (38–43 °C)

Pump oxygenator with Ringer's lactate and 95% O_2 and 5% CO_2 with drugs added and perfused at ~200–400 ml/min

Direct arteriotomy and venotomy for placement of catheters

Flush out solution at the end of the procedure and replace with 1 unit blood

Repair vessels

Avoid synchronous lymphadenectomy

Death, amputation and life-threatening leukopenia all <1%

TNF + melphalan + IF-γ = complete response rate of 90%

Elective ILP: melanomas of 1.5–3.0 mm – locoregional control advantage; no survival benefit

Reduces local recurrence rate of subungal MM but does not influence survival

Management of in-transit melanoma of the extremity with isolated limb perfusion

Fraker. *Curr Treat Options Oncol* 2004

- limited number of in-transit metastases (1–3 nodules) managed by simple surgical excision with minimal negative margins and primary closures plus staging of distant disease
  - no role for wide excision of in-transit lesions
- indications for isolated limb perfusion (ILP)

- rapid recurrent in-transit disease
- disease out of local surgical control
- ILP is a regional administration of high-dose chemotherapeutics within an extremity using an extracorporeal circuit2
- Once isolation is obtained
  - The limb is heated to mild hyperthermia (38.5–40 °C)
  - chemotherapeutics administered at high concentrations for 60–90 minutes
  - At the end of the treatment period, the limb circulating blood volume containing toxic levels of the chemotherapeutic agent is flushed from the extremity and normal perfusion is re-established
  - Typical treatment regimen
    - melphalan @ 10 mg/l limb volume for lower extremities
    - melphalan @ 13 mg/l limb volume for upper extremities
- results
  - response rates between 80% and 90%
  - complete response rates between 55% and 65%
    - 20% to 25% of the total patient population have sustained complete responses
  - duration of response is typically 9 to 12 months
- side effects
  - skin erythema
  - myopathy
  - peripheral neuropathy

Isolated limb infusion

Contralateral limb vessels cannulated using a radiological technique and sited in affected limb

Manual infusion >15–20 min

LA plus sedation

Same efficacy as ILP but reduced side effects

Still need blood transfusion

Probably the way forward

Prognostic factors after isolated limb infusion with cytotoxic agents for melanoma

Lindner. *Ann Surg Oncol* 2002

Isolated limb infusion (ILI) is essentially a low-flow ILP performed without oxygenation via percutaneous catheters

- The outcome in 135 patients treated by ILI was reviewed.
  - The overall response rate in the treated limb was 85% (complete response rate 41%, partial response rate 44%).
  - Median response duration response was 16 months (24 months for patients with complete response)
  - Median patient survival 34 months
  - In those with a complete response, the median survival was 42 months.
- Complete response rate and survival time decreased with increasing disease TMN stage

- Patients aged >70 years had a better overall response than younger patients.
- Multivariate analysis, factors associated with an improved outcome with:
  - earlier stage of disease
  - final limb temperature > 37.8 °C
  - tourniquet time >40 minutes
- Conclusion
- The frequency and duration of responses after ILI were comparable to those achieved by conventional ILP. The ILI technique is particularly useful for older patients who might not be considered suitable for conventional ILP

Isolated limb infusion for melanoma: a simple alternative to isolated limb perfusion

Mian. Can J Surg 2001

- Initial experience with the new technique of isolated limb infusion (ILI) for in-transit melanoma
- Nine patients treated by ILI for extensive in-transit limb melanoma
- Morbidity
  - no peri-operative deaths
  - deep venous thrombosis and pulmonary embolism in one patient
- Control of the in-transit metastases was achieved to some degree in all patients and was complete in four patients

Conclusion

- ILI is an alternative treatment modality for patients suffering from multiple, advanced in-transit melanoma metastases
- provides effective palliation with limited morbidity
- offers a safe, quick, inexpensive alternative to isolated limb perfusion with comparable results

Melanoma and pregnancy

Management of patients with melanoma who are pregnant, want to get pregnant or do not want to get pregnant

Editorial. Schwartz. *Cancer* 2003

- management of patients with melanoma who are pregnant
  - prognostic factors same as for non-pregnant patients (sentinel node status, tumour thickness and ulceration)
  - SLNB may be performed as radiation doses involved (5 milli Grays exposure to the fetus) are far below levels known to induce fetal malformation (100 milli Grays), although the risk of anaphylaxis to isosulfan blue may preclude use of this dye
  - Transplacental metastases are extremely rare (19 cases reported) so termination is not indicated but submission of the placenta for histological evaluation is recommended
- management of patients with melanoma who want to get pregnant
  - advice on becoming pregnant following a diagnosis of melanoma is designed to avoid the development of metastatic disease during pregnancy and is therefore related to the prognostic indicators of the primary tumour

- hence patients with low risk lesions may be advised to wait longer than patients with high risk lesions (e.g. 3 years rather than 5 years from diagnosis)
- patients with a poor prognosis tumour are also advised to consider the effect of losing a mother in early childhood
- management of patients with melanoma who wish to use the oral contraceptive pill
  - no evidence to show that either the OCP or hormone replacement therapy adversely affects outcome in melanoma patients

Pregnancy and early stage melanoma

Daryanani. *Cancer* 2003

46 pregnant patients with stage I–II melanoma were age and AJCC stage matched with non-pregnant controls from the Groningen database

- 10-year disease-free survival and overall survival was similar in both groups of patients
- growth or change in pre-existing naevi during pregnancy, contrary to popular belief, is uncommon and should be treated as suspicious by expedient excisional biopsy

Melanoma and HRT

Jeffrey and Lewis. *Br J Plastic Surg* 2000

Short review of the risks relating to HRT in the context of melanoma

- Studies from Sweden and Denmark have failed to identify increased risk with HRT
- Review undertaken by Franceschi in 1990 also failed to find evidence of increased risk
- Women treated for melanoma should continue with HRT where indicated

Melanoma in children

Malignant melanoma in children

Naasan and Quaba, *PRS* 1996

4700 cases of MM in Scotland since 1979 (Scottish Melanoma Group)

50 in patients <18 years (1.04%); Male:female = 2.5:1

Of these, 15 in prepubertal patients, i.e. <14 years (0.03%); male:female = 1:1

Nine patients developed metastatic disease – all had lesions >1.5 mm thick

Of these, only one patient was prepubertal

8/9 patients died, maximum survival 4 years

23/50 families could provide a reliable history

8/23 described a pre-existing naevus

Classification of pre-pubertal MM:

- congenital MM acquired through transplacental spread
- MM arising *de novo*
- MM arising in giant congenital naevi

Errors in diagnosis due to histological similarity with Spitz naevi

Disease behaves similarly in children as in adults and the treatment should be the same

Malignant melanoma in children

Burd, *BJPS* 1997

47/3246 MM patients were <21 years (1.4%) at Frenchay, 1967–93

Female:male = 2:1

10/47 were pre-adolescent (<14 years) – 21%

83% SSM, 4% nodular, 2% acral lentiginous, the remainder unclassified

0.29–50.00 mm

Ulceration more common among post-adolescents

16 arose in pre-existing naevi (but no cases of giant congenital melanocytic naevus)

Thickness and ulceration independent prognostic variables

Conclusions: less nodular, acral and LMM in the young

Anorectal melanoma

Sphincter sparing local excision and radiotherapy for anal–rectal melanoma

Ballo. *J Clin Oncol* 2002

Uncommon aggressive tumour

Early metastatic spread

Poor prognosis

Presentation:

- fifth–sixth decade
- rectal bleeding
- pain
- palpable mass

Abdominoperineal resection may improve local control but not overall survival

- only indicated for bulky disease where local excision transgresses tumour

23 patients managed by local excision and radiotherapy

- hypofractionated regimen of 30 Gy (5 fractions over 2.5 weeks)
  - addresses potential submucosal spread via treatment to paracolic gutters
- three patients underwent lymph node clearance for palpable nodal disease
- four patients underwent successful SLNB
  - positive in one patient
- median primary tumour thickness 5 mm

15 patients died from melanoma within a median follow-up period 32 months

Actuarial 5-year disease-specific survival 31%

Actuarial 5-year local control 74% (nodal control 84%)

Anorectal melanoma

Pessaux. *Br J Surg* 2004

Melanoma accounts for <1% of all anorectal malignant tumours

- Present with bleeding
  - May be mistaken for haemorrhoidal bleed

20% of lesions are amelanotic

Poor prognosis – less than 20% 5-year survival

Review of 40 patients

No difference in overall survival between patients treated by wide local excision compared with patients who underwent abdominoperineal resection

- Hence WLE, not APR, recommended
- Median overall survival was 17 months

Soft tissue sarcoma

Incidence and aetiology

UK 2.5 per 100 000 population per year

- no clearly defined aetiology
- Genetic factors
  - Neurofibromatosis
  - Retinoblastoma
  - Li–Fraumeni syndrome
  - Familial polyposis coli
  - Gorlin's syndrome
    - fibrosarcoma
    - rhabdomyosarcoma
    - gene PTC (Chr 9q22.3)
  - alterations in cell regulatory genes, e.g. Rb-1 and p53 detected in substantial proportion of sarcomas
  - autosomal dominant gene in 8–9% of children with soft tissue sarcoma
  - translocation in Ewing's sarcoma
  - presence of TLS-CHOP fusion protein; now a definitive diagnostic tool for myxoid liposarcoma
- Chemical agents
  - Phenoxyacetic acids (herbicides)
  - Vinyl chloride
  - Arsenic
  - Chlorophenols (wood preservatives)
  - Thorotrast (radioactive contrast agent)
- Radiation exposure (incl. radioisotope implantation)
  - particularly breast Ca, cervical Ca, lymphoma.
  - poor prognosis
- Lymphoedema (lymphangiosarcoma), e.g. post-mastectomy, post-irradiation
  - sarcoma not radiation induced as found outside irradiated zone
  - also found in filarial lymphoedema
- Age and sex
  - males slightly more common than females
  - age
  - 40% > 55 yrs
  - 15% < 15 yrs
- Histopathologic subtypes
  - Malignant fibrous histiocytoma – elderly
  - Liposarcoma – middle age
  - Leiomyosarcoma – young
  - Rhabdomyosarcoma – children
- Anatomical site
  - most common extremity sarcomas
    - Liposarcoma, MFH, fibrosarcoma, tendosynovial sarcoma
  - retroperitoneal

- Liposarcoma, leiomyosarcoma
  - trunk wall
    - Desmoid tumour, liposarcoma

Referral to a soft tissue sarcoma service

(Standards and guidelines for the management of soft tissue sarcomas (2nd edn). South West Cancer Intelligence Service 2004)

1. Mass >4 cm
2. Deep mass
3. Enlarging mass
4. Painful mass

Tumours should not be biopsied prior to referral to a specialist sarcoma centre

Diagnostic pathway

1. Clinical assessment
   - Size of tumour (and likely defect)
   - Skin involvement (flap or graft?)
   - Pulses (vascular reconstruction?)
   - Sensation (nerve involvement? graft needed?)
   - Involved muscle groups (tendon transfer? vascularized muscle transfer?)
   - Age and fitness for surgery
   - Lifestyle (limb preservation?)
2. Radiological assessment
   - Ultrasound may exclude benign soft tissue swellings such as lipomata or Baker's cysts
   - Magnetic resonance imaging provides most information
     - Size of tumour
     - Relationship to surrounding structures
       - Planning of surgical/anatomical margins
     - Vascular reconstruction likely to be required?
     - Proximity to nerves (can they be preserved?)
     - Fatty tumours identified by suppression on T_2 images
   - CT required for assessment of bone involvement
   - Staging CT
     - Chest
     - Abdomen/pelvis
3. Biopsy
   - FNA
     - May successfully diagnose high-grade tumours
     - Can be undertaken prior to imaging
   - Core biopsy
     - Undertaken after imaging to avoid disruption of images by haematoma
     - Biopsy tract should be planned to avoid contamination of uninvolved compartments
       - excised at the time of definitive resection to avoid tumour seeding
   - CT guided core biopsy
     - Anticipate route of surgical excision (plan with operating surgeon)
     - Targets most suspicious or most representative area of the tumour
   - Open biopsy
     - Reserved for failed core biopsy
     - May upstage tumours by transgressing compartments

- Biopsy scar will need wide excision (may necessitate flap reconstruction)
- Provides ample tissue for diagnosis, often required for low grade and rarer tumours
- Can be combined with frozen section histopathology to facilitate completion of excision
  - Frozen section also used for histological control of margins
- Pathological considerations
  - Grade
  - Tumour type
- What is the potential for local recurrence
- What is the potential for distant recurrence
  - e.g. well-differentiated liposarcoma (atypical lipomatous tumour) may recur locally but highly unlikely to metastasize
  - Local recurrence after incomplete excision does not necessarily corellate with earlier development of distant disease

4. Planning
- Within a multidisciplinary team environment
- Consider neoadjuvant therapy (radio- or chemotherapy) for high grade tumours
  - Isolated limb perfusion with TNF-α may be considered to treat locally advanced and inoperable extremity tumours with poor prognosis instead of limb amputation
- Consider anatomical margins of planned excision (muscle groups to be removed, etc.)
- Consider requirement for flap reconstruction
  - Skin
  - Nerve
  - Functional muscle
- Consider risk of nodal metastases
  - Rhabdomyosarcoma, epithelioid, synovial
  - SLNB reported for these tumours
- Plan adjuvant therapy
  - Post-operative radiotherapy
    - Marginal excisions
    - High grade tumours >5 cm
    - Consider brachytherapy if near radiosensitive tissues
  - Post-operative chemotherapy
    - High grade tumours
    - Chemosensitive tumours

5. Follow-up
- Clinical assessment
  - Years 1 and 2   3 monthly
  - Years 3–5   6 monthly
  - then annually if appropriate until year 10
- Radiological follow-up
  - Local tumour site (MRI)
    - Deep tumours
      - Baseline postoperative cross-sectional imaging at 6–12 months
      - further imaging annually for up to 5 years
    - Superficial tumours – imaged if clinical suspicion of recurrent disease
  - Distant site imaging (high grade tumours)

- Plain chest X-ray at each clinical review
  - CT chest if any change from previous film
- Annual CT chest
- Distant site imaging (low grade tumours)
  - Rarely metastasize
  - Annual chest X-ray

AJCC staging of soft tissue sarcoma

T1	<5 cm	**Stage Ia** G1/2 T1a/b
T1a	Superficial to fascia	
T1b	Deep to fascia	
T2	>5 cm	
T2a	Superficial to fascia	**Stage Ib** G1/2 T2a
T2b	Deep to fascia	**Stage IIa** G1/2 T2b
N1	Regional node involvement	**Stage IV** N1
M1	Distant metastases	**Stage IV** M1
G1	Well differentiated	
G2	Moderately differentiated	
G3	Poorly differentiated	**Stage IIb** G3/4 T1a T1b
		Stage IIc G3/4 T2a
G4	Undifferentiated	**Stage III** G3/4 T2b

Tumours of fibrous tissue

Nodular fasciitis

Benign subcutaneous tumour due to reactive proliferation of fibroblasts

Incidence
Any age, commonest in middle age

Pathology
Spindle-shaped fibroblasts in a myxoid stroma
Infiltrate fat or muscle bundles

Clinical
Rapidly growing masses beneath the skin (<2 weeks)
Mainly found in the forearm
1–3 cm diameter
Often tender

Treatment
Excision
Resolution may follow incomplete excision

Histiocytoma

Histiocytes

monocytes derived from the bone marrow that populate areas of acute or chronic inflammation of the skin. Closely related to foreign body giant cells and epithelioid cells

Pathology

Histiocyte, fibroblast and vascular endothelial cell proliferation
Iron inclusion bodies
Foam cells

Clinical

Predilection for lower extremities
~20% preceded by trauma or insect bite
Firm brownish nodules with smooth or warty surface up to 3 cm diameter
Females > males
Dermatofibroma: a histiocytoma with maturation of cells towards fibroblasts
Malignant histiocytoma may represent malignant change in a benign histiocytoma or may arise *de novo*

Treatment

Excision
Resolution may follow incomplete excision but 5–10% may recur

Desmoid tumour

Firm, irregular tumour arising from the muscular aponeurosis of the abdominal wall
Fibroblast proliferation and mucoid degeneration
Mainly parous women third–fifth decades
Subumbilical area
Association with **Gardner's syndrome**
An aggressive fibromatosis prone to local invasion but unlikely to metastasize
Local recurrence high following inadequate excision

Extra-abdominal desmoid tumour of the breast

Godwin. *Br J Plastic Surg* 2001
- Case report of a 58-year-old female presenting with a desmoid tumour of the breast necessitating mastectomy with full thickness chest wall resection and reconstruction, followed by a further dorsal chest wall lesion 1 year later requiring similar excisional and reconstructive surgery
- Extra-abdominal desmoid tumours peak in incidence between 25 and 35 years of age
- May arise primarily in musculoaponeurotic tissue or elsewhere (e.g. breast)
- May be multifocal
- Histologically identical to abdominal desmoids
  - Spindle cells
  - Abundant collagen
  - Few mitoses

- Possible aetiological factors:
  - trauma
    - reports of desmoid tumours arising in scars
    - desmoid reported in the capsule surrounding a breast implant
  - hormonal factors
    - extra-abdominal desmoids may express oestrogen receptors
    - increased growth observed during pregnancy
    - peak incidence in post-pubertal and pre-menopausal women
  - genetic factors
    - Gardner's syndrome
    - Familial multicentric fibromatosis
- Surgery
  - Wide local excision recommended
    - Positive histological margins increase risk of local recurrence but this is not inevitable
    - Younger patients more prone to local recurrence
    - Musculoaponeurotic lesions more likely to be multifocal

Dermatofibrosarcoma protruberans

A locally malignant tumour of dermal fibroblasts

Incidence
- Uncommon
- Male = female
- Occasionally preceded by trauma
- Hormone sensitive – accelerated growth during pregnancy

Pathology
A well-differentiated fibrosarcoma
Potential for progression to high grade MFH
Masses of fibroblasts extending from the dermo-epidermal junction into subcutaneous tissues
Wide lateral spread

Clinical
Front of the trunk, extremities, head
Onset early adult life, rarely diagnosed during childhood (congenital DFSP also reported)
Red dermal nodules which coalesce and become bluish
Some lesions become painful, ulcerated and show rapid growth
Others become irregular protuberant swellings
Metastasis very rare

Treatment
Excision with a wide (3 cm) margin
Local recurrence common if inadequately excised

Fibrosarcoma

Malignant tumour consisting of cells resembling fibroblasts

Incidence and aetiology
- Uncommon
- Males > females
- From birth onwards but most common from age 30–60 years
- Burns scars and xeroderma pigmentosum

Pathology
- Atypical fibroblasts
- Generous blood supply
- May produce large amounts of mucin (low grade fibromyxoid sarcoma)
- Less well-differentiated tumours best described as anaplastic sarcomas

Clinical
- Most commonly affects the deep tissues of the thigh, then trunk
- Red–purple nodule
- Smooth surface
- Slow or rapid growth
- Readily metastasizes via blood or lymphatics
- Anaplastic lesions ulcerate
- Fluctuance due to intralesional haemorrhage

Treatment
- Wide excision
- Radiotherapy

Epithelioid cell sarcoma

- Malignant connective tissue tumour comprised of epithelioid cells
- Extremities mainly, especially palm/flexor surface of fingers
- Nodules associated with fascia, periosteum, tendon and nerve sheaths
- May ulcerate
- Local recurrence common
- Metastases frequent
- Commonly mistaken for ulcerated SCC

Atypical fibroxanthoma

Locally aggressive cutaneous tumour of the head and neck
Superficial variant of pleomorphic malignant fibrous histiocytoma
Has invasive potential, may recur locally after excision, and rarely metastasizes
Most commonly on the ears and cheeks of elderly people
Sun-damaged skin, previous radiotherapy
Red, fleshy granuloma-type appearance

Often ulcerated

History <6 months

Fibroblasts, histiocytes and multinucleate giant cells

Treat by excision >1 cm margins

Malignant fibrous histiocytoma (MFH)

- Commonest overall soft tissue sarcoma – 20% of all diagnoses
- Commonest sarcoma of late adult life
- Histiocyte and fibroblast-derived cells
- Subcutaneous nodule
- May arise in burn scar
- Treat by wide excision but local recurrence and metastases are common
- Storiform-pleomorphic, myxoid, giant cell and inflammatory subtypes

Liposarcoma

Malignant tumour of mesenchymal cells resembling fat cells

Incidence
- Rare
- Middle age onwards
- Males > females (benign lipomas: females > males)

Pathology
- Uniglobular and multiglobular fat cells
- Undifferentiated sarcoma cells
- Well differentiated liposarcoma can de-differentiate to high grade MFH

Clinical
- Diffuse nodular swelling of subcutaneous fat
- Most commonly lower limb or buttock
- Retroperitoneal and mesenteric fat
- Haematogenous spread

Treatment
- Excision with a wide margin (3–5 cm)
- Radiotherapy
- Local recurrence common

Tumours of vessels

Glomus tumour

Glomus body: highly convoluted arteriovenous shunt richly innervated by sympathetic nerves controlling thermoregulatory activity. Consists of five parts:

- afferent artery
- arteriovenous channel
- neuroreticular tissue
- outer layer of lamellar collagen
- collecting veins

Glomus tumour: a tumour of proliferating glomus cells surrounded by nerves and vascular channels

Incidence and aetiology

- Late childhood onwards
- Female > male
- Familial inheritance (AD)
- Multiple tumours associated with limb malformations
- May have a preceding history of trauma

Pathology

Encapsulated dermal tumour

Epithelioid cells, derived from the pericyte of Zimmerman (also gives rise to haemangiopericytoma)

Alignment of glomus cells along vascular channels

Unmyelinated nerve fibres

Clinical (including glomus tumours of the hand)

van Geertruyden. *J Hand Surg* 1996

Pink–purple painful nodule

Usually on extremities, especially subungal

Larger tumours, situated elsewhere, may not be painful

Malignant change does not occur

Triad of pain, tenderness and cold sensitivity

Love's test: provoke with a pin head

One-third of patients have radiological evidence of indenting of distal phalanx

May have multiple tumours on one finger

Also metacarpals, wrist, neck, thigh, knee, leg

Average duration of symptoms before treatment was 10 years

Treatment

- Excision, if incomplete, leads to recurrence
- Remove nail first and repair nail bed afterwards
- Recurrence is usually within a few weeks

Pyogenic granuloma

Vascular nodule comprised of proliferating capillaries in a loose stroma

Often follows trauma

Reactive rather than neoplastic

Rapid evolution

Bleeds easily

Proliferating vessels extend deep into dermis, hence recurrence after cautery

May also treat by excision

Kaposi's sarcoma

Malignant, multifocal tumour of proliferating capillary endothelial cells and perivascular connective tissue cells

Incidence and aetiology
- *Type 1*: chronic – originally restricted to Eastern European Jews and Mediterranean races
- *Type 2*: lymphadenopathic
- *Type 3*: transplantation associated
- *Type 4*: related to HIV infection

Pathology
Spindle cells in a maze of vascular channels

Lymphocytic inflammatory response

Clinical
Multifocal blue–purple macular plaques which grow and coalesce

Usually on the extremities which become lymphoedematous

Lesions may involute or ulcerate and fungate

May develop in internal organs without skin manifestation

Lymphadenopathy

Develops in 50% of AIDS patients

Treatment
- Excision
- Radiotherapy
- Cytotoxic drugs

Angiosarcoma

- Least frequent soft tissue sarcoma
- Very poor prognosis generally
- Commonest non-rhabdomyosarcoma STS of childhood 930% present in under 20s)
- Four clinicopathological types
  - Cutaneous angiosarcoma
    - Elderly patients
    - Head and neck
    - Often well differentiated
  - Angiosarcoma of the breast
    - Occurs following radiotherapy for breast cancer
    - Associated with lymphoedema in the breast and extremeties
    - Often high grade
  - Angiosarcoma of the deep soft tissue
  - Angiosarcoma of the parenchymal organs, e.g. liver

Tumours of nerves

Neurofibroma (*Molluscum fibrosa*)

Benign tumour derived from peripheral nerves and supporting stromal cells including neurilemmal cells

Soft fleshy tumours, sessile or pedunculated

May become plexiform, usually in association with the fifth cranial nerve

Neurofibromatosis: multiple neurofibromas in association with café au lait spots, Lisch nodules (pigmented iris hamartomas), axillary freckles and acoustic neuromas

AD inheritance, frequently the result of mutation

Sarcomatous change (increase in size and pain) commoner in non-cutaneous lesions (<15%)

Cutaneous meningioma

Scalp and paraspinous region in children and young adults

Soft dermal or subcutaneous mass 2–10 cm in size

Histological features as for intracranial meningioma (psammoma bodies)

Merkel cell tumours (trabecular cell carcinoma, small cell carcinoma of the skin)
Al-Ghazal. *BJPS* 1996

Merkel disc: expanded cutaneous nerve ending responsible for mechanoreception An aggressive malignant tumour arising from dermal Merkel cells

Incidence
- Females > males (4:1)
- Elderly

Pathology
- Mass of small dark cells
- Immunostaining for neuro-endocrine differentiation

Clinical
Reddish-blue nodules

Any body site, particularly head and extremities

Aggressive tumour with early lymphatic spread

Spontaneous regression has been reported previously

Treatment
Wide excision

High recurrence rate after surgical excision: radiotherapy after resection

Combined chemotherapy followed by radiation therapy for advanced locoregional Merkel cell carcinoma and metastatic disease

Amenable to sentinel lymph node biopsy

Malignant peripheral nerve sheath tumour (malignant schwannoma)

Arise de novo or in pre-existing neurofibromas

Most are associated with the major nerves of the extremeties or trunk

Affects adults between 20 and 50 years of age

Clinically aggressive with *high metastatic potential*

Tumours of muscle

Leiomyoma

Benign smooth muscle tumour arising from erector pili muscle (leiomyoma cutis), tunica media of blood vessels (angiomyoma) or panniculus carnosus of the genitalia or nipple (dartotic myoma)

Familial lesions often multiple

Proliferation of smooth muscle-derived spindle cells

Presents as a collection of painful/tender pinkish dermal nodules

Adjacent nodules coalesce to form a plaque

Cutis lesions most commonly on the extremities

Distinguish from histiocytoma or glomus tumour

Excision is curative

Leiomyosarcoma

Malignant tumour of smooth muscle

- Most frequent site is uterine wall
- Also found in retroperitoneum
- Cutaneous leiomyosarcoma a distinct entity presenting as a reddish dermal nodule (see below)

Presents >60 years of age

Spindle-shaped cells containing myofibrils

Cytological atypia

May be painful/tender

Invades muscle and spreads along fascial planes and blood vessels

Haematogenous and lymphatic metastases

May present as a metastatic deposit of retroperitoneal leiomyosarcoma

Treat by wide local excision and adjuvant therapy where indicated

Cutaneous leiomyosarcoma

Porter. *Plastic Reconstruc Surg* 2002

Accounts for 1–2% of all soft tissue sarcomas

Present as smooth skin-coloured nodules

Mainly caucasians, male = female

Associated with premalignant leiomyomas, physical trauma, radiation

Arises from dermal smooth muscle

- Arrector pili
- Smooth muscle surround eccrine glands

High risk of local recurrence but metastases never reported

- *Sub*cutaneous leiomyosarcoma may have a metastatic potential – distinct biologically from cutaneous leiomyosarcoma

Retrospective review of eight patients over 12 years, mean follow-up 5 years

Mean patient age 62.2 years (range 39–84 years)

Four lesions located on head and neck, remainder on extremities

No local or distant recurrence observed despite narrow margins in some patients

Rhabdomyosarcoma

Incidence and aetiology

Most common soft tissue sarcoma in children <15 years

- 40% arise in children <5 years

Association with Li–Fraumeni syndrome and Beckwith–Wiedemann syndrome

- Most RMS sporadic

Increased risk in children to parents using marijuana or cocaine

Most frequently head and neck (approximately one-third)

- GU tumours approximately one-quarter (bladder, prostate, paratesticular)
- Extremity tumours 20%

Painless enlarging mass plus localized symptoms and signs

Head and neck RMS:

- Orbital
- Parameningeal
  - Middle ear, nasal cavity, paranasal sinuses, nasopharynx, infratemporal fossa
- Non-parameningeal
  - Scalp, parotid, oral cavity, larynx

Pathology

Some tumours may exhibit skeletal muscle and nerve differentiation (Triton tumours)

Pathological subtypes

- Embryonal (70%, primitive spindled rhabdomyoblasts)
- Alveolar (20%, increasing in proportion with age, common in extremities)
- Botryoid (5%, myxoid stroma, genitourinary tumours)
- Pleomorphic (1% rarest form, pleomorphic rhabdomyoblasts, adult RMS)

Treatment

Complete surgical resection, if not mutilating or cosmetically unacceptable (often the case), is the treatment of choice in combination with adjuvant treatments

- Includes elective or therapeutic dissection of regional nodes

Where surgery is not possible according to these criteria:

- Biopsy
- Definitive radiotherapy
  - But complicated by growth disturbance and induction of secondary tumours

- Adjuvant chemotherapy
  - Multiagent chemotherapy: the **Intergroup Rhabdomyosarcoma Study III**
    - Mainstay of adjuvant chemotherapy is VAC (Vincristine, Actinomycin D, Cyclophosphamide)
  - **IRS-IV** compared cyclophosphamide (VAC) with Ifosfamide (VAI) but showed no difference

5-year disease-free survival up to 65%

Advances in the surgical management of sarcomas in children

Andrassy. *Am J Surg* 2002

Soft tissue sarcoma accounts for approximately 7% of all childhood cancers

- Rhabdomyosarcoma accounts for over half of these

Synovial sarcoma

- Most common non-rhabdomyosarcoma (NRSTS) soft tissue sarcoma in children (30% of all patients with synovial sarcoma are under 20 years of age)
- Commonest location on lower extremity
- Lymph node metastases occur in up to 15% of cases
  - SLNB used to assess nodal status
- Distant metastatic disease mostly to the lungs
- All tumours essentially regarded as high grade
- Chemotherapy generally ineffective
- Adequate negative surgical margins essential plus adjuvant radiotherapy
- Late relapse possible therefore long-term follow-up advocated

Malignant fibrous histiocytoma (MFH)

- Second most common NRSTS in children after synovial sarcoma
- Surgical excision is the mainstay of treatment
- Poor prognostic indicators included size >5 cm and involved surgical markers

Fibrosarcoma

- Usually low grade in children
- Present as painless slow growing masses, usually on the extremeties in children over 8 years of age
- Prediliction for local recurrence even after apparent complete excision with negative margins

Extraosseus Ewing's sarcoma

- Closely related to peripheral neuroectodermal tumours (PNET)
- Highly chemoresponsive
  - Neoadjuvant chemotherapy commonly used
- Aggressive surgical resction after chemotherapy offers a good prognosis

Neurofibromatosis

- Patients especially under 10 years of age at risk from the development of malignant peripheral nerve sheath tumours
- Hence rapid growth of a cutaneous neurofibroma, or increasing pain, regarded as suspicious of malignant transformation

Rhabdomyosarcoma

- Botryoid RMS has best prognosis
- Alveolar RMSD has a poor prognosis (may be site specific – prediliction for extremity, trunk and perineal tumours)
- Li–Faumeni syndrome (inherited germ line P-53 mutation) associated with 20–30 $\times$ increased risk of STS or bony sarcoma

- Head and neck primaries in around 35% of patients
- Genitourinary RMS accounts for around 26% of primary tumours
- Extremity RMS (19%) associated with inguinal node involvement in up to 50% of patients

Treatment

- wide local excision and regional node staging
  - Complete excision, if possible, is desirable
  - Node staging by SLNB
  - Orbital, vaginal and bladder RMS treated by neoadjuvant chemotherapy shows good response and facilitates more limited surgery
  - Solitary lung metastases are very rare – confirmation of diagnosis by biopsy is required
- Postoperative chemotherapy and/or radiotherapy

Miscellaneous sarcomas

Synovial sarcoma

Most common in adolescents and young adults

Arises from soft tissues in the vicinity of large joints of the extremeties

Pathological subtypes:

- Biphasic with epithelial and sarcomatous cells
- Monophasic fibrous
- Monophasic epithelial

Poor prognosis with local and distant (including lymphatic) recurrence

Epithelioid sarcoma

Prominent epithelioid tumour cells

Adolescents and young adults

Subcutaneous and deep tissues of the hand and forearm predominantly

- Ulcerated nodules, often multifocal
- Deep lesions may adhere to tendon or fascia

Poor prognosis with local and distant (including lymphatic) recurrence

Clear cell sarcoma

Mainly young adults

Typically presents as a subcutaneous mass around the knee

S-100 and HMB45 positive – variant of malignant melanoma

Poor prognosis with local and distant (including lymphatic) recurrence

Positive resection margins, local recurrence and survival

- Relationship between local tumour recurrence and survival yet to be fully defined
- Local recurrence is a marker of an aggressive tumour that is more likely to metastasize

Classification of positive margins following resection of extremity soft tissue sarcoma and risk of local recurrence

Gerrand. *J Bone Joint Surg* 2001

A positive surgical margin may occur after limb sparing excision of soft tissue sarcoma for the following reasons:

1. *low grade liposarcomas*
   - often present as large tumours
   - planned marginal excision to protect vital structures such as blood vessels and nerves
   - seldom recurs locally and rarely metastasizes
   - a separate biological entity from soft tissue sarcomas of other histological types
2. *planned positive margins*
   - deliberate marginal resection of tumours other than low grade liposarcoma to preserve vital structures
   - decision to accept positive margins agreed at MDT planning meeting
3. *positive margin at re-excision of an incompletely excised and previously unrecognized sarcoma*
   - previously unrecognized sarcoma
   - attempted excision by a non-sarcoma surgeon with positive margins
   - re-excised by the sarcoma team, again with positive margins
4. *unplanned positive margin*
   - primary surgery performed by the sarcoma team but surgical margins found to be histologically positive
   - further excision always considered

Retrospective review of database of 566 soft tissue sarcoma patients at Mount Sinai Hospital, Toronto

- 87 patients had positive margins after limb sparing surgery for extremity soft tissue sarcoma
- all had had neoadjuvant radiotherapy and a post-operative radiotherapy boost
- most common histological types in groups 2–4 were MFH and liposarcoma
- High:intermediate grade approximately 2:1 for groups 2 and 3 and 1.3:1 for group 4
- Local recurrence at mean follow-up of 5.4 years:
  - Group 1 4.2%(1/24 patients)
  - Group 2 3.6%(1/28 patients)
  - Group 3 31.6%(6/19 patients)
  - Group 4 37.5%(6/16 patients)
- Risk of local recurrence must be compared with morbidity during limb sparing surgery for soft tissue sarcoma
- Low rate of recurrence following excisional surgery with planned positive margins

High grade extremity soft tissue sarcoma: factors predictive of local recurrence and its effect on morbidity and mortality

Eilber. *Ann Surg* 2003

Retrospective review of 753 patients treated for intermediate to high grade extremity sarcoma at UCLA

- 704 had limb sparing surgery
- 49 had primary amputation
- 498 had neoadjuvant chemotherapy plus radiation
- 607 patients were treated for primary tumours
  - 95% limb salvage
  - 63 patients developed locally recurrent disease (10%)
    - 24 required amputation to control disease
    - 7 had no further treatment due to development of systemic disease
- 146 patients were treated for locally recurrent tumours
  - 87% limb salvage
  - 29 patients developed locally recurrent disease (20%)
    - 11 required amputation to control disease
    - 6 had no further treatment due to development of systemic disease
- 18 patients overall had microscopically positive margins (2%), treated by:
  - amputation (3)
  - additional local excision (5)
  - additional radiotherapy (8)
  - no further treatment (2)
- 92 patients overall developed locally recurrent disease
  - 5 had positive resection margins (none subsequently amputated)
  - 87 had negative resection margins
    - positive resection margin was not a significant risk factor for the development of local recurrence
  - 25% of recurrences developed within 8 months
  - 50% of recurrences developed within 16 months
  - 75% of recurrences developed within 36 months
  - 13% of recurrences developed beyond 5 years
- Significant risk factors for development of local recurrence in order of hazard ratio:
  1. MPNS
  2. High histological grade
  3. Age >50 years
  4. Failure to receive neoadjuvant treatment was the only risk factor in patients treated for already locally recurrent disease
- Significant risk factors for decreased survival in order of hazard ratio:
  1. Local recurrence
  2. High histological grade
  3. Leiomyosarcoma
  4. Size
  5. Age >50 years
  6. Lower extremity location
  7. Male gender a risk factor in patients treated for already locally recurrent disease
- Overall survival in the primary tumour group:
  - 71% at 5 years
  - 62% at 10 years
- Overall survival in the already recurrent tumour group:
  - 67% at 5 years
  - 52% at 10 years

Re-resection of soft tissue sarcoma

Zagars. *Cancer* 2003

MD Anderson Cancer Centre experience of 666 patients in whom macroscopic tumour clearance had been achieved *prior to* tertiary referral

Histological margins were defined as:

- negative
  - if tumour was not actually present at the inked margin, the distance from it was not regarded as significant and the margin was judged to be negative
- positive
  - presence of microscopic disease at the surgical margin
- uncertain
  - no comment upon margin of clearance on the pathology report from the referring centre

Re-resection undertaken only when the primary surgery was judged as inadequate and when re-resection could be undertaken without significant functional morbidity

- 295/666 patients underwent re-resection
  - 9% of patients with negative margins ($n = 12/129$)
  - 53% of patients with uncertain ($n = 220/427$) or positive margins ($n = 63/110$)
- residual tumour identified in 46% of patients overall
  - 33% of patients with negative margins (but small group)
  - 45% of patients with uncertain margins
  - 55% of patients with positive margins
  - 25% of re-resections revealed macroscopic tumour
- when re-resection was not undertaken megavoltage radiation therapy was administered (371 patients)

Local control at 5, 10 and 15 years was greater in the re-resection group at each time point

Most significant predictors of local recurrence:

- patient age >64 years
- positive or uncertain resection margins (negative margins may be achieved by re-resection)
- recurrent tumour at presentation to the specialist unit
- tumour size >10 cm

Predictors of lymph node recurrence:

- histopathological tumour type
- epitheliod sarcoma, rhabdomyosarcoma, clear cell sarcoma

Predictors of distant metastases:

- tumour size >5 cm
- tumour grade
- margin status (negative margins may be achieved by re-resection)
- no evidence to suggest that local tumour recurrence in patients who did not undergo re-resection mediated in the development of distant metastases

Disease free and overall survival (where initial surgical margins were uncertain or positive):

- patients in whom negative margins were not achieved by re-resection had shorter disease free and overall survival compatred with patients who underwent re-resection
  - most significant for tumour of the extremeties or superficial trunk, least significant for head and neck tumours
- also significant were:
  - tumour size
  - tumour grade

Major amputation for soft tissue sarcoma

Clark and Thomas. *Br J Surg* 2003

Retrospective review of 40 major amputations undertaken at the Royal Marsden Hospital for soft tissue sarcoma over a 10-year period

- 18 forequarter
- 17 hind quarter
- 5 through hip
- 31/40 performed for recurrent disease following limb sparing surgery
- 37/40 performed with curative intent
- 25 high grade tumours, 18 > 10 cm diameter, 6 multifocal

Median hospital stay 10.5 days

20/40 patients (50%) disease-free survival at 12 months

- 9/40 (23%) alive and disease free beyond 2 years

Phantom pain or sensation after operation in 30/40 patients

- severe in 8 patients
- mild in 22 patients

Flap reconstruction in extremity soft tissue sarcoma

Lohman. *Cancer* 2002

Review of 100 patients requiring resection of an upper extremity soft tissue sarcoma at the MD Anderson Cancer Centre and the University of Alabama, Birmingham USA

- 71 patients required no reconstruction, defect closed primarily
- 29 patients required soft tissue reconstruction
  - two amputations reconstructed with free fillet flaps
  - more recurrent tumours
  - more tumours >5 cm
- 29% underwent intralesional (positive histological margins) or marginal (within the tumour pseudocapsule) resection
  - 70% of patients underwent wide excision (cuff of normal tissue) or compartmental resection
- indications for flap reconstruction included:
  - insufficient soft tissue for primary closure
  - cover of neurovascular structures or implant material
  - fill dead space
- free flaps used most commonly for reconstruction of the elbow region
  - gracilis, latissimus dorsi, rectus abdominis
- pedicled flaps used most frequently at the junction of the upper extremity with the trunk
  - latissimus dorsi, pectoralis major
- wound complications common in both groups of patients
  - primary closure group 24%
  - flap reconstruction group 38%
    - 1/29 total flap failure
- local recurrence
  - average margin for patients with local recurrence 9 mm
  - average margin for patients without recurrence 10 mm
    - not statistically significant

- recurrence rates similar for primary closure and flap reconstruction groups
- size of the resection margin is often dictated by the proximity of vital structures when undertaking limb sparing surgery

Soft tissue sarcomas of the upper extremity

Popov. *Plastic Reconstruc Surg* 2004

Retrospective review of 95 upper extremity soft tissue sarcomas treated at the Helsinki University Hospital over a 12-year period

80 patients underwent surgery with curative intent

- 67 high grade tumours
- 15 patients referred with local recurrence
- reconstructions included pedicled and free flaps

Definition of surgical margins:

- **compartmental** (entire compartment resected *en bloc* with tumour)
  - included 'myectomy' for intramuscular tumours
- **wide** (nearest margin >2.5 cm or <2.5 cm but intact anatomical barrier, e.g. fascia)
- **intralesional** (macroscopic or microscopic disease at margin)
- **marginal** (<2.5 cm but negative histological margins)

Aim of surgery:

- preservation of function
- wide excision
- if wide excision impossible then planned marginal excision supplemented by adjuvant radiotherapy
- amputation only when a major nerve, bone or joint was infiltrated by tumour (ten patients)
- reoperation following intralesional excision where possible

Results of treatment at 5 years:

- 79% overall local control rate
  - prognostic indicators for local recurrence was extracompartmental site (excludes cutaneous, subcutaneous or intramuscular tumours)
    - no difference in local recurrence rates when extracompartmental tumours treated by wide excision compared with marginal excision plus radiotherapy
      - radiotherapy should be considered following excision of all extracompartmental sarcomas
    - local control rate for extracompartmental tumours was 69%
- overall metastases-free survival 68%
  - prognostic indicators for metastases included extracompartmental primary and large tumour size

Cutaneous metastatic malignant tumours

Order of frequency: breast, stomach, lung, uterus, large bowel, kidney, prostate, ovary, liver, bone

Histologically usually poorly differentiated

May resemble primary lesion

Foreign body type inflammatory reaction

Trunk and scalp most affected

Para-umbilical metastases secondary to intra-abdominal malignancy (Sister Joseph's nodule)

Treat by excision or laser to prevent fungation

Miscellaneous conditions

Hyperhidrosis

Hyperhidrosis: a review of current management
Plastic Reconstruc Surg 2002

Excessive sweating from eccrine sweat glands affecting axillae, palms and soles of feet

Stains clothing, embarrassing socially

Primary hyperhidrosis:

- Affects up to 1% of the population
- Young adults predominantly

Secondary hyperhidrosis, due to:

- endocrine disorders, e.g. hyperthyroidism, menopause
- neurological disorders, e.g. syringomyelia
- drugs, e.g. antidepressants
- neoplastic disease, e.g. Hodgkin's lymphoma, carcinoid, phaeochromocytoma

Conservative treatment

- topical agents
  - Aluminium chloride hexahydrate in alcohol (Driclor)
- Systemic agents
  - Anxiolytic drugs, e.g. benzodiazepines to reduce anxiety-provoked symptoms
  - Glycopyronium bromide (anticholinergic side effects)
- Iontophoresis
  - Useful for palmar and plantar disease
  - Mechanism of action not fully understood
  - 15 treatments on average required to achieve euhydrosis
- Botulinum toxin
  - Temporary relief of symptoms
  - Multiple injections injected intradermally in a grid pattern
  - General anaesthesia required for palmar and plantar injections
  - 50 units of BoTox per treated area
- Surgery
  - Excision of skin and/or subcutaneous tissue (direct closure, Z-plasty or S-shaped closure)
    - Iodine-starch test used to define most affected areas
    - Wound infection, dehiscence, haematoma, delayed healing common
  - Axillary liposuction
    - Superficial (subdermal) liposuction
  - Thoracoscopic sympathectomy
    - more suited to palmar than axillary hyperhidrosis – good response rates
    - Horner's syndrome, thoracic duct injury and phrenic nerve injury reported

- Compensatory sweating on trunk, limbs or face in up to 50% of patients, especially if sympathectomy bilateral (treat dominant hand only)
- Vasodilated, dry fissured skin

Management of axillary bromidrosis – axillary bipedicled flap (modified Skoog procedure)

Wang. *Plastic Reconstruc Surg* 1996

Bromidrosis is an offensive odour due to the bacterial degradation of excessive apocrine sweat gland secretion

- Eccrine sweat glands
  - Entire body surface
  - Salt secretion
  - Cholinergic sympathetic nerves
- Apocrine sweat glands
  - Axilla, periareolar area, perianal area, eyebrows
  - Fat, cholesterol and salt secretion on to hair shafts
  - Ten times larger than eccrine glands
  - Adreneric sympathetic nerves
  - Present in equal numbers as eccrine glands in the axilla

Technique:

- Parallel incisions made in the axilla and a bipedicled strip of skin is raised
- Bipedicled flap turned over and careful thinning undertaken with scissors
- Divides sweat gland ducts and generates fibrosis between gland and skin surface
- Further parallel incisions can be made to extend treated area
- Technique similar to that originally described by Skoog, 1963 – raised four flaps (staggered + shape)

Good resolution of hyperhidrosis and bromidrosis

- reduction in sweating in 92% of operated axillae at 30 months

Hidradenitis suppurativa

Inflammatory disease of apocrine sweat glands

Recurrent deep abscesses in axillae and groins

Mostly young females

Excise to fascia under antibiotic cover, SSG if primary closure impossible

Delayed wound healing common

Hidradenitis suppurativa: pathogenesis and management

Slade. *Br J Plastic Surg* 2003

Disease associated with obesity, acne and hirsutism (i.e. androgen related) but not diabetes

- Weight loss can help control symptoms

Strongly linked with smoking, smokers should be advised to stop

May be familial (autosomal dominant inheritance)

Female:male 3:1

Peak incidence second and third decade

Non-surgical management

- Oral clindamycin 300 mg twice daily (including peri-operative infection prophylaxis)

- Cyproterone acetate (anti androgen) improves symptoms in females
- Acetretin 25 mg twice daily (retinoids reduce sebaceous gland activity)
- Laser treatment
  - CO_2 laser
  - Heal by secondary intention

Surgical management

- Incision and drainage of acute abscess formation
- Excision of hair/gland bearing skin
  - Healing by secondary intention
  - Primary closure of small defects
  - Reconstruction of larger defects
    - Split skin graft $+/-$ VAC dressings
    - Flap reconstruction

Excision and flap reconstruction for axillary hidradenitis

Soldin. *Br J Plastic Surg* 2000

59 patients (94 axillae) treated surgically for hidradenitis supprativa in two centres

Surgery

- Limited local excision
- Excision of hair bearing skin
- Wide excision including a 2 cm margin around hair bearing skin

Reconstruction

- Primary closure
- Split skin graft
- Flap reconstruction (Limberg – including fasciocutaneous – and parascapular flaps)

Less disease recurrence observed wih more radical excision although no significant advantage to wide excision with a margin over excision of all hair bearing skin only

Wound breakdown observed in all modalities of closure

Scar contracture observed in one third of axillae reconstructed with skin grafts

Pyoderma gangrenosum

Intense dermal inflammatory infiltrates composed of neutrophils

Little evidence of a primary vasculitis

Aetiology: altered immunologic reactivity

Diagnosis is based on clinical and histopathological findings

Cutaneous ulceration with a purple undermined border

Multiple skin abscesses with necrosis, often pretibial

~50% of cases of pyoderma are associated with a specific systemic disorder: inflammatory bowel disease, rheumatoid arthritis, non-Hodgkin's lymphoma, Wegener's granulomatosis (especially head and neck lesions) and myeloproliferative disorders

4% of patients are children

Gram-negative streptococci frequently cultured from wounds

Treat with steroids, azathioprine and cyclosporin

Surgery may exacerbate the disease

Pyoderma gangrenosum has been reported in a lower limb fasciocutaneous flap and complicating breast reduction (3 back-to-back reports, *Br J Plastic Surg* 53 (5), 2000).

Pyoderma gangrenosum

Callen. *Lancet* 1998

Classical PG may be associated with symptoms of fever, malaise, myalgia and arthralgia and has also been described in early childhood

Variants include

- parastomal PG
  - occurs in patients with inflammatory bowel disease following abdominal surgery
- genital PG
  - may be associated with Behçet's disease
- pyostomatitis vegetans
  - intraoral PG, linked with inflammatory bowel disease
- atypical (bullous) PG
  - superficial ulceration
  - blue–grey bullous margin
  - arm and face most affected
  - linked with haematological disease

2 Principles of plastic surgery (local and free flaps, skin grafts, wound healing)

Adult wound healing
Classification of skin grafts
Blood supply of the skin
Blood supply of muscles
Individual flaps

Adult wound healing

Wound repair proceeds through stages of:
- inflammation
- tissue formation (fibroplasia)
- remodelling (maturation)

Phases that are not mutually exclusive but overlap

Inflammatory phase

Upon wounding haemorrhage ensues and **haemostatic cascades** are activated to produce a
platelet clot, adherent to type II collagen, exposed by endothelial disruption

Platelet plug is a source of prepackaged
- **growth factors** – PDGF, TGF-α and -β
- **inflammatory vasoactive** and chemotactic cytokines

Fibrinogen, fibronectin, thrombospondin and von Willebrand factor

Subsequent **fibrin–thrombin mesh** traps more platelets to perpetuate the cycle

After an initial period of vasoconstriction there is active vasodilatation due to inflammatory
mediators (histamine, kinins, complement)

Macrophages are attracted to the wound where they synthesize and release further cytokines
and growth factors

Dermal **fibroblasts** migrate into the wound by forming cell–matrix contacts with provisional
matrix proteins such as **fibronectin**, vitronectin and fibrinogen

Integrins expressed by fibroblasts are predominantly α-1-integrins for attachment to
fibronectin and α-5-integrins for attachment to vitronectin

Within **12 h** of wounding, **neutrophils** and **monocytes** appear in the wound, attracted by chemotaxins including fibrin degradation products, complement proteins, leukotrienes, TGF-β and PDGF

Translocation of marginating neutrophils through capillary endothelium and basement membrane is facilitated by secretion of collagenase

Unless there is a continuing inflammatory stimulus, the neutrophil response and wound population declines after a few days, whereupon dead cells are cleared by macrophages

T-lymphocytes migrate into wounds following the influx of macrophages and persist for up to 1 week – anything less than this $\rightarrow$ poorer wound healing

Role of T-lymphocytes is to mediate in fibroblast recruitment and activation

Re-epithelialization begins within hours of wounding by crawling of marginal keratinocytes over matrix but beneath eschar

There is a phenotypic conversion of differentiated keratinocytes into non-polarized cells expressing basal cytokeratins (K5/14) and reminiscent of **cultured keratinocytes** or psoriatic skin

Restitution of the basement membrane induces these cells to adopt their previous morphology and form anchoring junctions with fibronectin

EGF mRNA levels increase rapidly after wounding to promote re-epithelialization, and although EGFR transcripts are similarly elevated, the EGFR protein appears to be functionally down-regulated in response to high EGF levels

Abnormalities of EGF expression are thought to impair wound healing

Glucocorticoids suppress EGF expression in cutaneous wounds but have less effect on EGF receptor levels

Increased mobility of wound keratinocytes is afforded by the dissolution of anchoring junctions and reorganization of the cortical actin cytoskeleton to form lamellipodia

Altered gap junction connexin expression, mainly an up-regulation of connexin 26, has been detected within 2 h of epidermal wounding and may coordinate these keratinocyte movements

In addition to growth factors, keratinocyte-specific cytokines have also been identified in cutaneous wounds

Melanocyte growth-stimulating activity, or growth-related gene (MGSA/GRO), is normally expressed by suprabasal, differentiated keratinocytes and is up-regulated in regenerating human epithelium

MGSA/GRO is a ligand for the type B IL-8 receptor which is also up-regulated both in proliferating keratinocytes and in dermal fibroblasts, macrophages and smooth muscle, suggesting that this cytokine may act as an autocrine or paracrine factor-mediating cutaneous wound repair

Insulin-like growth factor-1 (IGF) and IGF-binding protein-1 have been demonstrated to act synergistically to accelerate the healing of adult skin wounds suggesting a similarly important role in healing

Fibroplasia

Begins about day 4 and may last up to 2–4 weeks depending upon the site and size of the wound

Neovascularization of the wound and formation of a **type 3 collagen scaffold** (features of mature **granulation tissue**) are observed after $\sim$4 days

Activin A has been implicated in stimulating formation of granulation while activin B mRNA has been localized to hyperproliferative epithelium at the wound edge

Secretion of glycosaminoglycans (hyaluronic acid, chondroitin sulphate, dermatan sulphate) which become hydrated to form an amorphous **ground substance** within which fibrillar collagen is deposited

Increased wound **tensile strength** occurs during this fibroblastic phase

Oxygen tension → 40 mmHg augments **fibroblastic activity** and is required for the hydroxylation of proline and lysine residues to form **cross linkages** in the collagen α-chain

Oxygen also facilitates **cell-mediated killing** of pathogens in the wound

Zinc, vitamins A (retinoids) and C are also required for normal collagen_synthesis

Remodelling

Composition of the extracellular matrix changes during healing and appears to modulate fibroblast activity

When fibronectin predominates in the matrix, fibroblasts actively synthesize hyaluronic acid and collagen, but in a maturing wound, when the amount of collagen formed in the wound reaches a certain, abundant level, fibroblast proliferation and collagen production ceases irrespective of any residual stimulation by TGF-β

At this point, usually ∼10 days, the wound becomes a relatively acellular scar

Residual fibroblasts mature into **myofibroblasts** and form cell–matrix and cell–cell contacts to **contract** the wound

Remodelling commences ∼3 weeks after injury

Type 3 collagen is gradually replaced by **type 1 collagen** by the activity of metallomatrix proteins released by macrophages, keratinocytes and fibroblasts

Normal type 1:type 3 ratio = 3:1

Initially disorganized but then becomes **lamellar** by the activity of fibroblasts and collagenases with permanent cross-links

Regression of abundant capillaries

Peak wound tensile strength is at ∼60 days and achieves ∼80% of unwounded skin strength

Other points

Increasing age → decreased rate and strength of healing

Tissue expansion → increased rate and strength of healing

Low serum protein → prolonged inflammatory phase and impaired fibroplasia

Increased ambient temperature (30°) → accelerated wound healing

Wound infection → prolonged inflammatory phase, reduced oxygen tension affecting fibroplasia, collagen lysis, inefficient keratinocyte migration

Most factors impairing wound healing may be attributed to a lowering of the oxygen concentration in the wound including radiotherapy and diabetes

Anticoagulation

Aspirin: prevents platelet aggregation

Heparin: forces thrombin to bind irreversibly with antithrombin III

Dextran 40: complexes with fibrinogen

Fracture healing

Formation of a coagulum between the bone ends which becomes invaded by macrophages and fibroblasts to form a fibrin clot

Periosteal reaction:

- invasion of capillaries from the periosteum into the fibrin clot
- differentiation of periosteal mesenchymal cells along osteoblastic pathways to become chondrocytes
- formation of a cartilaginous external or bridging callus
- the extent of callus formation increases where there is movement of the bone ends
- further differentiation of chondrocytes into osteoblasts
- endochondral ossification to form woven bone

Medullary reaction:

- inflammatory response from within the medullary cavity
- macrophages remove tissue debris while osteoclasts resorb necrotic bone
- osteoblastic deposition of new woven bone without a cartilaginous phase

Re-organization into lamellar bone

Primary cortical union

Occurs where bone ends are anatomically reduced and there is rigid fixation

Bone regeneration from within the opposed Haversian canals

Little or no external callus reaction

Tendon healing in the hand

Dense network of spiralling collagen fibres. Predominantly type 1, some type 3, some elastin

Relatively acellular but contains: tendon cells (tenocytes), fibroblasts and synoviocytes

Endotenon is continuous with perimysium and periosteum

Epitendon – a vascular, cellular outer layer of a tendon which runs through a synovial sheath (zones 1 and 2)

In zones 3+, where there is no tendon sheath, the outer vascular layer is called 'paratenon'

Blood supply to the tendon in zones 1 and 2 is via a mesentry ('mesotenon') called the vinculum – long and short

Synovial fluid also contributes to nutrition via imbibition

Healing by a process of inflammation, fibroplasia and remodelling

Intrinsic healing by cells within the tendon itself

Extrinsic healing by cells recruited from synovial sheaths and surrounding tissues → adhesions

Strength of healing and rate of healing are maximal in a tendon which is moving and stressed

Tendon repair weakest during period of collagen lysis at about day 14

Gene therapy and plastic surgery

Tepper *Plastic Reconstruc Surg* 2002

The introduction of genetic material into cells in order to modulate protein synthesis for clinical benefit

Getting the genes into cells:

- Non-viral method (physical or chemical transfer)
  - Direct injection of DNA

- Insert the desired gene into a commercially available plasmid vector and inject directly into cell
- But low transfection efficiency and unable to target specific cells
- Electroporation
  - Electrical pulses punch holes in cell membranes allowing genetic material to pass through
  - But low transfection rates, non-specific and need a mechanism for delivery of electrical pulses
  - Useful *in vitro* technique
- Particle bombardment
  - Bombardment of cells with gold particles coated in genetic material
  - But unable to reach internal organs, non-specific and may damage cells
- Cationic liposomes
  - Genetic material contained within a positively charged liposome
  - Liposomes injected intravascularly and pass into cells by phagocytosis
  - Positive charge allows for interaction with negatively charged cellular DNA
  - Simple technique but low, non-specific transfection
  - Aerosol form may be used to deliver genes to pulmonary epithelial cells
- Antisense oligonucleotides
  - Single stranded fragments of DNA that bind specifically to messenger RNA for a particular gene product
  - Block synthesis of an undesirable gene
- Viral method (higher transfection efficiency
  - Adenoviruses
    - Viral genome not incorporated into host chromosome therefore low risk of insertional mutagenesis but only short-term gene expression – unsuitable for diseases requiring longer-term therapy
  - Adeno-associated viruses
    - Attractive viral vector because not associated with any human disease
    - Can insert into the host genome for long-term expression
  - Retroviruses
    - Integrate into areas of the host genome controlling cell growth (oncogenes) so may be cause of malignant transformation
    - Hence made replication deficient by removal of viral genes at the time of construction of the recombinant viral vector
      - *gag* (viral core proteins)
      - *pol* (reverse transcriptase)
      - *env* (evelope protein)
    - desired gene inserted in to space that is left between long terminal repeats
    - Most vectors derived from murine leukaemia virus
    - Only transfect replicating cells
    - Stable and permanent integration of the desired gene
  - Herpes simplex virus
    - Useful for targeting central nervous system
    - But difficult to make replication deficient and potentially toxic

Application of gene therapy in plastic surgery
- Optimising or boosting levels of growth factors at wound sites

- Skin
  - Transfection of keratinocytes by genes encoding EGF, IGF-1, TGFβ1 and PDGF demonstrated *in vitro* and in animal models to increase growth factor expression and improve wound healing
- Ligaments
  - Introduction of the *lac Z* gene in to cells cultured from rabbit tendon and ligament cell cultures
- Blood vessels
  - Increased angiogenesis by modulation of expression of VEGF, FGF and nitric oxide demonstrated *in vitro* and *in vivo*
  - Implications for flap survival
- Nerves
  - Delivery of genes encoding neurotrophic factors such as NGF-3 and brain-derived neurotrophic factor (BDNF) to enhance nerve regeneration
- Bone
  - Success with transfection of marrow cells with the *bmp-2* gene in enhancing fracture healing in rats
- Cartilage
  - Increased synthesis of collagen observed *in vitro* following transfection of human chondrocytes with TGFβ1
- Cranial suture development
  - Premature suture closure related abnormal FGFR1 and FGFR2 expression and binding
  - regulated by interaction of suture cells with the underlying dura
  - Transfection of rat dural cells *in vivo* with a gene encoding a defective *fgfr2* gene, capable of binding FGF2 but incapable of signal transduction
  - prevented the programmed closure of cranial sutures shortly after birth

Cytokines, growth factors and plastic surgery

Rumalla. *Plastic Reconstruc Surg* 2001

Cytokines

- proteins required for cell defence
- secreted predominantly by immune cells
- mediate in protective and reparative processes
- also regulate cell growth and maturation
- proinflammatory cytokines
  - TNFα
    - Released by macrophages/monocytes
    - Release stimulated by interaction with pathogens, tumour cells and toxins
    - Mediates in chemotaxis of inflammatory cells
    - Up-regulation of cellular adhesion molecules at neutrophil target cell sites eg vascular endothelium (margination)
    - Appears at wound sites after 12 hours of wounding and peaks at 72 hours
      - Effects include haemostasis, increased vascular permeability and collagen synthesis (although may impair wound healing if persists at high levels beyond natural peak)
    - Excess TNFα associated with multi-system organ failure
- Interleukin 1

- Produced by macrophages/monocytes and keratinocytes at wound sites
- Neutrophil activation and chemotaxis
- Detectable at wound sites after 24 hours, peaks around day 2 then rapidly declines
- Increased collagen synthesis and keratinocyte maturation
- High levels at chronic non-healing wound sites
- Interleukin 2
  - Produced by T lymphocytes
  - Sustains the post-injury inflammatory response via T-cell activation
  - Also promotes fibroblast infiltration at wound sites
- Interleukin 6
  - Released by macrophages/monocytes, polymorphs and fibroblasts
  - Promotes stem cell growth, B- and T-cell activation and mediates in hepatic acute phase protein synthesis (involved in the immune response)
  - Detectable at wound sites within 12 hours (as polymorphs arrive) and persists for up to a week
  - Stimulates fibroblast proliferation
    - High IL-6 increases scarring
    - Low IL-6 in elderly patients with impaired wound healing
    - Low IL-6 at scarless fetal wound sites
  - High systemic IL-6 levels a marker of wound extent/severity (eg major burns) and a prognostic indicator for poor survival
- Interleukin 8
  - Released by macrophages and fibroblasts at wound sites
  - Neutrophil chemotaxis, adhesion (via up-regulated expression of endothelial cell adhesion molecules) and activation
  - Promotes keratinocyte maturation and migration
  - High IL-8 in patients with psoriasis
  - Low at fetal wound sites
- Interferon γ
  - Produced by T-cells and macrophages
  - Macrophage and polymorph activation
  - Mediates in wound remodelling, reduces wound contraction
  - Possible role for decreasing scar hypertrophy but may decrease wound strength
- Anti-inflammatory cytokines
  - Interleukin 4
    - Produced by T-cells, mast cells and B-lymphocytes
    - Promotes B-cell proliferation, IgE mediated immunity and inhibits the release of pro-inflammatory cytokines by macrophages
    - Promotes fibroblast proliferation and collagen synthesis at wound sites
      - High levels in patients with scleroderma
  - Interleukin 10
    - Produced by macrophages and T-cells
    - Inhibits production of pro-inflammatory cytokines at acute wound sites
    - But if persistent at high levels at chronic wound sites, e.g. venous ulcers, IL-10 contributes to impaired the wound healing response

Growth factors

- Polypeptides whose primary role is in regulation of cell growth and maturation

- Platelet-derived growth factor
  - Released from α granules within platelets and by macrophages
  - Recruitment and activation of immune cells and fibroblasts in the early post injury phase
  - Later stimulates the production of collagen and glycosaminoglycans
  - Thre isomers of PDGF (2 polypeptide chains 'A' and 'B'):
    - AA: elevated at acute wound sites
    - BB: most useful clinically, used for chronic and diabetic ulcers (Regranex®)
    - AB
- Transforming growth factor β
  - Released by macrophages, platelets and fibroblasts
  - Fibroblast maturation, collagen and proteoglycan synthesis
  - Inhibition of proteases
  - Three isomers:
    - TGF-β1
    - TGF-β2
    - TGF-β3
  - TGF-β1 and 2 associated with hypertrophic and keloid scarring
    - Neutralizing antibodies decrease scarring at adult rat wound sites
    - Low TGF-β at fetal wound sites
  - TGF-β3 shown to decrease scarring
    - Ratio of TGF-β1 and 2:3 determines nature of scar
- Fibroblast growth factor
  - Regulates angiogenesis and keratinocyte migration at wound sites
  - Two main forms:
    - Acidic FGF (FGF-1)
    - Basic FGF (FGF-2)
      - Binds the same receptors as aFGF but ten times more potent
      - Apllication of exogenous bFGF to wound sites accelerates re-epithelialization
  - Eight other isoforms complete the family
    - FGF-7 and FGF-10 known as keratinocyte growth factor 1 and 2
      - Released from fibroblasts and endothelial cells
      - Important for keratinocyte maturation and migration
      - KGF-1 low in diabetics and steroid immunosuppression
      - Recombinant KGF shown to improve re-epithelialization at wound sites
- Epidermal growth factor
  - Released from keratinocytes to promote epithelialization
  - Also promotes collagenase release from fibroblasts (remodelling)
    - Decreased fibroblast EGF receptor expression during ageing
    - EGF inhibits wound contraction at fetal wound sites
- Vascular endothelial growth factor
  - Released mainly from keratinocytes, also macrophages and fibroblasts
  - Promotes angiogenesis at wound sites
  - Mediates in the formation of granulation tissue
- Insulin-like growth factor
  - At wound sites released by macrophages, neutrophils and fibroblasts
  - Promotes fibroblast and keratinocyte proliferation
  - Possible role in angiogenesis

- Two isoforms IGF-1 and IGF-2
- Levels rise to peak within 24 hours of wound and persist for several weeks
- Low IGF observed in diabetic and steroid-suppressed wounds

Classification of skin grafts

Autograft
Allograft
Xenograft
Split thickness, full-thickness, composite

Skin graft take

Adherence
- fibrin bond between graft and bed (especially if the bed is composed of granulation tissue)
- easily disrupted by shear forces and subgraft haematoma/seroma (adherence stronger on fascia)
- day 3 – in-growth of vascular tissue and collagen laid down by fibroblasts
- fibroblasts in a SSG are derived from circulating monocytes or perivascular mesenchymal cells
- bacterial proteases impair adherence

Plasmic imbibition – graft swelling and oedema
- breakdown of intracellular proteoglycans in graft cells into more osmotically active subunits
- absorption of interstitial fluid by osmosis
- may contribute to graft nutrition

Revascularization (inosculation)
- circulation restored after 4–7 days (thicker grafts take longer)
- vascular connections differentiate into afferent and efferent vessels
- re-innervation
- lymphatic circulation restored after a week
- full-thickness grafts establish a new dermal circulation
  - can bridge small areas of avascular graft bed
  - tolerate ischaemia poorly
    - may lose appendages
    - need a well-vascularized bed overall

Skin graft non-take

Shear
Haematoma
Infection
Unsuitable bed (avascular)

Graft maturation

Increased mitoses from day 3 onwards
Epidermal hyperplasia (scaling and desquamation)

Regeneration of appendages – sweat glands and hair follicles. Hair noticeable after 14 days in well-vascularized FT grafts

Re-innervation

- nerves enter neurilemmal sheaths
- sympathetic innervation of sweat glands
- sensory innervation of PT grafts (from 4 weeks) faster than FT grafts

Pigmentation – SSG

SSG vs. FTSG

SSG

- more contraction at the recipient bed
- less donor site morbidity
- survives better during the phase of plasmic imbibition – can wait longer for revascularization

FTSG

- less contraction at the recipient bed
- donor site morbidity in the form of a linear scar
- pigment changes but can be a good colour match with carefully selected donor site. Hyperpigmentation reduced by avoiding stimulation of melanocytes by sunlight
- less guaranteed take
- adnexal structures maintained
  - hair transplantation
  - lubricate grafts until return of sebaceous activity
  - sweating activity parallels the recipient rather than the donor site due to sudomotor re-innervation of the graft:
    - palms, soles and axillae stimulated by emotion
    - other sites stimulated by temperature

Re-innervation of SSG and FTSG occurs from the margins and from the graft bed

Final sensation may approximate that of adjacent skin unless bed is severely scarred

Sensory return begins at 3 weeks and can continue to improve for 2 years

Skin graft contraction

Primary

Immediate contraction of the graft due to the elastin fibre content of the dermis, i.e. graft shrinks

- FTSG shrinks by ~40%
- SSG shrinks by ~10%

Secondary

Recipient bed, not the skin graft, is the site of contracture

Factors that decrease graft contracture:

- thicker graft (FTSG)
- more rigid recipient site (e.g. periosteal bed leads to little contracture)
- greater percentage take (other areas heal by secondary intention)

Commences at day 10 and continues for up to 6 months

Some contracture may be beneficial, e.g. grafts on the fingertip contracting to draw sensate skin over the tip – hence choose SSG

Bone graft

Cortical bone
- **non-viable scaffold matrix**
- osteocytes within lacunae die leaving an intact Haversian canal system
- take by a process of **osteoconduction**
- osteoclastic resorption and osteoblastic bone deposition
- initially high strength, decreases with resorption, regained after remodelling

Cancellous bone
- **viable osteoblasts**
- morcellized pieces of bone readily vascularized from surrounding tissues
- **osteogenesis** by viable osteoblasts
- **osteo-induction** by bone morphogenetic proteins. Undifferentiated mesenchymal cells differentiate along osteoblastic pathways
- initially low tensile strength but increases as bone is incorporated

Distraction osteogenesis

Bone is resorbed when exposed to compressive forces and laid down when exposed to tension forces – principle of orthodontic treatment

Fibrovascular matrix between bone ends

Zones of bone formation and remodelling

Cartilage graft

Low metabolic requirements

Vascularized by surrounding tissues

Fat graft

Fat cells become digested by histiocytes, which then form new fat cells

Alternatively receive nutrient from surrounding tissues

Dermis included in the graft adds collagen bulk and improves take

Self assessment: outline of the process of healing of a skin wound

Four phases:

Coagulation – clotting cascade/complement along with activation of platelets → prepackaged growth factors (PDGF, TGFβ) and inflammatory cytokines → thrombin–platelet plug

Inflammation – days 0–4 – activation of mast cells (histamine) and influx of neutrophils (inflammatory mediators and cytokines), macrophages (remove debris, release TGFβ) and T-lymphocytes (recruit and activate fibroblasts), phenotypic conversion of differentiated keratinocytes to immature cells with lamellopodial crawling over the wound surface which begins within hours of injury

Fibroplasia – day 4 to 3 weeks – influx of fibroblasts over fibronectin scaffold (synthesize type III collagen) accompanied by blood vessels to form granulation tissue

Remodelling – 3 weeks to 18 months – differentiation of fibroblasts into myofibroblasts (scar contracture), remodelling of type III collagen into type I; maximum tensile strength by day 60 (80% of normal)

Self assessment: How does a fracture heal?

Four phases:

Haemorrhage – activation of clotting cascade, macrophage influx, formation of granulation tissue

Inflammatory phase – formation of an external bridging callus – differentiation of undifferentiated mesenchymal cells in the periosteum to form chondroblasts, laying down of cartilage to form a fibrin–cartilage callus; this undergoes endochondral ossification

Medullary reaction – debris cleared by osteoclasts and new bone laid down by osteoblasts without passing through a callus stage

Remodelling of woven bone to lamellar bone

Also primary cortical union – rigid internal fixation, regeneration of bone from Haversian canals

Self assessment: Outline the process of graft take

Four phases:

Adherence – fibrin bond between graft and bed

Plasmic imbibition – breakdown of matrix gags into osmotically active units, fluid enters by osmosis (graft swells) to provide nutrition

Revascularization – days 4–7 – blood vessels link up with graft vessels to restore circulation, alternatively there is neo-angiogenesis; lymphatic circulation restored by 1 week

Remodelling – from day 7 – from superficial to deep: epidermal hyperplasia, regeneration of adnexal structures, re-innervation, pigmentation changes, contracture of the graft bed

Collagen synthesis

Triple helix formed from three α-helical chains

25 different α-chains have been identified, each encoded by a separate gene

15 different types of collagen

Types of collagen:

- fibrillar
- network-forming
- fibril associated

90% of body collagen is type I

In normal skin the ratio of types I:III $= 3:1$

Type	Number	Distribution
Fibrillar	I	Bone, skin, tendon, ligaments, cornea (deficient: OI)
Fibrillar	II	Cartilage (deficient: chondrodysplasia)

Type	Number	Distribution
Fibrillar	III	Skin, blood vessels (XS: early wound, early DD, hypertrophic scar; deficient: Ehlers–Danlos)
Network-forming	IV	Basal laminae
Fibrillar	V	As for type I (active stage DD)
Fibril	IX and XII	
associated		Decorate fibrillar collagen

Synthesis:

- gene translation to form pro-α-chains
- post-translational modification – hydroxylation of proline and lysine residues (requires vitamin C and iron)
- assembly of pro-α-chains → pro-collagen
- pro-collagen secreted in secretory vesicles
- cleavage of pro-peptides on α-chains → collagen
- covalent cross links form between collagen molecules → fibril
- aggregation of fibrils → fibre

Regeneration

Formation of lost tissue without scarring

Labile cells – divide and proliferate throughout life, e.g. epithelia, blood

Stable cells – normally quiescent but can be stimulated to replicate, e.g. liver cells, bone cells

Permanent cells – once lost are never regained, e.g. neurones, cardiac muscle

All tissues heal with some degree of scarring in adult life except perhaps liver and the blood

Immunology

Major histocompatability Ags (in humans called human leucocyte antigens – HLA) – types 1 (all nucleated cells and platelets) and 2 (antigen-presenting cells – Langerhans cells, etc. – macrophages and lymphocytes)

Antigen-presenting cells present alloantigen to T-cells and express IL-1

IL-1 → T-helper (CD4 +) cells → IL-2

IL-2 → clonal expansion of T-helper cells and B-lymphocytes

IL-2 also → activation of Tc-cells and NK cells (cellular immunity)

B lymphocytes → antibody-mediated cell lysis (humeral immunity)

Allograft rejection

Hyperacute rejection:

- preformed antibodies
- rejection response begins immediately

Acute rejection:

- 7–10 days, due to T-cell infiltrate (cellular immunity)
- may be delayed in immunocompromised patients until the immunodeficient state has passed, e.g. recovery from a burn or stopping immunosuppressant drugs

Late rejection – Ab-mediated cell lysis (humeral immunity)

Graft versus host – occurs when allograft containing lymphoid tissue reacts against an immunocompromised host

Immunosuppressant drugs

Cyclosporin → blocks IL-2 → blocks clonal expansion of Tc-cells
Azathioprine → inhibits T-cell-mediated rejection by preventing cell division
Prednisolone → blocks the generation and release of T-cells

Factors influencing a fine scar

Surgical factors

Atraumatic technique
Eversion of wound edges
Placement of the scar:

- parallel to relaxed skin tension lines (facial wrinkles)
- adjacent to or within contour lines (e.g. nasolabial fold)
- within or adjacent to hair bearing areas (e.g. facelift, Gilles lift)

Shape of the scar:

- 'U'-shaped scars become pin-cushioned, e.g. bilobed flap
- ellipse length should be $4\times$ its width to avoid dog ears

Choice of suture:

- absorbable vs. non-absorbable:
  - absorption by proteolytic enzymes
  - mucous membranes absorb faster than muscle
  - rate of absorption also related to size of the suture
  - vicryl = polygalactic acid (polymer of glycolic acid – AA):
    - tensile strength gone by 30 days
    - absorbed by 90 days
    - braided, hence infection risk
  - PDS = polydioxanone:
    - loses tensile strength at 60 days
    - absorbed by 180 days
    - i.e. both double that for vicryl
    - monofilament
- non-absorbable sutures cause less tissue inflammation
- monofilament vs. braided
- cutting versus non-cutting needle

Patient factors

Age – infants and the elderly – good scars
Region of the body
Skin type – glabrous skin results in more scar hypertrophy
Individual's scar forming properties – hypertrophic/keloid scar former

Factors that contribute to suture marks

Length of time the suture is left in place

- sutures removed within 5–7 days do not leave stitch marks

- sutures removed at 14 days do leave stitch marks
- subcuticular sutures also avoid stitch marks

Tension on the wound edges

- sutures tied too tightly
- wound tension relieved by subcuticular stitches

Region of the body

- hands rarely affected by stitch marks
- face also rarely affected
- trunk, upper extremities more commonly affected

Infection

- remove infected sutures or will leave a mark
- braided sutures harbour more bacteria (*Staphylococcus*)
- minimize the number and weight of sutures

Propensity to keloid formation

Hence note that the suture itself (silk vs. ethilon vs. staples, etc.) is not so important

Abnormal scars

Abnormality of collagen metabolism – increased synthesis or decreased degradation

Fibroplasia into the third week without resolution

?Sustained levels of TGF-β (ratio of TGF-β1 and -2 to -β3)

High content of type III collagen

Numerous Langerhans cells

Not distinguishable by light microscopy although there are ultrastructural changes in collagen chains discernible by EM

Sensitivity symptoms due to release of neuropeptides from nerve endings in the scar

- substance P
- neuropeptide Y
- CGRP

Axsain® cream – contains capsaicin → neutralizes substance P → less itching/sensitivity

Hypertrophic scars

Limited to the initial boundary of the injury

Occur soon after injury

Spontaneous regression over years

Related to wound tension and delayed healing

- pull in multiple directions → hypertrophic scar
- pull in one direction → stretched scar (Langer's technique

Meyer and McGrouther *BJPS* 1991)

Sites of predilection include anterior chest, shoulders, deltoid

Young age

Keloid scars

Extension beyond the original boundary

Occur later after injury (months)

No regression

Better correlated with dark skin colour (15× more common in black people)

Young age

Significant familial tendency

Wounds do not have to be under tension – face, earlobes may also be affected in addition to the above

May represent an autoimmune phenomenon

Accelerated growth during pregnancy, may resolve after the menopause

Management

Intralesional steroid, pressure, topical silicone, surgery

Theories:

- pressure → decreased collagen synthesis, increased collagen lysis
- silicone → hydration of the wound
- steroids → decreased collagen synthesis

Keloid scars worsened by surgery and less success with topical silicone

Surgery may be contemplated in conjunction with postoperative radiotherapy (in keloids, 25% recurrence surgery plus radiotherapy, surgery alone >50–80% recurrence)

Retinoic acid (vitamin A) → decreased fibroblast DNA synthesis – some benefit in keloids

5% Imiquimod has been used to prevent recurrence after surgery (see below)

- an immune response modifying agent
- an imidazoquinolone compound that stimulates the production of Interferon α, TNF and IL-2 by binding to surface receptors (e.g. Toll 7) on macrophages and other inflammatory cells including T-cells
- Interferon α impairs collagen synthesis
- the generation of a T-cell mediated immune response and proinflammatory cytokines is used clinically to treat viral infections (including anogenital warts, HSV and *Molluscum contagiosum*) and non-melanoma skin cancers
  (Stanley. *Clin Exp Dermatol* 2002)
- reports also on the use of imiquimod in the treatement of lentigo maligna
  Powell. *Clin Exp Dermatol* 2002

Effect of imiquimod on keloid scars

Berman. *Am J Dermatol* 2002

5% imiquimod cream (Aldara) used topically following excision of keloid scars trialled in 12 patients with stable keloids

applied once daily from the day of surgery for 8 weeks

no recurrence observed at 24 weeks

- 7 scars showed mild hyperpigmentation

recommended as an adjuvant treatment for excised keloid scars

International clinical recommendations on scar management

Mustoe. *Plastic Reconstruc Surg* 2002

Evidence-based overview on scar management, citing over 300 published articles

Classification of scars:

- mature

- pale and flat
- immature
  - red and lumpy
  - itchy or painful
  - matures to become pale and flat (occasionally hyper- or hypopigmented)
- linear hypertrophic
  - post surgery or trauma
  - arise within weeks of surgery and grow over 3–6 months
  - rope-like appearance
  - maturation within 2 years
  - due to excessive tension or delayed wound healing
    - external taping used to reduce risk of hypertrophic scar
- widespread hypertrophic
  - widespread raised, red itchy scar
  - typically a burns scar – remains within the borders of the burn
- minor keloid
  - focally raised, red, itchy scar that extends beyond the borders of the original injury
  - may take up to a year to develop
  - fails to resolve, excision complicated by recurrence
  - genetic and anatomical influence
- major keloid
  - as for minor keloid but may continue to extend over years

Therapies:

- keloid scars
  - intralesional steroid first-line treatment option
    - triamcinolone 40 mg/ml
    - side effects dermal atrophy, telangiectasia and depigmentation
    - topical steroid generally less efficaceous
  - topical silicone gel sheeting
  - surgery alone = recurrence in 45%–100%
  - surgery + intralesional steroid = recurrence <50%
  - surgery + radiotherapy = recurrence 10%
    - risk of cancer induction
    - reserved for resistant keloid in adults
  - laser
    - recent reports of success using Nd:YAG for flattening keloid scars
    - pulsed dye laser reduces redness
- hypertrophic scars
  - silicone gel sheet first-line treatment option
    - commenced within days of wound healing
    - minimum 12 hours per day (ideally 24 hrs)
    - twice daily washing
  - intralesional steroid
  - pressure therapy
    - 24–30 mmHg for 6–12 months
  - surgery + external splintage + silicone gel sheet
- experimental therapies

- intralesional interferon injections
- intralesion 5-FU
- intralesional bleomycin

Blood supply of the skin

Cutaneous arteries

Direct branches of segmental arteries (concentration of direct cutaneous perforators near dorso-ventral midlines and intermuscular septae)
Perforating branches from nutrient vessels to deep tissues, especially muscle

Anastomoses between cutaneous arteries

Plexuses:
- subepidermal
- dermal
- subdermal
- fascial
- subfascial

True anastomoses, no change in calibre
Choke vessels, reduced calibre vessels which dilate to restore blood flow to areas of flap ischaemia

Cutaneous veins

Valved or avalvular oscillating veins in subdermal plexi
Bidirectional flow between adjacent venous territories
Equilibration of flow and pressure
Valved channels directing blood away from a venous plexus or towards a central draining vein
Interconnecting system of choke veins, tend to be oscillating

Concept of angiosomes

Taylor and Palmer. *BJPS* 1987
3D blocks of tissue supplied by a single artery and its venae commitantes (source vessels)
Adjacent angiosomes connected by true anastomoses or small calibre choke vessels
Choke vessels allow perfusion of an angiosome when raised with an adjacent angiosome and its source vessels
Angiosome composed of an arteriosome and a venosome
Junctional zone tends to occur within muscle, hence muscle choke vessels dilate to provide collateral circulation to an adjacent angiosome

An individual muscle may be included in two or more angiosomes, hence skin paddle from one angiosome may be raised on a muscle with a source vessel in the adjacent angiosome

If one source vessel is small, the adjacent source vessel is large – 'law of equilibrium'

Delay phenomenon

Useful for expanding the territories of random pattern flaps

Conditions the flap to survive with reduced blood flow

Partially sympathectomizes the flap to facilitate opening of choke vessels and angiogenesis

Choke vessel hypertrophy and hyperplasia maximal at 48–72 h

Longitudinal vascular orientation in a random pattern flap

Increased tolerance to ischaemia

Maximally augmented blood flow at 2–3 weeks

New A–V circulation established within 7 days

Optimal if delay is carried out in stages by elevating flap from base to tip

Delay phenomenon exploited for flap prefabrication

Tissue expansion is considered a type of delay

Testing vascularity with fluorescein:

- inject 20 ml 5% fluorescein IV ~20 min after the flap has been raised
- observe pattern of yellow–green fluorescence under UV light (Wood's lamp) in a darkened room

Skin flaps – Mathes and Nahai classification

Direct cutaneous flaps:

- axial cutaneous arteries, e.g. breast, groin, scapular area
- horizontal cutaneous vessels travel in loose connective tissue rather than on the deep fascia
- soft tissue laxity

Fasciocutaneous flaps:

- horizontal cutaneous vessels lie on the deep fascia
- difficult to separate off fascia so safest to include fascial layer in the flap
- skin relatively immobile over deep fascia, e.g. limbs, scalp

Septocutaneous flaps – perforators from the subfascial source vessel course along intermuscular septae, e.g. lateral arm flap ('in-transit perforators')

Musculocutaneous flaps – occasionally perforators arise as indirect branches from muscle branches off the source vessel (gluteal area)

Relationship of vessels to nerves

Cutaneous nerves travel parallel to vessels; hence, many fasciocutaneous flaps are neurosensory

Venous freeways (long saphenous, cephalic)

Long single arteries (lateral intercostal) or a series of perforators linked by true anastomoses

Classification of flaps according to their blood supply

Random pattern flap is a flap which relies for its vascularity upon the vessels of the **dermal and subdermal plexuses of the skin**

Axial pattern flap is vascularized **by vessels running longitudinally within it**:

- direct cutaneous A
- fasciocutaneous A
- septocutaneous A
  - intermuscular septum
  - muscle perforators

Types of local flap

Flaps that move about a pivot point

Rotation flap:

- **semicircular flap that rotates about a pivot point through an arc of rotation into an adjacent defect**
- donor site either closes directly (buttock rotation flap) or with a skin graft (e.g. scalp rotation flap)

Transposition flap:

- **triangular, square or rectangular flap that moves laterally about a pivot point into an adjacent defect**
- Z-plasty, Limberg flap, bilobed flap
- other examples include a posterior thigh flap for ischial sore
- hatchet flap is probably a combination of rotation and transposition – could be likened to a rotation with a large back cut

Interpolation:

- **flap that moves laterally about a pivot point into a defect which is not immediately adjacent to it**
- examples include nasolabial island flap to the nasal tip and a deltopectoral flap to the head and neck

Advancement flaps

Flap that moves forwards without rotation or lateral movement

V–Y, Y–V, Reigler flap on the nasal dorsum, lip advancement techniques

Rectangular flaps require excision of Burrow's triangles

Z-plasty

Technique involving the transposition of two adjacent triangular flaps

All limbs of the 'Z' must be of equal length

Angles do not have to be the same

At the completion of the transposition the 'Z' has rotated by 90°

Angled limbs extend from the central limb with angles of between 30 and 90°

In clinical practice, 60° permits a maximal length gain **while allowing transposition of the two triangles**

Actual length gain is less than the theoretical length gain due to the visco-elastic properties of skin

Actual length gain is proportionately less as the lengths of the limbs become smaller

Angle (°)	Theoretical gain in length (%)
30	25
45	50
60	75
90	100

Tension required to close a 90–90 Z-plasty is $10\times$ that required to close a 30–30 Z-plasty

- but a 90–90 Z-plasty can be divided into four flaps, each with an angle of 45° to reduce this tension

Greater gain in length is achieved by one large Z-plasty than multiple small Z-plasties whose total central limb length is equal (but the lateral skin availability may be limited so a single large Z-plasty may not always be practical)

Uses:

- Transpose normal tissue into a critical area, e.g. return a vermilion step into alignment
- Change the direction of a scar
  - break up an ugly scar contour on the face
  - re-orientate a scar around the knee
- Lengthen a scar, e.g. burn scar contracture, lip lengthening with the Tennison cleft repair

The Z-plasty made simple

Hudson. *Plastic Reconstruc Surg* 2000

Multiple Z-plasties in series

- Length gain is additive (equating to a single large Z-plasty i.e. 75% for 60 degree flaps) but the tissue recruited from the parallel axis is equivalent to that of one small Z-plasty alone
- The field of tension exerted by each Z-plasty affects the neighbouring flaps and thereby reduces actual overall length gain
- Central flaps tend to develop a square shape and do not interdigitate easily
- Better applied to a long scar with less tissue available parallel to the direction of lengthening (e.g. correcting volar skin shortage associated with Dupuytren's contracture)

Double opposing Z-plasty

- Z-plasty plus Z-plasty-in reverse
- Advantaged by flaps remaining as triangles so interdigitate easily
- Length gain is equivalent to two Z-plasties in series or one large Z-plasty, i.e. 75%

Four Flap Z-plasty

- Either 90 degree or 120 degree Z-plasties, with each angle divided into two flaps
- Length gain equal to that of two individual 45 degree or 60 degree Z-plasties (100% and 150%) but flaps are easier to transpose as triangles
- Represents two Z-plasties in parallel
- Better applied to a short scar with a greater amount of tissue available to recruit from parallel to the direction of lengthening (e.g. deepening a web space)

Five flap Z-plasty

- A double opposing Z-plasty that incorporates a V–Y advancement – 'jumping man flap'
- Provides an additional 50% of scar lengthening over a double opposing Z-plasty alone i.e. 125% in total
- But less lengthening than a four flap Z-plasty for a given scar length

Single limb Z-plasty
- Used to introduce a triangular flap of skin in to an area of skin shortage
- Breaks up the contracted scar but does not offer the mechanical advantages of the Z-plasty

Blood supply of muscles

Mathes classification

Dominant pedicle:
- whole of the muscle may be perfused on this vessel
- if only one dominant vessel then this is critical to muscle survival
- where more than one vessel is dominant, these are **major** vessels

Minor pedicle – non-dominant vessel, may be variable

Segmental supply:
- multiple segmental vessels such as the intercostal branches
- flap will not survive if too many vessels are divided

I – one dominant pedicle, e.g. **TFL, gastrocnemius**

II – dominant pedicle(s) plus minor pedicle(s), e.g. gracilis, soleus
- delaying a type II muscle flap by ligation of the dominant vessel improves survival
- a portion of the muscle can be based on minor pedicle but the whole muscle will not survive

III – two dominant pedicles, e.g. pectoralis minor, serratus, rectus, temporalis, gluteus maximus
- type III muscles suited to segmental design, e.g. pectoralis minor facial reanimation, slips to orbit and angle of the mouth
- free or pedicle TRAM breast reconstruction

IV – segmental supply, e.g. **sartorius**

V – one dominant plus segmental, e.g. **latissimus dorsi, pectoralis major**. Such flaps will survive if the dominant vessel is ligated but segmental vessels preserved, e.g. pectoralis major turnover flap for sternal defects

Taylor classification of muscle innervation

I – single nerve, branches within the muscle – latissimus
II – single nerve, branches before entering the muscle – vastus lateralis
III – multiple nerves from the same nerve trunk – serratus
IV – segmental nerve supply – rectus

Free and pedicled flaps and their application
A free flap is a composite block of tissue that may be removed from a donor site to a distant recipient site where its circulation is restored by microvascular anastomosis

Flap selection
Replace like with like:
Types of tissue required

Volume of tissue required

Sensate or insensate

Donor site

Ease of raising/speed/positioning

Length of pedicle

Anaesthesia

Keep patient well filled

Hct 0.30–0.35

Keep patient warm

Monitor urine output

Muscle relaxation

Prevention of pressure sores

Flap monitoring

Colour

Refill

Temperature (δ-T) – beware warming of core temperature to peripheral temperature, a time when the peripheral vasculature vasodilates and perfusion pressure falls (need extra fluid)

Bleeding on pinprick

Doppler pulse

Transcutaneous oxygen saturation/thermography/laser Doppler

Causes of free flap failure

Mechanical

- anastomosis problem (technical failure)
- pedicle problem (kinked, twisted, stretched, compressed)

Hydrostatic

- inadequate perfusion (hypovolaemia, spasm, hypothermia)
- inadequate venous drainage (inadequate sized vein, dependency, shunting via a superficial system)

Thrombogenic

- vessels in a zone of injury
- traumatic pedicle dissection
- hypercoagulable state
- ischaemia–reperfusion injury (prolonged ischaemia time)

Antispasmodics

Papaverine (adrenoceptor blockade)

Verapamil (calcium channel inhibitor)

Lignocaine (membrane stabilization by sodium channel blockade)

No reflow phenomenon

Failure of a flap to perfuse after anastomosis

Possibly due to endothelial injury or platelet aggregation

Ischaemia–reperfusion

Kerrigan. *Microsurgery* 1993

Pathophysiology of ischaemia

Tissue and cellular hypoxia → build up of products of anaerobic metabolism, e.g. lactate (the greater the metabolic activity of the tissue, the more vasoactive metabolites are formed)
This causes disturbance to membrane transport systems resulting in the **influx of calcium** into the cell
Calcium influx triggers the production of inflammatory mediators (heparin, kinins, PGs) by tissue mast cells (second messenger)

Pathophysiology of reperfusion

Restoration of perfusion provides oxygen for formation of oxygen free radicals by neutrophils – 'respiratory burst' (xanthine oxidase pathways)
Further influx of calcium into cells increases the generation of inflammatory mediators

Cigarette smoking and microsurgery

Chang. *J Recon Struc Microsurg* 1996
Thrombogenic state due to effects on:
- dermal microvasculature
- blood constituents
- vasoconstricting prostaglandins – nicotine → increased TXA_2 and decreased PGI_2

Carbon monoxide $= Hb →$ carboxyHb → tissue hypoxia and increased platelet adhesiveness
Adverse affect on procedures
- involving extensive undermining, e.g. facelift surgery – relies upon subdermal and dermal plexuses
- where a block of tissue depends upon a vascular pedicle for survival, e.g. breast reduction, pedicled TRAM flaps

No proven adverse affect on free tissue transfer although smoking may compromise the flap-recipient tissue interface and healing at the donor site. Due to denervation of the flap – not subject to central sympathetic tone?
Smoking one cigarette → 42% decrease in blood flow velocity to the hand lasting for up to 1 h: hence, digital replants at risk in smokers
Advise stopping smoking for 3 weeks pre- and post-operatively

Muscle flaps

Advantages
- Can provide large surface area and volume coverage
- Donor site closes directly
- Well vascularized – combats infection
- Muscle split allows customizing
- May retain motor function (reanimation)

Reanimating flaps

Match size of donor and recipient nerves
Leave donor nerve short to minimize re-innervation time

Allow for 50% loss of motor power following transfer

Match size and shape of donor muscle to available pocket

Fasciocutaneous flaps

Pontine

Length:breadth ratio = 3:1

Thin, pliable, sensate

Little donor morbidity, often closed directly

Perforator flaps

Perforator flap terminology: update 2002

Blondeel. *Clin Plastic Surg* 2003; Direct and indirect perforator flaps. Hallock. *PRS* 2003

- Perforator flap
  - a flap of skin/fat supplied by a perforating branch (indirect) of the source vessel, passing through deep tissues and fascia to supply the flap
- Indirect perforators: perforating vessel passes through muscle and fascia before supplying the flap tissue
  1. Muscle perforator = perforating vessel passes through muscle and fascia before supplying the flap tissue (a musculocutaneous perforator flap), e.g. DIEP flap, SGAP flap, DCIP flap
  2. Septal perforator = perforating vessel passes along a fascial septum before supplying the flap tissue (a septocutaneous perforator flap), e.g. anterolateral thigh flap
- Direct perforators:
  - Perforator passes from the source vessel directly through fascia to supply the overlying tissue (most axial pattern fasciocutaneous flaps of the extremities)

Flaps based on nerves

Sural flap

- sural nerve
- short saphenous vein
- arterioles perfusing sural nerve and overlying skin island

Cephalic flap

- lateral cutaneous nerve of the arm
- cephalic vein

Bone flaps

Endosteal and periosteal circulation maintained

Healing as for fracture healing

Wedge osteotomies to conform donor bone to defect

Hypertrophy to meet mechanical loading

Consider donor defect

Toe and joint transfers

Replaces composite functioning tissues

Sensory potential

Close donor defect primarily

Preserve first metatarsal head

Toe pulp may be transferred independently

Gastrointestinal flaps

Upper and lower GI tract

Include two vascular pedicles for greater length

Keep ischaemic time to a minimum to avoid mucosal sloughing

Omental flaps, free jejunum

Caution in patients with a history of GI surgery

Specialized tissues

Vascularized nerves

Vascularized tendons

Leeches

Annelid worm

'V'-shaped mouth parts. Three jaws each with >100 teeth

Secrete hirudin in saliva – prevents fibrinogen → fibrin

Aeromonas hydrophila in gut

- induction of vomiting (salt water) increases transmission to the patient
- prophylactic augmentin

Used once only

Surrounding circle of paraffin prevents migration

Cost ~£5 each or £9 if requested out of hours

Individual flaps

Workhorse flaps

Latissimus dorsi

Anatomy

Dominant pedicle: thoracodorsal A, continuation of subscapular A (from the third part of the axillary A) after giving off the circumflex scapular A – this passes through the triangular space (when viewed from the front: subscapularis/teres major/long head of triceps) to gain the posterior axilla

Both A and single V are ~2 mm diameter

Extends from T7 to posterior superior iliac crest, angle of the scapula and lower four ribs, converges upon the bicipital groove of the humerus beneath the tendon of teres major and forms the lower border of the posterior axilla

Innervated by the thoracodorsal nerve – C6,7,8 – posterior cord of brachial plexus

Action: extension and adduction at the shoulder and medial rotation of the humerus

Test by palpating the lower border during resisted adduction

Surface markings

Mark out lower border during test as above; apex via angle of scapula for upper border; vertebral midline C7 to iliac crest

Vessel enters on the deep surface of the upper border of the muscle at the apex of the axilla with the thoracodorsal nerve

Transverse or oblique skin paddle usually up to 8 cm in width

Type of flap

Type V muscle flap

Myocutaneous

Megaflap with serratus ± rib

Common uses

As an islanded flap may be used for chest wall, breast, shoulder, back and neck reconstruction

Functional muscle flap for proximal upper limb reconstruction

As a free flap used for defects of the scalp and lower limb

Technique

Mid-lateral position with arm abducted to 90°

Circumcise skin paddle, bevelling edges outwards

Develop upper border first and sweep anteriorly/inferiorly towards the lower/free anterior border – this avoids inadvertent elevation of serratus

Divide paravertebral perforators and vertebral attachments

Serratus intimately associated with deep surface of the muscle from its scapular attachment to the ninth rib

Identify and preserve the long thoracic nerve and serratus vessels, although branch to serratus, off the thoracodorsal A, may be divided along with the circumflex scapular A for greater pedicle length

Inferior fascial blood supply may be precarious

Other points

Quilting technique for reducing donor site seroma

Skin paddle may be orientated obliquely at 90° to the axis of the pedicle for breast reconstruction

May also be pedicled on its segmentally vascularized origin – the reversed latissimus dorsi – if the subscapular A is then divided, reverse flow up the thoracodorsal A and then along the circumflex scapular A can allow perfusion of a scapular flap.

This scapular flap can be used for reconstruction of the lower trunk and perineum

Donor site morbidity – no difference in shoulder strength when one muscle has been harvested (Laitung, *BJPS* 1985)

Rectus abdominis/TRAM

Anatomy

Embryologically derived from anterior mesodermal somites, hence innervated segmentally T7–12

Fused at tendinous intersections: one intersection at the umbilicus, one at the xiphisternum and one in between (occasionally also below)

Muscle fibres arranged in three layers to represent external oblique, internal oblique and transversus abdominis – these blend together at tendinous intersections, a site where the anterior rectus sheath is firmly adherent

Attached superiorly to the fifth–seventh costal cartilages and inferiorly by two heads to the pubic symphysis and upper border of the pubic crest

Pyramidalis arises from the pubic crest and blends with its counterpart at the linea alba 4 cm above its origin

Superior epigastric A (terminal branch of internal mammary) and deep inferior epigastric A (branch of the iliac A) **plus** small segmental branches entering the deep surface from the lower six intercostal As (accompanying intercostal Ns)

Accompanying VCs

Deep inferior epigastric vessels measure 2–4 mm in diameter and 6–8 cm in length (superior epigastric vessels are of a smaller diameter at 1–2 mm)

Acts to flex the trunk (first 30–40°), depress the ribs with the pelvis stabilized, raise intra-abdominal pressure

Surface markings

Midline, lateral border of rectus muscle, iliofemoral axis

DIEA arises 1 cm above the inguinal ligament, enters the muscle on its deep lateral surface midway between the umbilicus and the pelvic crest (i.e. at the level of the arcuate line)

Type of flap

Type III muscle (two dominant pedicles) or myocutaneous

DIEP flap – skin/fat flap – discard zone IV

Common uses

Defects requiring a muscle between gracilis and latissimus dorsi in size

Lower and upper limb defects as a muscle flap (myocutaneous flap is too bulky)

Breast reconstruction (TRAM)

Perineal reconstruction (inferiorly pedicled)

Technique

Vertical paramedian incision for raising a rectus muscle flap

Transverse ellipse for a TRAM, vertical ellipse for a VRAM, or oblique

TRAM: elevate without fascia until approaching para-umbilical perforators on the pedicle side – include these in a strip of anterior rectus sheath

If a muscle-only flap is needed, bipolar para-umbilical perforators

Bipolar intercostal branches, preserve Ns if a functional segment is needed

Isolate and divide superior pedicle

Follow inferior pedicle along the lateral side of the flap to origin

Isolate and divide inferior pedicle

Other points

Muscle measures ~30 ∞ 10 cm *in situ* but only 20 ∞ 8 cm after raising

Caution following previous intra-abdominal surgery, caesarean section is not a contraindication

TRAM: mesh repair if unable to close rectus sheath directly

TRAM: zones of perfusion 1–4 may amputate zone 4 electively

Obese patients may be unsuitable for a TRAM because of unreliability of para-umbilical perforators

Segmental nerve supply limits transplantation as a functional muscle but small strips can be used for facial reanimation

Convenient to raise – supine for anterior defects

Delay by dividing inferior pedicle and superficial inferior epigastric vessels. Venous valves become incompetent

Radial forearm flap

Anatomy

Forearm superficial musculature from radial to ulnar includes brachioradialis, FCR, PL, FDS, FCU

Tributary to the cephalic vein from one of the VCs often communicates with the cephalic vein near the antecubital fossa (hence, this can drain the whole flap)

Surface markings

Palpate radial A at the wrist and trace beneath brachioradialis to the antecubital fossa

Mark out tributaries of the cephalic vein

Mark out desired shape of skin paddle

Type of flap

Fasciocutaneous

Osseofasciocutaneous with $1 \propto 10$–12 cm of lateral cortex of radius

Free or pedicled

Distally based flap shows reversed flow from the ulnar artery

Common uses

Indications include head and neck surgery, resurfacing of the dorsum of the hand, penile reconstruction

Technique

Tourniquet

Begin elevation on the ulnar side and work radially

Preserve paratenon on FCR

On the radial side of FCR the dissection proceeds from superficial to the tendon to a deeper plane to ensure fascial continuity between vessels and skin paddle

Tie off the radial vessels distally or temporarily clamp to check hand perfusion with the tourniquet down

Then dissect beneath the vessels raising the flap up from distal to proximal

When raising bone, do not dissect beneath the vessels but maintain septocutaneous continuity and a cuff of FPL muscle origin

Other points

'Chinese flap'

First described for mandibular reconstruction by Soutar in 1983

First described by Chang for penile reconstruction

Non-dominant forearm preferred

May be innervated with medial or lateral cutaneous nerves of the forearm

May include palmaris longus

Contraindicated where Allen's test indicates poor perfusion by the ulnar artery – may consider reversed cephalic or saphenous vein grafting

Complications include stress fracture of the radius in postmenopausal women if an osseocutaneous flap is harvested

Poor donor defect in young or obese patients

Other complications include non-take of graft on FCR and injury to the superficial branches of the radial N

Ulnar A may be superficial in ∼9% of patients – beware devascularizing the hand!

Communicating channels between venae commitantes allow for bypass of venular valves when venous blood flows in reverse – distally based flap

Alternatively valves may become incompetent

Can also be used as a flow through flap

Commonly used flaps

Scapular flap

Anatomy

Based upon circumflex scapular A, terminal branch of the subscapular A

Horizontal and descending branches (parascapular flap)

Descending branch courses down the lateral border of the scapula, the transverse branch divides the scapula into upper and lower equal halves

Emerges through the triangular space formed, when viewed from the back, by the long head of triceps superolaterally, teres minor superomedially and teres major inferiorly

Average pedicle length 4–6 cm

1.5–3 mm diameter A plus ×2 large thin-walled VCs

Surface markings

A horizontal ellipse drawn over the centre of the scapula, apices in the posterior axilla and within 2–3 cm of the midline

Maximum dimensions ∼10 × 20 cm

Type of flap

Adipocutaneous

Fasciocutaneous – inclusion of the thoracic fascia may enlarge the territory perfused

Osseocutaneous

Common uses

Upper and lower limb resurfacing, facial reconstruction

Technique

Elevate medial to lateral in a bloodless plane superficial to the deep fascia

Transillumination may aid identification of vessels

Fat fills the triangular space between teres minor and major

Small flaps may be passed anteriorly through the triangular space on the subscapular axis

Other points

First described by Gilbert, *PRS* 1982

Thin versatile flap

Easy to raise

Donor site may be closed directly provided flap not >10 cm in width

Elevate with the patient prone or in mid-lateral position

May be raised along with other flaps on the subscapular A axis such as latissimus dorsi or serratus ± rib for large composite defects

Can also raise a bilateral scapular flap but this requires two anastomoses

DCIA

Anatomy

Pedicle is deep circumflex iliac A, a branch of the external iliac A above the inguinal ligament, along with the deep inferior epigastric A and proximal to the superficial circumflex iliac, superficial epigastric and deep and superficial external pudendal arteries (and veins) which emerge below the inguinal ligament as branches of the femoral A

Vessels skirt the inner pelvic rim deep to the fascia overlying iliopsoas muscles

VCs run lateral to the external iliac A then cross either in front of (50%) or behind (50%) the artery as they ascend medially to join the external iliac V

An ascending muscular A and V lie 1–2 cm medial to the ASIS but do not contribute to the skin territory of the flap or the bone

Pedicle length 5–8 cm

Vessel diameter is large at 1.5–4 mm

Skin perforators emerge in a row just above the inner lip of the iliac crest, commencing near the ASIS and emerging at 2 cm intervals

Largest skin perforator (terminal branch of DCIA) arises 6–8 cm beyond the ASIS

Iliacus and psoas lie on the inner surface of the bone and gluteus maximus and minimus and TFL on its outer surface

Surface markings

Cutaneous paddle is centred on the iliac crest

Two-thirds of its area above the iliac crest

Extends medially to the femoral vessels

Extends laterally to a point 8–10 cm away from the ASIS

DCIA branches from anterolateral or posterolateral aspect of the external iliac A 2 cm above the inguinal ligament

Type of flap

Osseocutaneous flap with cuff of muscle

Common uses

Perhaps most suited to the reconstruction of curved bone (fibular for straight bone)

Mandible and composite intra-oral defects

Pelvic reconstruction

Tibial defects – use step osteotomies to straighten the bone

Technique

Raise the medial upper part of the flap first, along with a segment of the anterior abdominal wall (external oblique/internal oblique/transversus abdominis) to identify and preserve the superficial circumflex iliac A and V

Elevate the flap by following the DCIA laterally but maintaining a cuff of iliacus between the vessels and the bone

Raise the flap from its inferior incision, cutting through TFL and the glutei as an outer muscle cuff

Superficial circumflex A and V may be anastomosed to the ascending muscle vessels as an internal shunt

Repair the upper cut edge of abdominal wall muscle to the pelvic side wall using a strong nylon suture anchored through bone

Other points

Described by Taylor in 1979

Bone graft size up to $7 \times$

Skin paddle size up to 14×27 cm

Use the ipsilateral hip for hemimandible reconstruction – right curvature

Can rotate the skin flap at $90°$ to the bone segment

Inconspicuous donor site

Poor colour match and often bulky

Since the bone is supplied from its medial cortex, it can be split to harvest this cortex alone while preserving the outer cortex

Free fibula

Anatomy

Common peroneal nerve crosses the neck of the fibula from posterior to anterior and divides in the substance of peroneus longus into superficial (to the peroneal compartment) and deep (to the anterior compartment) peroneal nerves

Popliteal A divides into anterior and posterior tibial As at the level of politeus muscle; the peroneal A is a branch of the posterior tibial A 2.5 cm below its origin

This runs beneath the attachment of FHL posteromedial to the fibula (placing the peroneal A in the **posterior** compartment along with the posterior tibial A) and gives off muscle branches to FDL and tibialis posterior

Other muscle branches wind around the fibula to supply peroneus longus and brevis and a nutrient branch is given off to the fibula itself

Terminates as the lateral calcaneal A and a perforating branch which penetrates the inter-osseus septum to reach the anterior compartment

Four septocutaneous perforators run in the septum between peroneus longus and soleus at the junction between the upper and middle thirds of the fibula

Occasionally these perforators arise from muscular branches of the source vessel (peroneal A) necessitating intermuscular dissection of soleus

After entering the fibula at the same upper/middle third junction as the septocutaneous perforators, the nutrient branch gives off ascending and descending branches

Surface markings

Mark the fibula head and lateral malleolus

Palpate and mark the common peroneal N

Mark 8 cm distal to the fibula head as site of proximal osteotomy (distal to common peroneal nerve but proximal to peroneal vessels)

Maintain the distal quarter of the fibula and at least 5 cm proximal to the lateral malleolus

Axis of the skin paddle placed along the posterior border of the fibula based upon the septocutaneous perforators (upper/middle third), also the point of entry of the nutrient branch

Maximum skin paddle dimensions 22–25 × 10–14 cm

Type of flap

Bone only

Myo-osseus

Osseocutaneous

Myo-osseocutaneous

Common uses

Segmental long bone defects

Mandibular reconstruction

Technique

Raise the skin paddle by preserving the intermuscular septum and thus septocutaneous perforators

Maintain a posteromedial cuff of muscle on the fibula

Perform the distal osteotomy first, ligating the peroneal vessels emerging from the lower border of FHL

Allow 2 cm extra bone than required to fit the defect at either end and flaps of periosteum for wrapping around the fixation

Continue dissection proximally preserving the vascular pedicle

Skin paddles >8 cm need a SSG

Other points

Can be used to bridge bone defects up to 22 cm

First used by Taylor in 1975

Straight, tubular and good for weight bearing

May be osteotomized to provide two struts of bone on a single pedicle

Large vessels and easy to raise

Cosmetically acceptable donor site

Beware injury to the common peroneal nerve

Ankle joint may be disrupted if bone is harvested too distally

Detachment of FHL, FDL and tibialis posterior may adversely affect ankle movement

When used for tibial reconstruction support by casting for up to 18 months to avoid mid-shaft fracture (up to 30%)

Serratus

Anatomy

Lateral thoracic A (second part of the axillary A) supplies the upper part of the muscle while a continuation of the thoracodorsal–subscapular axis supplies the lower part ('serratus branch')

Arises from first to ninth ribs

Upper slips – innervated C5, next two by C6 and lower slips by C7 fibres within the long thoracic nerve

Lies anterior to the A but still deep to the deep fascia, joining the A at the level of the sixth rib

Lower slips (seventh, eighth, ninth ribs) thus have an independent nerve and blood supply

Vessels enter at the junction of middle and posterior third of the muscle

Inserts into the angle of the scapula

Action: protrusion of the scapula and rotates the scapula upwards and outwards

Test by pushing the outstretched hand against a wall – absence or denervation produces winging

Surface markings

Incision parallels the eighth rib on the lateral chest sidewall, curving superiorly to the axilla

Type of flap

Type III muscle flap – two dominant pedicles (lateral thoracic A plus serratus branch of thoracodorsal)

Myo-osseous flap (raised with rib)

Myocutaneous

Myo-osseocutaneous

Common uses

Coverage of head and neck defects

Facial and hand reanimation

Closure of soft tissue defects on the extremities

Technique

Identify the anterior border of latissimus dorsi and raise this muscle off the underlying serratus in its posterior part

Anterior part is exposed by elevation of the overlying skin

Elevate the lower slips of serratus off their rib origins, tie off multiple intercostal perforators unless underlying bone and/or overlying skin are required

Trace the pedicle superiorly

Preserve the long thoracic N unless an innervated muscle is required – can then separate out a discrete bunch of fascicles to the lower part of the muscle only; a nerve graft can be inserted if the long thoracic N is harvested on a long pedicle

Tie off thoracodorsal A to the latissimus dorsi and the circumflex scapular A to provide an extremely long pedicle (whole of subscapular A)

Other points

Lends itself to easily splitting

Long pedicle so may obviate the need for vein grafts

Lateral arm flap

Anatomy

Based upon the posterior radial collateral A (plus VCs) that passes from the profunda brachii A behind the lateral malleolus to anastomose with the radial A

Innervated by the **lower lateral cutaneous N**, a branch of the radial N which pierces the belly of triceps; the radial N also gives off the posterior cutaneous N of the arm, which runs through the flap but innervates only the skin on the back of the arm, while the upper cutaneous N of the arm is a terminal branch of the axillary N

Skin paddle centred upon lateral intermuscular septum

Anterior to septum from above down are biceps, brachialis, brachioradialis and ECRL

Posteriorly are lateral (above spiral groove) and medial (below groove) heads of triceps

Pedicle diameter 1–2 mm, maximum length 8 cm (need to spilt lateral head of triceps)

Surface markings

Skin paddle lies on the axis of a line drawn between deltoid insertion and lateral epicondyle

Type of flap

Sensate fasciocutaneous

Fascia-only flap

Osseofasciocutaneous

Common uses

Soft tissue defects of the dorsal and volar surfaces of the hand

Foot and anterior surface of tibia

Facial defects

Intra-oral defects

Technique

Narrow sterile tourniquet

Posterior incision first, elevating flap in a subfascial plane

Then repeat from anteriorly

Ligate distal PRCA and detach fascial septum from bone unless bone is also to be harvested

Dissect pedicle proximally preserving radial N lying between brachialis and brachioradialis

Donor site of up to 6 cm width will close directly

Other points

Thin, innervated fasciocutaneous flap

Large posterior cutaneous N of the arm must be taken in the flap even though it does not innervate it

Protect the radial N in the spiral groove

Additional proximal exposure may be gained by incising the lateral head of triceps

Excellent for covering tendons because deep surface is fascia

Thin and hair-free

Can cut flap at midpoint, between perforators to form two paddles for intra-oral/facial skin reconstruction

Area of numbness along lateral forearm

Groin flap
Anatomy
Pedicle is superficial circumflex iliac A, branch of the femoral A

Diameter usually ~1 mm (similar to the superficial temporal or facial vessels, hence these used as recipient vessels in the head and neck)

Venous drainage by VCs and by a direct cutaneous vein draining into the saphenous bulb, ~2 mm diameter, which drains the whole flap

Surface markings
ASIS, pubic tubercle, saphenous bulb/femoral sheath

Long axis of the flap parallels the inguinal ligament

SCIA branches from the femoral A at the medial border of sartorius

Type of flap
Adipocutaneous, free or pedicled

Common uses
Head and neck defects

Chest and extremity defects

Technique
Begin raising laterally

In the flank the full-thickness of fat need not be elevated – can thin to dermis at this point

Preserve the lateral cutaneous nerve of the thigh

As sartorius is approached include fascia in the flap since this transmits a number of cutaneous perforators

Visualize the SCI vessels on the underside of the flap

Preserve the inferior epigastric vein as it runs beneath the medial part of the flap since this has a sizeable tributary from the groin skin

Other points
Inconspicuous linear donor site scar

Pedicle short and inconsistent – expect anatomical variations

Poor donor area in obese patients

Liposuction can be used to reduced bulkiness

Flaps 15 × 30 cm can be raised and closed directly

May be de-epithelialized to fill out contour defects of the face

Described by McGregor and Jackson 1972

Gracilis
Anatomy
After giving off four small branches below the inguinal ligament, the femoral gives off the profunda femoris A which passes behind the femoral A, behind adductor longus

Profunda then gives off medial and lateral circumflex femoral As and four perforating branches which supply the adductor muscles and the hamstrings (semimembranosus, semitendinosus, biceps femoris)

Femoral A continues into the subsartorial canal and emerges from the adductor hiatus (free aponeurotic edge of adductor magnus) as the popliteal A

Dominant artery is the medial circumflex femoral A, accompanied by (usually) two veins

One or two minor pedicles are muscular branches off the superficial femoral A, distal to the origin of the medial circumflex femoral A

Gracilis arises as a flat sheet from the inferior pubic ramus, narrowing inferiorly to insert into the subcutaneous surface of the tibia, just below sartorius on the medial side

Bounded anteriorly by adductor longus and by sartorius (in the distal part of the thigh) and posteriorly by semimembranosus and semitendinosus

Long saphenous vein crosses lateral to medial

Innervated by the obturator nerve which enters the muscle lying just superior (2 cm) to the vessels, entering the muscle on its medial side

Adductor of the hip, flexor of the knee, medially rotates the flexed knee

Surface markings

Pubic symphysis, inferior pubic ramus, ischial tuberosity and medial condyle of femur

Incision to run from midpoint between symphysis pubis and ischial tuberosity superiorly to the medial femoral condyle inferiorly

Dominant pedicle enters the muscle from its deep surface (upper third)

Type of flap

Type II muscle flap:

- major pedicle – medial branch of circumflex femoral A
- minor pedicle – branch from superficial femoral A

Common uses

Long thin defects following lower extremity trauma and osteomyelitis

Facial and hand reanimation

Contour restoration in the head and neck

Technique

Incision as above keeping the long saphenous vein anteriorly

Raise the muscle from inferiorly, ligating multiple perforators to overlying adductor longus from the gracilis pedicle

Retract adductor longus to expose the full length of the pedicle right up to its origin

Other points

Can be used for closure of defects up to 5×20 cm

Well vascularized muscle for use at sites where bulk is a disadvantage

Pedicle 6–8 cm long

10–12 cm of nerve available

Skin paddle may be unreliable

Since the obturator nerve trifurcates at its entry point to the muscle, gracilis can be split to provide slips for facial reanimation

Rectus femoris myocutaneous flap

Flap of choice in most situations of perineal reconstruction

Can also reconstruct defects of the lower abdominal wall and greater trochanter

Greater length and arc of rotation compared with TFL (pivot point anterior thigh rather than lateral thigh)

Arises by two heads – anterior inferior iliac spine and upper part of acetabulum

Heads unite to contribute to the patellar tendon along with the vasti (= quadriceps femoris)

Pedicle is the descending branch of the lateral circumflex femoral artery

Enters the flap 8 cm below the inguinal ligament

Three-to-four perforators supply the skin proximally and should be included in the skin paddle

Flap can be raised as a musculocutaneous flap with a skin paddle of 15 × 40 cm

Can also be split to form a muscle flap and a fasciocutaneous flap and used to fill separate defects

Centralize vasti after raising the flap

Can be freed from proximal attachments to increase arc of rotation

Tensor fascia lata flap

Supplied by a transverse branch of the lateral femoral circumflex artery. Vessel enters 6–8 cm below the ASIS

Segment of muscle in the proximal third of the flap

Suitable for reconstruction of perineal, ischial and lower abdominal/groin defects

Arises from the ASIS and greater trochanter of the femur

Inserts as fascia lata into the iliotibial tract (lateral tibial condyle) – maintains lateral knee stability

Distal extent of skin paddle is 8 cm above the lateral femoral condyle

Can be freed from proximal attachments to increase arc of rotation

Donor site can be closed directly or skin grafted

Pectoralis major

Anatomy

Sternocostal (upper six ribs) and clavicular heads

Inserts into the bicipital groove of the humerus

Acts as a powerful adductor and medial rotator of the humerus

Supplied by the medial and lateral pectoral nerves

Blood supply from the thoraco-acromial and lateral thoracic arteries

Surface markings

Demonstrated by resisted adduction of the arm

Forms the anterior border of the axilla

Pectoral artery runs along a line drawn from the acromion to the xiphisternum

Type of flap

Myocutaneous

Common uses

Head and neck reconstruction

Technique

First described by Ariyan in 1979

Skin paddle medial to the nipple

Oblique or horizontal back cut over the chest wall

- horizontal back cut preserves the deltopectoral flap as a salvage flap
- direct closure with an element of rotation in small flaps

Dissect out the inferior border, lift up the muscle to observe pedicle

Wide muscle cuff encompassing the thoraco-acromial vessels

Other points

Palmer and Bachelor modification: the functional island flap

- more suited to large volume defects than a radial forearm flap
- reduces shoulder dysfunction following radical neck dissection in which trapezius is denervated

Sternocostal and clavicular heads left intact

Pectoral branch of the thoraco-acromial axis dissected off overlying muscle from which it is separated by loose areolar tissue

Islanded flap delivered through a button hole in the clavicular head of the muscle

Increased pedicle length ($\sim$3 cm), greater arc of rotation, less compromise of shoulder function

Superior gluteal flap

Anatomy

Gluteus maximus lies most superficially, passing from the gluteal surface of the ilium, the lumbar fascia, the sacrum and sacrotuberous ligament to the gluteal crest of the femur and the iliotibial tract

Muscle is a broad, flat sheet which crosses the gluteal fold at $45°$

Action is to extend and externally rotate the femur; acting through the fascia lata it also supports the extended knee

Supplied by the inferior gluteal N only

Supplied by both the superior gluteal A and the inferior gluteal A

Superior gluteal A is from the posterior branch of the internal iliac A while the inferior gluteal A is one of three parietal branches off the anterior branch, along with the pudendal A and obturator A

Superior gluteal A emerges from the greater sciatic foramen with the superior gluteal N, passing between gluteus medius above and piriformis below, and divides into deep and superficial branches

Deep branch sinks between gluteus medius and minimis before further dividing into an upper branch and lower branch which form anastomotic links around the hip joint

Superficial branch supplies gluteus maximus and the overlying skin

Inferior gluteal A emerges from the pelvis below piriformis, and hence through the lesser sciatic foramen, along with the lesser gluteal N, the sciatic N, the N to obturator internus and the pudendal N and vessels

Sciatic N thus lies deep and caudal to piriformis

Surface markings

Surface marking of the lower border of piriformis: from the midpoint of a line connecting the PSIS and the tip of the coccyx, to the greater trochanter

Pedicle lies on a line connecting the PSIS and the greater trochanter

Superior gluteal A emerges from the pelvis at a point between the upper third and lower two-thirds of this line, 6 cm below the PSIS and 4 cm lateral to the midline of the sacrum

Flap may be drawn horizontally based upon this pedicle to conform to bikini line

Type of flap

Type II muscle flap

Myocutaneous flap

Common uses

Breast reconstruction

Pedicled S-GAP flap for sacral pressure sores

Technique

Circumcise flap through skin and deep fascia

Divide the upper third of gluteus maximus in line with the upper skin incision

Develop the plane between gluteus maximus and gluteus medius

Identify the superior gluteal pedicle emerging from between gluteus medius and piriformis

Complete the inferior incision and elevate the flap from lateral to medial

Dissect along the pedicle to the pelvic side wall

Other points

Inconspicuous donor site, no functional deficit

Need to turn the patient

Skin paddle 25–35 × 9–13 cm

Thickness of fat ~8 cm, thickness of muscle 4 cm, flap volume ~800 ml

Pedicle length 3 cm

Vessel diameter 2–3 mm

Anastomose to internal mammary vessels or via vein graft into the axilla

S-GAP flap (perforator flap) now described and recommended as a sensate flap for autologous breast reconstruction (Blondeel, *BJPS* 1999)

Temporoparietal fascial flap

Anatomy

Pedicle is the superficial temporal vessels

Superficial temporal A is a terminal division of the external carotid A, along with the maxillary A

At the level of the zygoma the superficial temporal A gives off the middle temporal A that supplies temporalis muscle

Other branches, beyond the middle temporal A, include the frontal and occipital As

Large thin fascial sheet which covers the temporal, parietal and occipital areas of the scalp

Extension of the SMAS layer, passing from face to scalp, and continues above the temporal line as the galea aponeurosis, densely adherent to overlying skin/fat via connective tissue and separated by loose areolar tissue from pericranium beneath it (SCALP)

Temporalis muscle and temporalis fascia (deep temporal fascia) lie deep to the temporoparietal fascia inferior to the temporal line

A and V ascend anterior to the ear with the V lying superficially

Auriculotemporal N lies posterior to the pedicle (sensation to the scalp)

Surface markings

Frontal branch of the facial N passes from a point 0.5 cm below the tragus to 1.5 cm superior to the lateral brow

Superficial temporal A can be palpated or identified by Doppler

Type of flap

Free or pedicled fascial flap

Fasciocutaneous

Osteofascial flap (carrying underlying parietal cranial bone)

Common uses

Head and neck reconstruction

Upper limb reconstruction – allows tendon gliding

Technique

Incision posterior to the pedicle

Begin elevation of skin flaps at the level of the tragus, identify the pedicle and trace superiorly

Other points

Very thin flap

Cosmetic donor site unless there is male pattern baldness

Large, anatomically consistent vessels

Can carry facial skin, hair-bearing scalp and calvarial bone together

A up to 2 mm; V > 2 mm in diameter

Skin paddle up to 3 cm wide may be closed directly

Transient alopecia has been observed

Omental flap

Anatomy

Pedicle is the right gastro-epiploic A (and V), a terminal division of the gastroduodenal A (off the hepatic A – coeliac trunk) along with the superior pancreaticoduodenal A

Attaches along the greater curvature of the stomach as far as the first part of the duodenum and loops down and backwards to attach to the transverse colon

Separates the greater from the lesser sac that communicate via the foramen of Winslow (epiploic foramen)

Type of flap

Free fat flap

Common uses

Reconstruction of scalp defects

Contour deformities (Romberg's disease)

Radiosclerosis of the brachial plexus

Technique

Separate from its attachments to the greater curvature of the stomach and the transverse colon, ligating multiple vessels to each

Other points

Contraindicated by previous abdominal surgery

Requires laparotomy or endoscopic harvest

Provides an extensive vascular film to restore moving tissue planes

Advocated in the past for augmenting lymphatic drainage in lymphoedema

Pedicle length 3–4 cm

Anterolateral thigh flap

Anatomy

Based upon septocutaneous or myocutaneous perforators from the descending branch of the lateral circumflex femoral artery

Surface markings

Line drawn from ASIS to midpoint of lateral border of patella – this marks the lateral intermuscular septum between vastus lateralis and rectus femoris (septocutaneous perforators)

Common uses

Intraoral reconstruction, extremity reconstruction

Technique

Incision medial to marked line of septocutaneous perforators to reach fascia overlying rectus femoris

Lateral dissection towards the intermuscular septum – identification of perforators (septal or intermuscular)

Ligation of the descending branch of the LCFA distal to the most distal perforator

Complete flap raising by division of fascia and skin lateral to the intermuscular septum

Main pedicle traced to its origin from the LCFA

Other points

Minimal donor site morbidity

Large skin paddle

Can be used as a flow through and sensate flap

Approximately 10% of perforators arise from the profunda femoris artery

General points

Pedicle length generally correlates with vessel diameter

Upper limb flaps of smaller vessel diameter except latissimus dorsi and radial forearm

Facial artery is ~2 mm in diameter – recipient A in head and neck reconstruction

Safest when estimating vessel size to ± 0.5 mm

Flap	First described	Pedicle	Length (mm)	Maximum diameter (mm)
DCIA	Taylor 1979	Deep circumflex iliac	8	4
TRAM	Pennington 1980	DIEA	8	4
DIEP	Allen 1994	DIEA	10	4
TFL	Hill 1978	Lateral and medial	6	3
Fibula	Taylor 1975	Peroneal	6	3
Gracilis	Harii 1978	Circumflex femoral	8	3
S-GAP	Allen 1995	Superior gluteal (P)	8	3
Radial forearm	Yang 1981	Radial	15	3
Latissimus dorsi	Tansini 1906	Thoracodorsal	8	3
Scapular	Gilbert 1982	Circumflex scapula	6	2
Lateral arm	Song 1982	Posterior radial Collateral	8	2
AL thigh	Song 1984	Lat circumflex fem	10	4

Hypospadias (embryology, anatomy and clinical management of hypospadias)

3

Embryological development of the penis and urethra
Anatomy of the penis
Anatomy of the male urethra
General points
Techniques and papers
One-stage repair
Two-stage repair
Other papers
Gonadal dysgenesis

Embryological development of the penis and urethra

Langman's Medical Embryology

Hypospadias results from incomplete closure of the urethral folds during the twelfth week of development and may represent abnormal fusion between endodermal and ectodermal processes
Third week of development – primitive streak mesenchymal cells migrate around cloacal membrane to form the **cloacal folds** which fuse cranial to the membrane to form the **genital tubercle**

Sixth week of development

Fetus sexually indeterminate until sixth week of gestation
- Cloacal membrane divides into urogenital and anal membranes
- Cloacal folds also divide into **urethral folds** anteriorly and anal folds posteriorly and **genital swellings** arise lateral to them – form scrotal swellings in the male and labia majora in the female
Sixth to eleventh week
- Under the influence of androgens, (leydig cell secrete testosterone), the genital tubercle elongates to form the **phallus**. Sertoli cells secrete a testosterone analogue, which acts as a Mullerian (paramesonephric) duct inhibitory factor. The Wolfian or mesonephric duct in the male forms the epididymis, vas deferens and seminal vesicles.
- As the phallus develops, it pulls forward the urethral folds to form the lateral walls of the **urethral groove**

- Urethral groove extends only up to the distal part of the phallus – here the epithelial lining is of endodermal origin and is known as the **urethral plate** (glandular urethra)

Twelfth week

- Urethral folds close over the urethral groove and plate to form the penile urethra
- Penile urethra at the level of the urethral plate (i.e. glans) is not canalized at this stage

> Thirteenth week

- Glandular urethra becomes canalized by the inward migration of ectodermal cells to form the **external urethral meatus**
- Genital swellings enlarge to form each half of the scrotum, separated by the scrotal septum

Anatomy of the penis

Root of the penis

Attached to the inferior surface of the perineal membrane

Consists of the **bulb** of the penis (posterior part of the corpus spongiosum) and the **lateral crurae** (posterior ends of the corpora cavernosa)

Ischiocavernosus muscles are attached to the perineal membrane and ramus of the ischium, passing forwards to insert into the upper part of the corpus cavernosum, and act to move the erect penis

Bulbospongiosus muscles are attached to the perineal body and pass forwards to attach to the corpus spongiosum, with some fibres passing around to the corpus cavernosum

Bulbospongiosus muscles empty the urethra of semen and urine

Bulbourethral glands enter the urethra at this point – mucous secretions which lubricate the urethra before ejaculation

Body of the penis

Between the root and the glans

Urethra runs through the ventral **corpus spongiosum**, which is related on its dorsolateral surface to the **corpora cavernosa**

A fibrous sheath surrounds the two corpora cavernosa and corpus spongiosum – the **tunica albuginea** of the corpus

Penis is suspended to the under surface of the symphysis pubis by a **suspensory ligament**, a reflection of the tunica albuginea

Enveloping the tunica albuginea and the three corpora is a continuation of Colles fascia, the deep fascia of the penis (Buck's fascia), beneath which lie the dorsal arteries, deep dorsal vein and dorsal nerves

Loose areolar tissue (Dartos fascia), containing the superficial dorsal vein, covers Buck's fascia which is then enveloped by skin

Glans penis

Expanded end of the corpus spongiosum

Surrounded by prepucial skin

Blood supply

Three pairs of arteries, all branches of the internal pudendal A (off the anterior division of the internal iliac A)

Artery to the bulb: supplies the corpus spongiosum as far as the glans

Dorsal artery of the penis: supplies the corpus cavernosum, skin, fascia and glans (hence an anastomosis between the artery to the bulb and the dorsal artery)

Deep artery: supplies corpus cavernosum, sole function is erectile

Venous drainage is by venae commitantes to the arteries, draining into internal pudendal veins, but mainly via the deep dorsal vein, draining into the prostatic venous plexus

Superficial dorsal vein drains skin only and joins with the superficial external pudendal and great saphenous veins

Lymphatic drainage

Lymphatic channels accompanying the superficial dorsal vein, drain into the superficial inguinal nodes

Glans and corpora drain to the deep inguinal nodes, and later to the internal iliac nodes

Nerve supply

Skin of the penis supplied by the posterior scrotal and dorsal branches of the pudendal nerves (sacral plexus, S2,3,4)

Ischiocavernosus and bulbospongiosus muscles supplied by perineal branch of the pudendal nerves

Ejaculation is mediated by sympathetic nerves (L1 root from the sacral ganglia) via the superior and inferior hypogastric plexuses

Erection is mediated by parasympathetic pelvic splanchnic nerves (nervi errigentes) from the sacral plexus (S2,3,4) via the superior and inferior hypogastric plexuses

Anatomy of the male urethra

Prostatic and membranous (posterior urethra), and spongy or penile (anterior) parts

Lined by transitional epithelium except that part proximal to the external urethral meatus, the navicular fossa, which is lined by stratified squamous epithelium

Navicular fossa has blind-ending lacunae

Urethral glands of Littré open into the urethra on its anterior and lateral aspect, against the stream, with a similar function to the bulbo-urethral glands

The empty urethra is horizontal in cross section while the external meatus forms a vertical slit, hence urine spirals

Three constrictions: internal meatus (bladder neck), proximal end of navicular fossa, external meatus

Three dilatations: prostatic urethra, bulb, navicular fossa

General points

Hypospadias is characterized by:

- ventral position of the meatus (ventral meatal dystopia)
- dorsal hooded foreskin
- ventral curvature on erection – chordee
- deficiency of ventral skin
- clefting of the glans
- in the most severe cases scrotal bipartition

Aetiology of hypospadias

Environmental (oestrogenic chemicals)
Androgen hyposensitivity (especially if associated with micropenis, severe hypospadias, hypogonadism, undescended testis and inguinal hernia)
Genetic: father–son 8%, sibs 14%; Bauer, *Urol Clin N Amer* 1981
- But identical twins do not necessarily both have hypospadias, hence multifactorial
Link with cleft palate and hypertelorism – Scilbach–Rott syndrome
Joss. *Am J Med Genet* 2002

Congenital penile curvature

Abnormal fixation of penile skin or Dartos fascia
Corporal disproportion
Preserve the urethral plate
Need tunica albuginea plication ± excision (Nesbit)
Torsional deformity is always counter-clockwise – correct by degloving procedure

Chordee

A fibrous remnant of the corpus spongiosum causing ventral penile curvature in association with hypospadias
Dissection of the urethral plate alone will not correct
In >90% of cases chordee is due simply to ventral skin shortage

Hypospadias classification

Classification is based on the position of the abnormally proximal opening of the urethral meatus from distal to proximal:
glanular
coronal
subcoronal
distal shaft
mid-shaft
proximal shaft

penoscrotal
scrotal or perineal

Incidence

One in every 100–300 live male births and increasing
17 % of cases have associated urogenital abnormalities including undescended testis and inguinal hernia
Patients with proximal hypospadias should be screened for abnormalities of the urinary tract (renal USS, isotope renogram)

Aims of correction of hypospadias

Allow micturition while standing with a non-turbulent stream
Achieve a natural appearance with slit-like meatus located at the distal extent of the glans
Allow normal sexual function

History and examination of the hypospadias child

Has erection been witnessed, was it straight?
Urinary stream
This should include general examination and exclusion of intersex state in severe anomalies
Presence of inguinal hernia
Position of testis
Position of the meatus
Presence of para-urethral sinus (represents abnormal ectodermal ingrowth)
Depth of urethral groove
Presence of urethral bar (may determine one-stage or two-stage repair)
Prepucal involvement (circumcision or prepucal reconstruction)

Timing of surgery

Stage 1–12 months
Stage 2–18 months
Single stage–12 months
Opinion regarding timing of surgery vary but it is generally accepted that earlier repairs will reduce psychological impact of the condition as young children will have little memory of their hospital stay

Surgical techniques

Techniques to repair hypospadias can be divided in to one-stage and two-stage repairs.
One-stage repairs can be classified as:
urethral advancement techniques
onlay techniques in which vascularised tissue is transposed onto the urethral defect to close the tube
inlay techniques in which a tubed flap of vascularized tissue is transposed into the defect to reconstruct the whole circumference of the tube

History

Ancient Greeks: amputation of the penis distal to the meatus and tip remoulding with glowing cautery

First unsuccessful attempt at repair (Dieffenbach, 1838)

First successful repairs (Mettauer, 1842, Anger, 1874)

Duplay, 1874 (prepucial skin flaps for ventral release then urethral reconstruction)

Nové-Josserand, 1897 (use of skin grafts for hypospadias)

Described repairs

Mathieu, *J Chir* 1932 (flip–flap one stage)

Browne, *Proc Roy Soc Med* 1949 (modified Duplay)

Ceceil-Culp, *J Urol* 1952 (modified Duplay)

Cloutier, *PRS* 1962 (two-stage prepucial FTSG)

Devine and Horton, *J Urol* 1963 (modified Mathieu)

Mustarde, *BJPS* 1965 (modified Mathieu)

Van der Meulen, *PRS* 1977 (modified Duplay)

Duckett, *Urol Clin N Am* 1980 (transverse prepucial island flap)

Duckett, *Urol Clin N Am* 1981 (MAGPI)

Harris, *BJPS* 1984 (split prepucial flap technique)

Elder and Duckett, *J Urol* 1987 (onlay island flap)

Snodgrass, *J Urol* 1994 (tubularized incised plate)

Bracka, *Br J Urol* 1995 (modified Cloutier)

Turner Warwick, *J Urol* 1997 (bulbar elongation and anastomotic meatoplasty – BEAM)

Commonly used modern techniques

Single stage glanular reconstruction and prepucioplasty or circumcision

Snodgrass technique

Two-stage repairs as popularized by Bracka

Anaesthesia

Dorsal penile block – fails to fully anaesthetize ventral skin/glans

Penile ring block – full penile block

Caudal block – also anaesthetizes mucosa, less bladder neck spasm, lighter general anaesthetic, fewer opiates but causes semi-erection

Post-operative management

Urinary diversion for 2–6 days – size 8–10F silicone catheter, 15 mm diameter in children

25 mm/size 12 catheter in adults – fix catheter carefully

Paediatric drainage system – adult bags can give rise to air locks and obstruction

Ketoconazole 400 mg tds – rapid control of erections

Treat bladder neck spasm with oxybutinin 1 mg 8 hourly

0.75% plain marcain continuous dorsal penile block, 1 ml 4 hourly

Follow-up

Monitor for stenosis primarily

Also fistula and aesthetics

Urodynamics: onset of spraying indicative of stenotic process

See patient regularly for ~3 years then intermittently until after puberty

Other points

Ventral skin flap techniques may give rise to a hairy urethra – nidus for calcification

Prepucial flap techniques are impossible following prior circumcision

May have urethral valve → infection

If there are two meati, the more distal meatus tends to represent the opening of a paraurethral sinus

Techniques and papers

Benefits of a one-stage repair over a two-stage repair:
- fewer operations for the patient
- less expensive
- less psychological trauma

Advantages of a two-stage repair over a one-stage:
- better versatility to deal with a wider spectrum of hypospadias
- hence, less need to master a greater number of techniques
- technically easier
- more reliable results
- avoids a circumferential anastomosis, a potential site of stricture
- achieves a more natural-looking slit-like meatus
- psychosexual adjustment more related to appearance than number of operations

Suture materials

PDS dissolves quickly when exposed to the urinary tract – avoid

Subcuticular 6/0 to glans, 7/0 to skin

7/0 vicryl suture of choice

Vicryl rapide also useful, lasts ~2 weeks

One-stage repair

Flip–flap one stage

Mathieu. *J Chir* 1932

Mid-shaft to coronal hypospadias

No chordee, broad flat glans

Turnover of a ventral penile skin flap, distally based at the meatus and with parallel incisions, into the glanular groove to form the neo-urethra

Modified by Devine and Horton

Relies on using abnormal urethral plate in the repair which is scar-like tissue and therefore prone to problems with wound healing

modified Mathieu

Devine and Horton. *J Urol* 1963

Subcoronal incision extended on to ventral surface of penis, encircling native urethra

Release of chordee

Tripple glans flaps raised, central 'V'-shaped flap with its apex at the native urethra

Distally based 'V'-shaped ventral penile skin flap raised and tubularized to the 'V'-shaped central glans flap.

Lateral glans flaps cover the neo-urethra, shaft skin defect closed by prepucial flaps

If the native meatus is more proximal, FTSG is used to reconstruct the anterior urethra beyond the limits of the flip–flap

Again relies on repair from abnormal tissue

modified Mathieu

Mustarde. *BJPS* 1965

Operations performed within 12 months

Release of chordee

Distally based ventral skin flap, with its base at the ectopic meatus, is elevated

One or two catgut sutures to minimally tubularize the flap

Flap is fed through a tunnel created in the glans

Dog ears excised

Prepuce opened out and button-holed (Ombrédanne, 1932)

Glans fed through button-hole to allow reconstruction of the ventral skin defect

Diverting perineal urethrostomy

Historical repair

Transverse prepucial island flap

Duckett. *Urol Clin N Am* 1980

Suitable for anterior urethral defects of 2–6 cm

Suprapubic catheter

Subcoronal incision

Release of chordee and erection test

Transverse prepucial rectangle is marked out on inner prepucial skin, as long as the anterior urethral defect and 12–15 mm in width

Island flap tubularized around a catheter and raised with Dartos fascia

Anastomosis to the native urethra

Neo-urethra channelled through glans

Ventral skin closure by splitting the prepuce vertically in the midline and rotating two prepucial skin flaps ventrally around either side of the penis (i.e. same as Duplay)

Magpi

Duckett. *Urol Clin N Am* 1981

Subcoronal hypospadias, especially where the glans is broad and flat

Gives the appearance of a more terminally located meatus

- incision in the cutaneomucosal junction of the prepuce
- deep vertical incision in the glans groove with advancement of the meatus
- transverse closure of the glans incision
- ventral lip of meatus lifted up with a stay suture
- closure of glans flaps beneath the elevated meatus

Split prepucial flap technique

Harris. *BJPS* 1984

Similar to Duckett's transverse prepucial island flap technique

Penile block, perineal urethrostomy

Subcoronal incision and develop plane between Dartos fascia and tunica albuginea to enable release of chordee

Elevation of one central (inverted 'V') and two lateral glans flaps

Back cut the prepucial skin to allow this to rotate ventrally to the right of the shaft of the penis

Incise the free edge of the prepuce and separate the internal skin from the external skin based on a vascularized flap of Dartos fascia

Tubularize the inner prepucial flap around a catheter and anastomose proximally to the native urethra and distally to the central glans flap

Drape the external prepucial skin over the neo-urethra to reconstruct ventral skin shortage

Silicone foam dressing, decreases haematoma and oedema

Fistula rate 6%

Onlay island flap

Elder and Duckett. *J Urol* 1987

Preserve urethral plate by 'U'-shaped incision around hypospadic meatus and along glandular groove lines (no midline chordee)

Mobilize penile skin and Dartos fascia around the urethral plate, removing chordee tissue

If curvature persists need dorsal tunica albuginea application

Excise proximal thin/hypoplastic urethra

Raise a transverse prepucial island flap but instead of tubularizing inset into the 'U'-shaped incision as an onlay island flap

Close lateral glans flaps and ventral penile skin using prepucial skin flaps

Too much skin laid on causes development of diverticulae

Tubularized Incized Plate

Snodgrass. *J Urol* 1994

Distal hypospadias

Subcoronal degloving incision

Chordee corrected by TAB (Nesbitt)

Parallel longitudinal incisions at edges of urethral plate to create glans wings

Midline incision in urethral plate

Ventral closure of epithelial strips – dorsal defect re-epithelializes

Waterproofing layer

Closure of glans wings

The Snodgrass technique of incising the urethral plate and tubularizing the ventral flaps, allowing the incision in the urethral plate to re-epithelialize can be used in conjunction with other modern techniques when urethral closure might otherwise be too tight.

Bulbar elongation and anastomotic meatoplasty. Beam

Turner Warwick. *J Urol* 1997

Relies upon mobilization of the bulbar urethra to gain sufficient increased length to allow advancement of the distal hypospadic urethra to the glans tip

Ventral penile curvature may result from over-ambitious stretching of the anterior urethra

2–2.5 cm in children and 4–5 cm in urethral length in adults may be gained

Bulbar urethra is first mobilized via a perineal approach and then mobilized anteriorly via a subcoronal incision

After mobilizing, the urethra should project, tension free, beyond the glans tip

Where the glans has little clefting, the urethra is tunnelled to a new terminal position

Where there is a significant glans cleft, the urethra is formally inset after raising glans flaps

Slit-like meatus may be achieved by a Parkhouse procedure (double spatulate the urethra at 6 and 12 o'clock positions and partially resuture, face to face)

Two-stage repair

Prepucial skin flaps for ventral release then urethral reconstruction

Duplay. *Arch Gen Med* 1874

Modified by Browne 1949, Cecil-Culp 1952, 1959 and van der Meulen 1977

Stage one

Subcoronal incision and dorsal slit

Release of chordee

Ventral skin closure, having split the prepuce vertically in the midline, by rotating two prepucial skin flaps ventrally around either side of the penis

Stage two

Vertical incisions to form free edges of neo-urethra continuous beneath the native meatus and up to the neomeatus at glans tip

Free edges sutured together to tubularize a neo-urethra

Direct ventral skin closure possible due to previously imported prepucial skin

Browne modification: buried skin strip

Allow a buried skin strip to tubularize itself by not suturing the free edges of the neo-urethra

Cecil–Culp modification: scrotal skin

Used for proximal hypospadias

At the second stage, a vertical incision is made from the native urethra on to the scrotum

Penis is turned down and ventral skin closure is achieved by insetting the penis into the scrotum

At a third stage, the penis is released with ventral closure using scrotal skin

Van der Meulen modification: one-stage correction

In the patient without chordee the anterior urethra can be reconstructed in one operation by using Duplay's second stage only, and incorporating Browne's modification (buried skin strip)

Two-stage prepucial ftsg

Cloutier. *PRS* 1962

First-stage
>18 months
Circumcision
Glans split and transverse coronal incision
Correction of chordee
Ventral FT prepucial skin graft

Second stage
>3 months later
Modified Dennis Browne procedure (FTSG overcomes the problem of skin shrinkage)
Vertical incisions to form free edges of neo-urethra continuous beneath the native meatus and up to the neomeatus at glans tip
Excision of mucosa on glans flaps
Lateral skin is undermined and edges are sutured over the skin strip, i.e. same as Browne modification
Dorsal relaxing incision and SSG

Modified Cloutier technique

Bracka. *Br J Urol* 1995

Stage 1
3 years of age
Tourniquet, 8F urinary catheter, erection test (Horton)
Subcoronal incision and dissection down to distal ends of corpora cavernosa to release chordee
Repeat erection test
Glans split and inner prepucial FTSG (buccal mucosal graft is preferred in the presence of BXO) and jelonet tie-over dressing
FTSG restores thin skin layer firmly adherent on to glans tissue, flap techniques cannot achieve this
Leave catheter 2 days, trimethoprim antibiotic prophylaxis
GA or sedation + EMLA change of dressing at 5 days
Keep patient in hospital until dressing change

Stage 2 – after 6 months
Tubularize the grafted skin around an 8F catheter, starting with a 'U'-shaped incision beneath the native meatus and allowing a width of 14–15 mm of skin for tubularizing
Close in two layers and cover with a waterproofing pedicled flap of Dartos fascia/subcutaneous tissue from the prepuce
In very proximal repairs, insufficient tissue may be available for the waterproofing layer; in this situation use an anteriorly based fascial flap from the scrotum
In most cases the penis is circumcised rather than reconstructing the foreskin which can often become tight and uncomfortable
Leave catheter for 6 days
Augmentin antibiotic prophylaxis

In adults or older children, cyproterone acetate is given to reduce erections – commence 10 days before admission

Alternatively, 'a sharp icy blast of PR freeze spray' can be 'kept on the bedside locker for emergency use'!

Complications

Fistulae: salvage surgery 10%; primary surgery 3%

Stricture: early 2%; overall 7%; late strictures mainly due to BXO developing in prepucial FTSGs

Revision of the first stage: 3.7% (further chordee release, meatoplasty, etc.)

Revision of the second stage: 5.5% (aesthetic adjustments)

Choice of repair

Distal meatal dystopia

Tubularized incized plate (Snodgrass)

MAGPI (Duckett)

Two-stage repair (Bracka)

BEAM (Turner Warwick)

Mid-shaft to coronal meatal dystopia

Ventral skin flip–flap (Mathieu)

Transverse prepucial island flap (Duckett)

Two-stage repair (Bracka)

Penoscrotal meatal dystopia

Transverse prepucial island flap (Duckett)

Two-stage repair (Bracka)

Two-stage repair (Cecil–Culp)

Other papers

Long-term review of series

Harris. *BJPS* 1994

10-year follow-up on 35 patients – split prepucial flap technique

Appearance – 80% objectively assessed as looking normal

Urinary function – 40% of patients had intermittent spraying, all had a forceful stream

Psychological adjustment – 80% felt confident in peer company, 20% felt penis was too small or abnormally shaped, one teased by the name 'purple willy'!

Sexual function – all patients 'masturbated to their satisfaction', 83% had straight erections, only 5/35 patients had any sexual experience (mean age at follow-up 16 years)

Analysis of meatal location

Fichtner. *J Urol* 1995

Analysis of meatal location in 500 men

55% 'normal' with meatus located in the distal third of the glans

32% had meatus located in mid-third of the glans

13% had hypospadias (glandular:coronal ratio = 3:1)

Two-thirds of coronal hypospadias men were unaware of a penile anomaly, all but one (homosexual) had fathered children and all were able to micturate from standing

Only one case of subcoronal hypospadias was associated with penile curvature

Given these observations, the need for meatal advancement for distal hypospadias, potentially complicated by meatal stenosis and fistula formation, is questioned

Satisfaction with penile appearance

Mureau. *J Urol* 1996

No correlation between patient and surgeon satisfaction

Patients less satisfied

Satisfaction did not correlate with penile length

Patients with a glandular meatus were more satisfied than those with a retracted meatus

Urodynamic investigation of hypospadias repair

Van der Meulen. *J Urol* 1997

No difference in flow between different operative techniques (including one- and two-stage)

Improvement in uroflowmetry with time

No relationship between flow rates and clinical obstruction

Review of one-stage techniques

Harris. *Rec Adv Plast Surg* 1997

One-stage repairs using dorsal prepucial flaps can be separated into two groups: those that transpose the whole prepuce as a double-faced flap (onlay island flap, Elder and Duckett 1987) and those that use two independently vascularized flaps (transverse prepucial island flap, Duckett 1980 and split prepucial flap technique, Harris 1984)

Internal prepucial skin is vascularized from the Dartos fascia while external prepucial skin is vascularized from the subdermal plexus (larger vessels) – a readily dissectable plane exists between these two layers

Hence, the internal prepucial skin may be islanded as a fasciocutaneous flap and tubularized to form neo-urethra while external skin may be raised as a cutaneous flap to resurface a ventral defect

Lateral chordee – urethral plate may be retained – onlay flap or ventral flap

Midline chordee – urethral plate excised – tubed flap

But from an embryological perspective, the urethral plate is always abnormal and should be EXCISED as is performed in Bracka's technique?

Corpus spongiosum extends to the apex of the corpora cavernosa:

- chordee is due to ventral skin shortage and condensed fascia **lateral** to the untubed urethra
- excise lateral tissue
- reconstruct ventral skin

Corpus spongiosum does not extend the full length of the corpora cavernosa:

- chordee is due to **midline** failure of differentiation
- excise along with urethral mucosa
- reconstruct a neo-urethral tube

Must divert the urinary stream away from the suture lines of the neo-urethral tube using a suprapubic catheter (give oxybutinin to prevent bladder spasm) – extravasation of urine causes fibrosis and stricture formation

Use a stent secured with an elastomer sponge dressing

Turbulence of the urinary stream causes fistulae and ballooning – must achieve good calibre match between native and neo-urethra

Review of series – Aesthetics of hypospadias repair

Coleman. *BJPS* 1998

Retrospective analysis in 157 repairs (both one- and two-stage; also see below) with particular emphasis upon aesthetics

Single-stage GRAP (glanular reconstruction and prepucioplasty, Gilpin 1993) repair for distal hypospadias if tourniquet erection test excludes chordee with a well-formed glans sulcus

Up to 40% of cases of hypospadias

Glans flaps are used to re-create the distal urethra around an 8F silicone catheter

Avoid if a dense bar of tissue is present between meatus and glans sulcus

Closed with a waterproofing fascial layer

Foreskin reconstruction (prepucioplasty) carried out

Natural looking meati, no suture marks, no stenosis

Bracka two-stage repair in >60% of cases of hypospadias

Suitable for a more proximally situated meatus with no appreciable glans sulcus

Foreskin reconstruction at the second stage

Learning curve for fistulae: rate halved after first 40 repairs (5% for all primary repairs but >20% for salvage procedures)

Natural looking meati, no suture marks, no stenosis

Treatment modalities for hypospadias cripples

van der Werff J, *Plastic Reconstruct Surg* 2000

Hypospadias cripples can be defined as patients with remaining functional complications after previous hypospadias repair

A retrospective follow-up study 94 patients

- major meatal dystopia (87%)
- 46% residual curvature of the penile body
- 20% meatal stenosis,
- 5% had one or more fistulae.

The techniques used to solve these problems were

- circumferential advancement of penile skin
- dorsal transposition flap of preputial skin
- distally based transposition flap of penile skin
- full-thickness skin graft.
- 1–9 further procedures (mean two operations)

Complications:

- fistulae
- meatal stenosis
- residual curvature

Functional complaints included spraying at micturition, dribbling and deviation of urinary stream

Recommends meticulous technique, delicate tissue handling, and advanced postoperative care

Grading system proposed for post-operative complications

Role of antibiotics in hypospadias repair

Meir. *J Urol* 2004

Prospectively randomized clinical trial evaluating role of oral cephalexin in hypospadias repair

101 boys in whom tubularized incised plate urethroplasty was undertaken

Urethral catheter for mean of 8 days post-operatively

- bacteruria in 11/25 patients receiving antibiotics
  - urinary tract infection in three patients
  - commonest pathogen was *Pseudomonas aeruginosa*
  - three fistulae
  - meatal stenosis in one patient
- bacteruria in 25/49 patients in the control group
  - urinary tract infection in 12 patients
  - commonest pathogen was *Klebsiella pneumoniae*
  - nine fistulae
  - meatal stenosis in four patients

Sexual function following hypospadias repair

Bubanj. *J Urol* 2004

Questionnaire-based study of 37 adult hypospadias patients and 39 controls

Self-reported libido was similar in both groups

No difference in achieving erection

- downward curvature noted in 40% of hypospadias compared with 18% of controls

Ejaculation difficulties in 13 patients following hypospadias repair (spraying/dribbling)

Hypospadias patients less completely satisfied with their sex life and fewer partners

Aetiology of hypospadias – role of maternal smoking/reproductive history

Kallen. *Teratology* 2002

Swedish health registry showed that, of 1 413 811 infants born between 1983 and 1996, 3262 had hypospadias

- Negative association was found between maternal smoking and hypospadias
- Positive association was found between primiparity and hypospadias

Long term results of buccal mucosal grafts in hypospadias surgery

Hensle. *J Urol* 2002

10-year review of 47 patients in whom buccal mucosal grafts were used in secondary surgery for hypospadias

overall complication rate was 32%

- All occurred within 6 months of surgery
- Three patients with BXO in the series – all developed complications (may not be indicated in these patients)

onlay grafts preferred to tubularized grafts

most patients benefited from a durable reconstruction

Hypospadias fistula

Healing under adverse conditions:

- continually bathed in urine under pressure
- skin may be under tension
- oedema
- erections
- post-operative haematoma
- friable or scarred tissues (multiple operations)
- infection

Early fistulae due to postoperative obstruction, extravasation, haematoma, infection

Late fistulae due to turbulent flow

90% detectable within 1 week of operation

Repair

Ensure no distal obstruction

Wait for softening of tissues and settling of inflammation

Close the hole in the urethra

Interpositional fascial flap (including elevation of glans and placement of fascial flap for coronal fistula)

Test integrity of repair at end of procedure

Avoid overlapping suture lines

NO catheter

> **Self assessment: A 3-month-old child is referred with hypospadias. What is hypospadias, what factors cause it and how is it managed?**

Hypospadias is characterized by ventral dystopia of the urethral meatus associated with a dorsally hooded prepuce, clefting of the glans, ventral curvature on erection (chordee) and ventral skin shortage

May also be associated with cryptorchidism and congenital inguinal hernia

Occurs ~1 in 300 live male births

Hypospadias is the result of incomplete closure of the urethral folds over the urethral tube during the twelfth week of embryological development

Aetiological factors include environmental oestrogens, intersex states, genetic influence (familial hypospadias)

Management:

- history
  - family history of hypospadias
  - any urinary tract infections or known abnormalities of the upper GU tract
  - any failure to thrive (UTI)
  - maternal drugs, occupation of the father, etc.
  - any witnessed erections – curvature?
- examination
  - penis – size, degree of meatal dystopia, chordee, dorsal hooding
  - testes – descended/undescended, size
  - hernial orifices

- investigations
  - U&Es, renal USS or isotope renogram if concerned about upper GU tract
  - investigation of cryptorchidism or intersex states
- treatment
  - middle third meatal dystopia → nothing or MAGPI
  - proximal third meatal dystopia → two-stage Bracka repair
    - timing either 12 and 18 months or beyond 3 years
    - versatile, easy to learn, good results (aesthetic, distal slit-like meatus, low fistula rate ~3%)

Complications

Early – haematoma, infection, dehiscence (all → fistulae)

Late – fistula (turbulent flow), stenosis, poor aesthetics

Alternative procedures

One-stage repair – transverse prepucial island flap (Duckett) or split prepucial flap (Harris) techniques

Onlay flap (Elder and Duckett) for lateral chordee but a normal
urethral plate

Older one-stage techniques based on Mathieu flip–flap procedure

Older two-stage techniques based on Duplay procedure – prepucial skin flaps to supplement ventral skin then tubularized (or buried – Dennis Browne) to form a neo-urethra

Epispadias and bladder exstrophy

Embryologically different from hypospadias

Developmental abnormality of abdominal wall

Reflects abnormal development of the cloacal membrane – failure of rupture and mesenchymal in-growth → abnormal abdominal wall development

Features:

- divarication of recti
- widening of the pubic symphysis
- low set umbilicus
- in males:
  - short penis
  - dorsal chordee
  - epispadic meatal dystopia
  - divergent corpora
- in females:
  - short vagina
  - wide separation of the labia
  - bifid clitoris

Three-to-four times commoner in males

Exstrophy plus epispadias (commonest combination) – 1 in 30 000

Epispadias proximal to the bladder neck → incontinence

Management goals:

- reconstruction of the genitalia – appearance and function

- where there is exstrophy:
  - reconstruct the bladder
  - reconstruct the abdominal wall defect

Surgery for epispadias is virtually the same as for hypospadias but conducted on the dorsal surface

- flip–flap type of procedure (Devine–Horton) or
- prepucial island flap (Duckett)

Exstrophy of the bladder

- Features:
  - abdominal wall defect
  - separation of the symphysis pubis
  - absent anterior bladder wall
  - eversion of the bladder
  - may → carcinoma risk if untreated
- Timing: staged functional reconstruction
  - bladder closed as a neonate – 1 week
  - epispadias repair at 1–2 years of age
  - bladder neck reconstruction at 3–4 years of age
- Surgery
  - iliac osteotomies to allow closure of the symphyseal defect
  - free bladder edges approximated and closed
  - abdominal wall closure – may need rectus muscle flap

Peyronie's disease

Majority have upward curvature with thickening on the dorsal surface of the tunica

Rare before 40 years of age

Tunica albuginea fibrosis extending into septum between corpora

Similar phenomenon to Dupuytren's disease

Repetitive trauma, especially to the semi-erect penis

TGF-β over-expression?

Medical treatment

Para-aminobenzoic acid

Vitamin E

Colchicine

Ultrasound

Tamoxifen

Steroid injections

Verapamil

Surgical treatment

Indicated if unable to have intercourse

Nesbit procedure to plicate the ventral tunica – but shortens the penis

Penile prosthesis if bordering upon impotence

Excision of plaque and grafting with dermis (also dura, fascia lata, alloderm, vein and gortex patch have been reported) but can resorb or produce ballooning of the corpora and compromise erection

50% spontaneous resolution may occur – do not operate within 1 year of presentation

Balanitis xerotica obliterans

Male genital form of lichen sclerosis

Unknown aetiology

Viral association

HLA association

Obese patients

Warm, moist uriniferous environment

Accounts for many hypospadias cripples

Early – dyskeratosis and inflammatory changes progressing to:

Late – fibrosis and skin atrophy, prepuce becomes adherent to glans

White stenosing band at the end of the foreskin and a haemorrhagic response to minor trauma leading to phimosis and distal urethral stenosis

Chronic BXO may lead on to SSC

Treat by circumcision (allows glans to dry out) and/or meatoplasty – meatotomy will restricture

May try steroid creams for early disease in children

Surgical excision of advanced disease and thick SSG

Need a substitution urethroplasty – buccal mucosal grafts

Bladder mucosal grafts fail to keratinize and retain an ugly fleshy appearance

Recurrence in:

- genital FTSG – 18 months–2 years
- PAWG – >5 years
- Buccal mucosa – none yet recorded

Penile enhancement

Liposuction of pubic fat pad

Partial/complete division of suspensory ligament (drops angle of erection)

V–Y skin advancement from pubic area

Dermofat onlay grafts around tunica to increase girth

Stretching with weights for prepucial advancement after circumcision

Vaginal reconstruction

Historical

Local labial flaps – Graves, 1981

SSG and stent – McIndoe

- poor graft take
- visible donor site
- requires daily dilatation
- multistage procedure
- neoplasia described
- 'U'-shaped incision in forchette to create shallow pocket for intercourse – Williams

Described using postage stamp grafts of buccal mucosa

Pathology

Congenital absence (Rockitansky syndrome) or segmental (imperforate hymen, long segment atresia)

Congenital malformation – female hypospadias

Surgical ablation – e.g. mid-section excision for prolapse

Radionecrosis – hostile tissues

Fistula – requires flap closure

Surgical options

Preferred tissues

- vagina
- vulva
- skin
- bowel (jejunum)

Distant flaps

- Wei Wei (bilateral groin flaps)
- TRAM, pedicled through the pelvis on IEA
- bowel, but tend to get stenosis at mucocutaneous anastomosis

Vulval tissue expansion

- appropriate tissue
- no donor defect
- high success rate
- two stages
- hospitalize for 6–7 weeks during expansion

Radionecrosis – need to import well-vascularized tissue on its own blood supply, TRAM, omentum, gracilis

Vagina construction in transsexuals

Van Noort. *PRS* 1993

Male → female 3 × commoner than female → male

Epithelium-lined cavity must be created between prostate/urethra/seminal vesicles and rectum

Urethra cut obliquely to avoid stenosis when reinserted into the introitus

Techniques:

- inversion of penile or penile **and** scrotal skin flaps
    - most commonly used technique
    - scrotal skin incorporated into neovagina or used to fashion labia
- split skin grafts (McIndoe – vaginal agenesis)
- perineal or abdominal pedicled skin flaps
- intestinal segments

Regular dilatation postoperatively by stent or vibrator and then intercourse

27 male → female transsexuals evaluated

Comparison of penile skin inversion with penile and scrotal skin inversion

Combined technique offers a more capacious neovagina but hair growth and skin prolapse more of a problem

Most patients in both groups could experience an orgasm

Gonadal dysgenesis

Enzyme deficiencies

Androgen-insensitivity syndrome: testosterone receptor insensitive to androgens, male karyotype but female genitalia

Congenital adrenal hyperplasia: female karyotype but ambiguous genitalia due to adrenal androgen excess

- 21-hydroxylase deficiency
- involved in the aldosterone pathway
- precursors diverted into androgen synthesis
- salt-losing type may → hyponatraemia, hyperkalaemia and dehydration 1 week post-natally

5-α-reductase deficiency: converts testosterone to dihydroxytesterone in the target tissues

17-α-hydroxylase deficiency: enzyme required for synthesis of androgens and oestrogens but all of these patients are phenotypically female regardless of karyotype. Impairment of glucocorticoid synthesis → adrenal hyperplasia

Karyotype problems

Mixed gonadal dysgenesis: usually a mosaic 45X/46XY with both male and female gonads (one of which is 'streak') and ambiguous genitalia. High risk of gonadal malignancy

Hermaphroditism: 46XY/XX, testes and ovaries, male genitalia or ambiguous. May be familial (Bantu population of South Africa). Most, but not all, patients are infertile

Turner's syndrome: 45XO, streak gonads, female genitalia, short stature and webbed neck, primary (congenital) lymphoedema

Klinefelter's syndrome: 47XXY, small testes, hypogonadism, gynaecomastia

Disorders of sexual differentiation

Endocrinology and Metabolism. Warne. *Clin. North Am*, 1998

SRY gene – **s**ex determining **r**egion of the **Y** chromosome is the testis determining factor

Absence of the *SRY* gene → no testis → female phenotype

Leydig cells in the developing testis secrete testosterone → confers male phenotype through action on wolffian ducts (epididymis, vas deferens, seminal vesicles)

Testicular Sertoli cells secrete Mullerian inhibiting substance (member of TGF-β family) → regression of Mullerian ducts (upper third vagina, uterus, oviducts)

Virilization of the external genitalia requires conversion of testosterone to dihydrotestosterone via 5-α-reductase

Intersex disorders:

- XY female
  - mutation in the *SRY* gene
  - 5-α-reductase deficiency
  - 17-α-hydroxylase deficiency
- XX male
  - resembles Klinefelter's
  - male phenotype due to *SRY* gene translocation from Y to X chromosome
- ambiguous genitalia
  - phallus intermediate in size between penis and clitoris
  - most likely diagnoses are:
    - CAH
    - 5-α-reductase deficiency
    - mixed gonadal dysgenesis
- XY male with persistent Mullerian duct structures – mutations in the *MIS* gene or its receptor
- XX female with absent Mullerian duct structures
  - Meyer–Rokitansky–Kuster–Hauser syndrome
  - activating mutation in the *MIS* gene or its receptor

Management:

- counsel the parents – defer registering or naming the child
- streak gonads → malignant change therefore must be removed
- androgen insensitivity syndrome → 9% risk of seminoma – remove testes before 20 years (phenotypically female)
- feminizing genitoplasty
  - timing and necessity?
  - **CAH → almost always reared as female and are fertile** therefore feminizing genitoplasty reinforces sexual identity

Ambiguous genitalia

45XO Turner's

47XXY Klinefelter's

SRY mutations:

- 46XX male
- 46XY female

Mixed gonadal dysgenesis

45XO/46XY mosaic

Intersex

Diagnostic approach to ambiguous genitalia

Karyotype	Possible diagnosis
46XY	Androgen insensitivity syndrome, 5-α-reductase deficiency
46XY	17-α-hydroxylase deficiency
46XX	Congenital adrenal hyperplasia (21-hydroxylase deficiency)
45XO	Turner's syndrome
47XXY	Klinefelter's syndrome
45XO/46XY	Mixed gonadal dysgenesis
46XY female	*SRY* gene mutation
46XX male	*SRY* gene mutation

Cleft surgery (embryology, anatomy and management of cleft lip, palate, pharyngoplasty, orthodontics)

4

Embryological development of the maxillofacial skeleton
Anatomy of the palate and pharynx
General considerations
Cleft lip repair
Cleft palate repair
Pharyngoplasty
Cleft nose
Orthodontics
Ear disease

Embryological development of the maxillofacial skeleton

Weeks 4–5 of development

Formation of ridges in the cranial mesenchyme, the pharyngeal arches
Pharyngeal arches are separated by pharyngeal clefts
Out-pouchings of the foregut are formed – pharyngeal pouches
Stomodeum is the cranial opening of the foregut (mouth and nasal aperture)
Five swellings are formed ventrally:
- left and right mandibular swellings (from first pharyngeal arch)
- left and right maxillary swellings (from first pharyngeal arch)
- fronto-nasal prominence (down growth from primative forebrain, not a pharyngeal pouch)

Skeletal components are formed by inward migration of neural crest cells
First pharyngeal arch of importance from a cleft perspective
Second pharyngeal pouch forms the tonsillar fossa
First pharyngeal cleft forms the external ear and eardrum

First pharyngeal arch
Artery
Maxillary artery from external carotid
Cartilaginous component
maxillary process (quadrate cartilage forms the incus and greater wing of the sphenoid)

and the mandibular process (Meckel's cartilage forms condyles of mandible)

During further development both of these disappear except for those parts forming the incus and malleus

Mesenchyme of maxillary process undergoes intramembranous ossification to form the premaxilla, maxilla, zygoma and part of the temporal bone

Mandible is formed by intramembranous ossification of mesenchyme surrounding Meckel's cartilage

Muscles of first arch are muscles of mastication:

- temporalis, masseter, pterygoids
- anterior belly of digastric, mylohyoid, tensors tympani and tensor veli palati

Nerve

Motor from mandibular branch of the fifth cranial nerve

Sensory all three divisions of Vth nerve

Mesenchyme of the first arch forms the dermis of the face

First arch syndromes

Treacher Collins (mandibulofacial dysostosis) Chr 5 5q31–33

Characterised by Tessier 6, 7 and 8 cleft centred around the zygoma

Failure of first arch neural crest

Abnormalities of external, middle and inner ear and macrostomia (7 cleft)

Absent or hypoplastic zygoma

Maxillary and mandibular hypoplasia

Defects of lower eyelid – loss of lashes or coloboma (6 cleft)

Cleft palate

Hypertelorism

Anti-Mongoloid slant

Hearing defects

Broad nasal bridge

Pierre Robin sequence

First described in 1822

One in every 8000 live births

Risk of further children being affected = 1–5%

Can often be part of a larger syndrome, the most common of which is Stickler syndrome

- mandibular hypoplasia
  - mandible will grow to more normal proportions between 3 and 18 months of age
  - normal profile by 6 years of age – mandibular advancement osteotomy rarely required
- cleft palate – closed at 12–18 months
- defects of ear and eye
- glossoptosis
- airway obstruction

Airway management

- infant suffers from airway obstruction during sleep and will die of exhaustion if not corrected
- try nursing face down
- emergency management: tongue stitch/towel clip, nasotracheal intubation

- more permanent techniques for managing the tongue – suture to inner surface of lower lip (Routledge) or pass a K-wire through the mandible to skewer the base of the tongue in a forward position
- definitive procedure is tracheostomy

Stickler syndrome (Hereditary progressive arthro-ophthalmopathy)
Autosomal dominant – linked to the type II procollagen locus on chromosome 12?

Described in the 1960s by Dr Stickler from the Mayo clinic

Severe progressive myopia, vitreal degeneration, retinal detachment

Progressive sensorineural hearing loss

Valvular prolapse

Scoliosis

Robin features: cleft palate and mandibular hypoplasia

Hyper- and hypomobility of joints

Variable epiphyseal dysplasia → joint pain, dislocation or degeneration

Consider in:
- any infant with congenitally enlarged wrists, knees or ankles, particularly when associated with the Robin sequence
- anyone suspected of Marfan syndrome who has hearing loss, degenerative arthritis or retinal detachment

Sequence (definition)
Single developmental defect results in a chain of secondary defects

Pierre Robin syndrome – mandibular hypoplasia → posterior displacement of the tongue → airway obstruction and precludes closure of the palatal arches → cleft of the secondary palate

Entire cascade of events is often known in a sequence

Syndrome (definition)
Groups of anomalies that contain multiple malformations and/or sequences

A given anomaly may be incompletely expressed or absent

Pathogenic relationship of the group of anomalies is frequently not understood

Second arch
Artery

Stapedial

Cartilage

Forms the stapes, lesser horn of hyoid and upper part of the body of the hyoid

Bone

Body and ramus of mandible

Nerve of the second arch is VII (Facial)

Muscles are stapedius, stylohyoid, posterior belly of digastric, muscles of facial expression (Möbius' syndrome – a failure of innervation of facial muscles)

Third arch
Cartilage is the greater horn and inferior part of the body of the hyoid

Nerve of the third arch is IX (Glossopharyngeal)

Muscles are stylopharyngeus, upper pharyngeal constrictors

Thymus and inferior III parathyroids (abnormal in Di-Georges or velo-cardio-facial syndrome)

Fourth and sixth arches

Thyroid cartilage, cricoid, arytenoid, corniculate and cuneiform

Nerve is the superior laryngeal branch of X

Muscles are cricothyroid, **levator palati**, palatopharyngeus, palatoglossus and lower constrictors of the pharynyx

Sixth arch intrinsic muscles are supplied by recurrent laryngeal branch of X

Superior IV parathyroids

Development of the tongue

Appears at ~4 weeks of development

Two lateral plus one median (tuberculum impar) lingual swellings of first arch mesenchyme form the anterior two-thirds of the tongue

Behind this a median swelling (copula or hypobranchial eminence) of second, third and fourth arch mesenchyme forms the posterior tongue

Part of the posterior fourth arch mesenchyme forms the epiglottis

Sensory innervation to anterior two-thirds by the mandibular division of V; to posterior third by IX and X

Motor innervation mainly XII – musculature derived from occipital somites all except palatoglossus innervated by the X nerve

Development of the nose and upper lip

Maxillary and mandibular swellings present by the fifth week of development

Maxillary swellings lie cephalad to the stromodeum, mandibular swellings lie caudal

Frontal process lies in the midline, cephalad to the maxillary swellings

On each side of the frontal process just above the stromodeum ectoderm thickens to form two nasal placodes

Swellings develop lateral and medial to each nasal placode which deepens to form the nasal pit

By week 7 the maxillary swellings advance into the midline, pushing the **medial** nasal swellings to the midline where they fuse to form the upper lip

Nasolacrimal duct is formed as the maxillary swellings fuse with the **lateral** nasal swellings

Development of the palate

Undersurface of the fused maxillary and medial nasal swellings forms the intermaxillary segment

Intermaxillary segment contributes to:
- philtrum of the upper lip
- part of the maxilla bearing the upper four incisors
- triangular primary palate

During week 6 the palatal shelves grow out from the maxillary swellings to lie lateral to the tongue

During week 7 the palatal shelves ascend (hydration of glycosaminoglycans) and fuse to form the secondary palate

Secondary palate fuses anteriorly with the primary palate, a junction marked by the incisive foramen

Epstein's pearls are cystic epithelial remnants of the zone of apoptosis between the fusing palatal shelves

Developmental abnormalities leading to cleft lip and palate

Divided embryologically into clefts of the primary palate – in front of the incisive foramen – and clefts of the posterior palate – posterior to the incisive foramen.
Whilst this is an embryological classification,

- the primary palate consists of the lip, alveolus and hard palate anterior to the incisive foramen
  - clefts represent failure of mesenchymal penetration between medial and lateral palatine processess and failure of fusion of maxillary and medial nasal processes (cleft nose, lip and alveolus between incisors and canines extending to incisive foramen)
- the posterior or secondary palate consists af both the posterior part of the hard palate behind the incisive foramen and soft palate
  - clefts represents failure of the lateral palatine processess to fuse with each other and the nasal septum/vomer

Anterior and posterior clefts may appear together or in isolation
Degrees of clefting observed for primary clefts (e.g. incomplete vs. complete cleft lip) and secondary clefts (wide cleft palate vs. cleft uvula)
Failure of fusion of medial nasal swellings gives rise to the rare median cleft
Failure of fusion of maxillary and lateral nasal swellings causes an oblique facial cleft

Anatomy of the palate and pharynx

Hard palate

Made up from the palatal processes of the maxilla and the horizontal plate of the palatine bone
Foraminae:
- incisive foramen
- greater palatine foraminae (level with last molar tooth)
- lesser palatine foraminae (just behind the greater)

Attachment of mucoperiosteum to bone by Sharpey's fibres
Blood supply via the greater palatine A (branch of the maxillary A) which enters at the greater palatine foramen and exits via the incisive foramen
Venous drainage via VCs to the artery and also to the tonsillar and pharyngeal plexuses
Lymphatic drainage to the retropharyngeal and deep cervical nodes
Sensory innervation via the pterygopalatine ganglion (branches of the maxillary N) – nasopalatine nerves to the premaxillary area (in front of the incisive foramen) and by the greater palatine nerve posteriorly

Soft palate

Five paired muscles:
- tensor palati (**tensor veli palatini**)
  - from the scaphoid fossa of the medial pterygoid plate, the lateral part of the cartilaginous auditory tube and the spine of the sphenoid

- passes around the pterygoid hamulus as a tendon
- inserts as a concave triangular aponeurosis to the crest of the palatine bone, blending in the midline with that of the opposite side
- acts to tense the soft palate (flattening it slightly) so that the other muscles may elevate or depress it
- opens the auditory tube during swallowing
- levator palati (**levator veli palatini**)
  - arises from the quadrate area of the petrous bone (anterior to the carotid foramen) and the medial part of the auditory tube
  - forms a rounded belly inserting into the nasal surface of the palatine aponeurosis between the two heads of palatopharyngeus
  - together the levator palati muscles form a 'V'-shaped sling pulling the soft palate upwards and backwards to close the nasopharynx
  - also opens the auditory tube
- palatoglossus
  - arises from the under surface of the aponeurosis
  - passes downwards to interdigitate with styloglossus
  - forms the anterior fold of the tonsillar fossa
  - acts as a sphincter to raise the tongue and narrow the transverse diameter of the oro-pharyngeal isthmus
- palatopharyngeus
  - anterior head arises from the nasal surface of the hard palate
  - posterior head arises from the nasal surface of the aponeurosis
  - two heads clasp the levator palati muscle insertion
  - muscle arches downwards over the lateral edge of the palate to form the posterior pillar of the tonsillar fossa and the innermost muscle of the pharynx
  - inserts into the thyroid lamina and blends with the inferior constrictor
  - anterior head (arising from bone) acts to raise the pharynx/larynx
  - posterior head depresses the tensed soft palate
  - some fibres, along with fibres from the superior constrictor, contribute to the palatopharyngeal sphincter (forms Passavant's ridge when the soft palate is elevated, hypertrophied in cleft palate patients and in 25–30% of normal individuals)
- muscle of the uvula
- blood supply by the lesser palatine As, the ascending palatine branch of the facial A and the palatine branches of the ascending pharyngeal A
- all muscles of the palate are supplied by the pharyngeal plexus (cranial accessory N and pharyngeal branch of X) except tensor palati (nerve to medial pterygoid – branch of the mandibular N)
- sensory innervation via the pterygopalatine ganglion via lesser palatine nerves

Pharynx

12 cm long muscular tube extending from the skull base to become the oesophagus at the level of C6

Invested anteriorly by prevertebral fascia

Nasal, oral and laryngeal parts

Wall consists of four layers:

- mucous membrane
- submucous (fibrous) layer
- muscular layer
- thin outer buccopharyngeal fascia

Muscles:

- overlapping superior middle and inferior constrictors
- stylo, palato and salpingopharyngeus

Pharyngobasilar fascia forms the posterior wall of the nasopharynx at the skull base

Superior constrictor attaches to the skull base and the pterygomandibular raphe (pterygoid hamulus to mylohyoid line of the mandible, buccinator passes anteriorly from this raphe) and sweeps posteriorly to insert into the pharyngeal raphe

Middle constrictor arises from the stylohyoid ligament and the greater horn of the hyoid and inserts into the pharyngeal raphe

Inferior constrictor has two parts:

- thyropharyngeus – from the oblique line of the thyroid cartilage to the pharyngeal raphe
- cricopharyngeus – from the cricoid cartilage passing posteriorly to form a sphincter with that from the other side
- between thyropharyngeus and cricopharyngeus is a weak area – Killen's dehiscence

Palatopharyngeus is described above

Salpingopharyngeus arises from the lower part of the auditory tube and blends with palatopharyngeus, assists in opening the tube

Stylopharyngeus arises from the styloid process and passes through a space between superior and middle constrictors (along with IX and the lingual N) to lie inside the middle constrictor, behind palatopharyngeus, inserting into the thyroid cartilage lamina

Blood supply by superior and inferior laryngeal As, ascending pharyngeal A, also from vessels supplying palate

All muscles supplied by pharyngeal plexus (motor fibres in pharyngeal branch of X, IX fibres are purely afferent) except stylopharyngeus (IX) and cricopharyngeus (recurrent laryngeal branch of X)

Tonsils:

- pharyngeal tonsil lies high on the posterior wall of the nasopharynx – enlarges to form the adenoids
- opening of the auditory tube (along with tubal tonsil) lies on the lateral wall of the nasopharynx
- palatine tonsils lie between anterior and posterior pillars in the oropharynx
- lingual tonsils plus tubal, palatine and pharyngeal tonsils form Waldeyer's ring

General considerations

Clinical variations

Cleft lip – A congenital abnormality of the primary palate and may be complete/incomplete/microform; unilateral/bilateral; ± cleft palate

Cleft palate – a congenital abnormality of the primary palate which may be unilateral/bilateral; or submucous cleft

Incidence and aetiology

~1.5 in 1000 in Europe

1 in 500 in Asia

1 in 1000 in Africa

Cleft lip ± palate is more common than cleft palate alone

Cleft lip and palate is the commonest variation (approximately 50%)

More cleft lip ± palate in boys

More isolated cleft palate in girls. Overall, cleft palate alone occurs in 30%

Cleft lip alone occurs in 20%

Left side affected twice as often as the right

Ratio left : right : bilateral 6: 3: 1

Possible link with maternal drugs including anti-epileptics, salicylates, tretinoin (retinoids), benzodiazepines and cortisone

Higher incidence in offspring of smoking mothers

Genetic predisposition

Combination of all of the above

Genetic counselling

Inheritance may be:

- chromosomal
- Mendelian
- sporadic

Chromosomal inheritance includes syndromes such as **trisomy 13 and 21**

Mendelian inheritance includes syndromes due to single gene defects that may be an autosomal dominant gene (**van der Woude** syndrome – CL/P, missing teeth, lip pits – and **Treacher Collins** syndrome), or passed on in a recessive or X-linked manner in a family

Sporadic cases may be associated with developmental abnormalities (e.g. **Pierre Robin** sequence) with a low risk of further affected children

Non-syndromic clefts display multifactorial inheritance – includes a genetic **predisposition** plus one or more of the above risk factors

	CL/P	CP
Chromosomal	Trisomy 13 (Patau), trisomy 21 (Down)	
Single gene	van der Woude (chromosome 1)	TCS (chromosome 5), VCF -(chromosome 22), Stickler (chromosome 12)
		Nagers syndrome (cleft and radial dysplasia)
		Opitz (Hypertelorism, cleft lip and palate)
		Syndromic craniosynostosis
Sequence		Pierre Robin
Sporadic	Yes	Yes

Habib, Z. *Obst Gyn Survey* 1978, **33**: 441–7

Non-syndromic clefts

Normal parents, risk of child with cleft lip is 1 in 750–1000

Second affected child – risk 4%

Third affected child – risk 10%

If one parent has cleft lip the risk of having a child with cleft lip is 4%

Second affected child – risk 17%

If a child is born with CP, the risk of CL/P is still 1 in 750

Fogh–Andersen figures relating to CL/P clinical genetics 1971

Overall risk 1 in 700 (=1.5 in 1000 live births)

If the father has CP the risk of a child with CL/P is the same

If the father has CL/P the risk of a child with CL/P is 4%

Second child 10%

Initial assessment of the baby with a cleft lip

Breathing

- if dyspnoeic nurse prone: tongue → falls out of airway
- check oxygen saturation
- nasopharyngeal airway
- tongue stitch

Feeding

- trial of breast feeding
- soft teat
- squeezy bottle
- CP babies have worse feeding problems

Cleft clinic – assessment, planning and treatment within a multidisciplinary team environment

Timing of repair

6 weeks–3 months

- lip and nose correction (McComb)
- vomerine flap to anterior hard palate only
- synchronous soft palate repair in wide clefts may make subsequent hard palate repair easier

3–6 months

- palate repair
- grommets

5 years

- pharyngoplasty
- nasal correction – Tajima
- lengthen columella – forked flaps (bilateral)

9 years – alveolar bone graft, when the canine teeth first appear radiologically to prevent their root from collapsing into the cleft

16 years – rhinoplasty

Delaire approach

Maxillofacial surgeon in Nantes

6 months: lip and soft palate repair – Delaire lip technique – 'functional' repair (more muscle dissection) – muscle better developed at 6 months

18 months: hard palate repair – medial relaxing incisions possible because palate has been narrowed by previous soft palate closure

(Guest editorial) CSAG report

Boorman. *BJPS* 1998

CSAG = Clinical Standards Advisory Group

57 units providing CL/P care

17 units assessed, 457 patients reviewed

Only two units judged good overall

Two sets of criteria:

- **the unit itself**
  - multidisciplinary team
  - use of protocols
  - data collection
  - experience of team members
  - morale
- **assessment of children treated aged 5–6 and 12–13 years at the time of the survey**
- appearance
- dental hygiene
- speech
- hearing
- growth
- jaw relationships
- patient/parent satisfaction

No significant differences demonstrated in treatment outcomes between plastic and maxillofacial surgeons

Very few high volume operators, 92/99 surgeons performed <10 new repairs per annum

Only 7/99 surgeons performed ~30 new repairs annually

Only demonstrable benefit of high volume surgery was in speech outcome

Recommendations:

- number of CL/P units should be reduced from 57 to 8–15. Reducing the number of units will enable better data analysis and facilitate treatment advances
- each surgeon should treat between 40 and 50 new patients annually

Cleft lip repair

Unilateral cleft lip categorized

Microform ('forme fruste' – vertical furrow or scar, notch in the vermilion and white roll, variable vertical lip shortness)

Incomplete (variable vertical lip shortness, nasal sill intact – Simonart's band)
Complete (complete separation of the lip, nasal sill and alveolus)

Technical aims

Reposition the displaced atrophic alar cartilages and alar base
Reconstruct the nasal floor
Lengthen the medial side of the lip
Reconstruct orbicularis oris (approximation of muscle in transverse alignment)
Reposition cupid's bow and lip vermilion
Reconstruct the buccal sulcus

Cosmetic aims

A cupid's bow
A philtral dimple
Symmetrical alae
A straight columella
A camouflaged scar
Pouting of the lower portion of the lip (avoiding whistle deformity)

Management of the protruding premaxilla

Lip repair or lip adhesion (excising edges of cleft and simply suturing together as an adjunct to/instead of presurgical orthopaedics)
Presurgical orthopaedics
Premaxillary setback (but sacrifices incisors and compromises growth – condemned)

Lip adhesion

Skin traction on the maxilla following closure of the cleft lip under tension helps to reduce the size of the alveolar cleft
Temporary direct closure of the lip (adhesion) achieves this aim without compromising the **definitive** lip repair
Edges of the cleft are freshened and the lip closed in three layers
Alternative to presurgical orthopaedics

Presurgical orthopaedics

Bad bilateral clefts
Pioneered by McNeil 1950s – maxillary obturator used to reduce alveolar and palatal cleft (passive)
Active techniques described by Latham
Does not enhance maxillary growth
Orthodontic benefits are limited
Non-surgical closure of palatal bone and soft tissue is impossible
Spontaneous retropositioning of the premaxilla may follow lip repair

Correction of nasal deformity with a nasal moulding plate and stent: columella becomes more vertical, improved nasal tip projection and alar cartilage symmetry

Commonly used in the UK and USA and instituted within 2 weeks of birth

Repair techniques – brief principles

Complete unilateral clefts of the lip

Millard. *PRS* 1960: Rotation–advancement repair

Relies upon rotation of a flap (A flap) in the philtrum (non-cleft side) downwards and advancement of a flap from the cleft side (B flap) to meet the A flap

As the A flap rotates downwards, a small triangular flap above it, the C, flap can cross the midline and inset between the B flap and the nostril sill

Unilateral cleft lip – stencil method

Tennison. *PRS* 1952

Avoids a straight line scar by fashioning a Z-plasty on each side of the cleft

Modified by Randall and Skoog – reduced the size of the inferior flap

More suited to wide unilateral clefts and very short lip, but leaves a transverse scar low down on the philtral column

Closure of bilateral cleft clip and elongation of the columella by two operations in infancy

Millard. *PRS* 1971

Principle of banking the fork flap

Presurgical orthopaedics to the premaxilla

Lip repair at 1 month and banking of forked flaps

Columellar lengthening at 3 months

Protruding premaxilla

Poorly formed or absent anterior nasal spine

Retruded area under the base of the septal cartilage

Recession of the foot plates of the medial crura

Broad, flat nose

Absent columella

Prolabium is deficient of white roll and vermilion

Prolabium lacks muscle, columella is short and premaxillary segment is suspended from the nasal septum

Use of bilateral advancement flaps from the lateral lip segments

Prolabial vermilion is turned down

Muscle sutured together from lateral lip segments in the midline

Prolabial vermilion used for lining behind the muscle repair – adds bulk and prevents whistle deformity

Advancement of vermilion and white roll from lateral lip segments, joined in the midline beneath prolabial skin

Bilateral fork flaps are derived from the lateral edges of the prolabium

Each fork flap is sutured end-on to the alar base to form a standing cone/pyramid

At a second stage an inverted 'V' incision is made in the columella to join the bases of the two fork flaps

Incision is closed as a V–Y to gain columellar length

Combines columellar lengthening with advancement of the alar base

Bilateral incomplete cleft lip

Near normal nose

Normally positioned premaxilla

Simonart's bands across the nasal floors

Clefts involving only the lip

Repair using the advancement–rotation technique as for unilateral repair in two stages, one side at a time

Functional cleft lip repair. Kernahan, Rob and Smith's *Operative Surgery* (Plastic Surgery) 4th Ed. 1986

Flap of skin-mucosa reflected off each side of the cleft and sutured together

Orbicularis is mobilized on the cleft side

Pockets created on the non-cleft side just beneath the inferior nasal spine and beneath the vermilion border of the lip

Mobilized orbicularis is split into an upper two-thirds and lower third and these strips are sutured into contralateral orbicularis in upper and lower pockets

Overlying skin is closed using Z-plasties for lengthening

Management of whistle deformity – inadequate red margin/vermilion

Mucosal V–Y advancement (Kapetansky, *PRS* 1971)

Free graft from lower lip

Mucosal advancement from the buccal sulcus

Abbé flap

Cleft palate repair

'The goal of cleft palate surgery is to close the palate with a technique and timing that produce optimal speech and minimize facial growth disturbances.'

Veau classification

Soft palate

Soft and hard palate

Soft and hard palate and unilateral prepalate

Soft and hard palate and bilateral prepalate

Other classifications

Kernahan's striped Y further modified by Millard and Jackson allows the cleft to be located anatomically 1–3 on the right, 3–6 on the left, from lip anteriorly to the incisive foramen, 7, 8 hard palate and 9 soft palate

LAHSAL classification

- used by the national database on clefts
- capital indicates complete cleft: lip, alveolus, hard palate, soft palate, alveolus, lip

Also submucous cleft palate:

- described by Caplan *et al.*
- submucous cleft ~1 in 1000
- bifid uvula ~1–2%
- palpable notch
- blue line
- most have normal speech, 15% have VPI
- present with:
    - feeding problems
    - hearing problems
    - VPI
    - routine paediatric examination
- if speech and ENT assessment are OK, then palatal or pharyngeal surgery can be avoided

Aims of cleft palate correction

Closure of oronasal fistula
Allow normal development of speech
Minimize maxillary growth retardation
Facilitate velopharyngeal closure

Techniques

General anaesthesia
South-facing ET tube
Dingman gag – do not catch the lips
Throat packs
Mark incisions
Infiltrate with local anaesthetic/adrenaline solution
Remove the throat packs and Dingman gag at the end of the procedure

Vomerine flap

Used to close the anterior hard palate/alveolus at the time of lip repair
Decreases frequency of alveolar nasal fistulae
May worsen maxillary growth retardation

Flap-less repair

Relies upon movement of mucoperiosteum off the arched palate to lie horizontally to gain enough length for primary closure in the midline without lateral releasing incisions
Narrow clefts
Closure under slight tension hence may expect slightly higher fistula rate

Straight line closure (von Langenbeck)

Moves tissues towards the midline using lateral releasing incisions, lateral to the greater palatine artery – identification of the site of the greater palatine foramen – forms an equilateral triangle with the posterior alveolus and the hamulus

Medial von Langenbeck repairs use a releasing incision medial to the greater palatine artery essentially creating random pattern flaps.

Technique

- incise along the cleft
- dissect out muscle from nasal and oral mucosa
- mobilize the muscle to the midline, sweeping it backwards off the hard palate
- close nasal mucosa and then muscle
- make releasing incisions as necessary and close the oral layer
- pack surgicel into the raw areas

Forms a midline scar

No increase in length of the soft palate

Medial flaps described by Delaire

- medial to greater palatine artery → reduces maxillary growth retardation
- but flaps under greater tension → more fistulae

Lengthen the palate (Gilles, Veau, Kilner, Wardill)

'Push-back' procedures

Slide the mucoperiosteum of the hard palate posteriorly while transposing myomucosal flaps towards the midline, leaving lateral donor defects

Fracture of the hamulus to release tensor palati no longer advocated

May be performed with or without dividing the nasal mucosa

Dividing the nasal mucosa at the hard–soft palate junction to allow greater movement leaves a raw area on the nasal surface which may be left to granulate or closed with a variety of local flaps including Z-plasty

Flaps moved on greater palatine neurovascular bundles

Although palatal musculature is detached from the hard palate, fibres still course **anteriorly** rather than *transversely*.

It has been postulated that the 'push back' techniques may have a greater detrimental effect on future maxillary growth

Realignment of the palatal muscle

Aim to reposition muscle fibres so that they lie more posteriorly and transversely

Intravelar veloplasty. Popularized by Sommerlad, with radical muscle dissection and posterior repositioning.

Wide dissection of the tensor muscle back to the pterygoid hamulus

Lengthen the soft palate and reconstruct palatal muscle sling

Double opposing Z-plasty (**Furlow**) This is a popular technique that raises two Z plasties, one on the nasal mucosal surface and the other on the palatal surface, drawn opposite to each other but designed so the posteriorly transposed flap contains the muscle layer. When the flaps are transposed, muscle is relocated posteriorly and the suture lines are at right angles to each other on the nasal and oral layers reducing the chance of fistula.

Complications

Fistula (0–34%)

Maxillary growth retardation may be less pronounced in late repair but at the expence of late correction of VPI and therefore delaying development of normal speech

Pharyngoplasty rate for troublesome post-palatoplasty VPI up to 20%

Nasal airway obstruction:

- early postoperative swelling
- late due to altered nasal morphology (25% decrease in pressure flow through nasal airway)

Growth retardation – Oslo cleft lip and palate growth archive

Cephalometric recording

Growth retardation related to age at surgery

Seniority of surgeon, type of lip repair and pharyngoplasty not prognostic

Alveolar bone grafting does not inhibit growth but provides a valuable matrix for the eruption of teeth

Palatoplasty and postoperative hypoxaemia. *BJA* 1998

Post-operative hypoxaemia potentiated by oedema of palate, pharynx or tongue

Inability to clear pulmonary and oral secretions

Higher oxygen consumption in children compared with adults

Low elastic recoil pressure of thorax and lungs

Treatment groups studied:

- von Langenbeck palatoplasty
- push-back palatoplasty
- push-back plus superior pharyngeal flap pharyngoplasty

Oxygen saturation dips to <85% were recorded most frequently in the combined procedure patients

Desaturation was most profound within the first 30 min of arrival in the recovery room

Von Langenbeck repairs were significantly less likely to cause hypoxaemia than either push-back or combined procedures

Cleft palate fistulae
Cohen, *PRS* 1991

Symptoms

Audible nasal escape during speech

Hypernasality

Nasal regurgitation

Deterioration in speech intelligibility

Retrospective review of 129 non-syndromic CL/P patients

Nasal–alveolar fistulae excluded

23% fistula rate

16% large fistulae (>5 mm), repaired early (speech problems)

47% small fistulae (1–2 mm), repaired at time of lip revision, nasal surgery or bone grafting

Multivariate analysis to determine causative factors:

- push-back palatoplasty (43% developed fistulae)
- Veau classification 3 and 4
- operating surgeon

Non-causative factors:

- age and gender of patient
- intravelar veloplasty

Surgical management:

- total revision of the palate repair
- local mucoperiosteal flaps
- vomerine flaps
- bone grafting plus soft tissue closure
- tongue flaps

Recurrent fistula (37%) was significantly more common in females

Second recurrences in 25%

Fistulae are mostly small and located in the anterior part of the hard palate

Neonatal repair of the cleft palate
Magee. *Cleft Palate–Craniofacial J* 1996

Against

Anaesthetic risk

Technical difficulty

Implications for facial growth

Chance of missing undiagnosed anomalies

Hypoglycaemia

Jaundice

For

Improved speech

Psychologically better for parents (especially fathers?)

Easier feeding

Can perform synchronous palate and lip closure under one anaesthetic

Cleft palate repair by double opposing Z-plasty
Furlow. *PRS* 1986

Z-plasty flaps create a muscle sling across the cleft

Soft palate lengthened without using tissue from the hard palate (needs Von Langenbeck repair)

No relaxing incisions hence only hard palate scar is in the midline, reducing interference with maxillary growth

Two soft palate Z-plasty flaps with their central limbs made by incising along the cleft

Anteriorly based flaps are composed of **mucosa**, the posteriorly based flaps are myomucosal to incorporate palatal **musculature**

Nasal flaps are transposed first, subsequent transposition of oral flaps creates an overlapping sling of palatal muscle

Importantly, the nasal Z-plasty is a mirror image of the oral Z-plasty

Anterior Z-plasty incisions should be placed along the posterior margins of the hard palate

Superior speech and less VPI compared with historical controls

Effect of Veau–Wardill–Kilner type of cleft palate repair on long-term midfacial growth

Choudhary. *Plastic Reconstruc Surg* 2003

Concerns that Veau–Wardill–Kilner type of cleft palate repair causes extensive denudation of the palate, resulting in inhibition of maxillary growth

- 25 non-syndromic complete unilateral cleft lip and palate patients
- Average 12 year follow-up

Midfacial growth studied using 12-year dental models and lateral cephalograms taken before definitive orthodontic treatment

- evaluated using the GOSLON Yardstick and digital cephalometric analysis
- 72% of the patients had a good or satisfactory outcome, with a GOSLON score of 1, 2, or 3,
- 28% obtained a poor score of 4 or 5.

The results suggest that satisfactory long-term midfacial growth can be obtained with Veau–Wardill–Kilner cleft palate repair

A technique for cleft palate repair

Sommerlad. *Plastic Reconstruc Surg* 2003

Technique of palate repair that combines minimal hard palate dissection with radical retropositioning of the velar musculature and tensor tenotomy.

- performed under the operating microscope
- 442 primary palate repairs performed between 1978 and 1992
- follow-up of at least 10 years
- 80% of repairs carried out through incisions at the margins of the cleft and without any mucoperiosteal flap elevation or lateral incisions

Secondary velopharyngeal rates have decreased from 10.2 to 4.9 to 4.6% in successive 5-year periods within this 15-year period.

Evidence suggests that this more radical muscle dissection improves velar function

Prenatal counselling for cleft lip and palate
Matthews. *PRS* 1998

Cleft lip and palate may be diagnosed incidentally during routine prenatal screening at 15 weeks

Prenatal ultrasound specifically looking for clefts has a low sensitivity but high specificity (high false-negative), low false-positive

Most ultrasound diagnoses are for bilateral clefts

No parents felt termination would be an option for an isolated cleft but 30% were against having a further pregnancy

High incidence of associated abnormalities – karyotyping advised

Majority of parents felt prenatal counselling with the cleft team was helpful

Anatomical approach to (intravelar) veloplasty
Kriens. *PRS* 1969

Detailed description of abnormal muscle insertions and directions of pull

Described dissection of individual muscles at operation to restore as near normal anatomy as possible

Self assessment: Discuss your **treatment** plan for a baby born with a unilateral complete cleft of the lip and palate

Plan treatment in a multidisciplinary team environment – cleft clinic

Priorities:

- ensure that there are no breathing difficulties; give CPAP if necessary (more relevant to PRS)
- treat any feeding difficulties with parent education, soft teat and squeezy bottle

First operation

- 6 weeks–3 months
- lip repair (Millard rotation–advancement for unilateral)
- vomerine flap to anterior alveolar cleft
- primary McComb nasal correction

Second operation

- 6 months
- palatal repair (von Langenbeck technique including intravelar veloplasty, vomerine flap to close nasal layer at the level of the hard palate)
- insertion of grommets if required

Speech therapy – commence 3–4 years

Third operation

- 5 years
- **pharyngoplasty** for post-palatoplasty VPI (superior pharyngeal flap preferred except where there is significant lateral wall immobility – then Orticochoea)
- Tajima secondary nose correction if required

Orthodontics – early dental management – age 6 onwards

Fourth operation

- 9 years (mixed dentition)
- alveolar bone graft

Orthodontics – management of permanent dentition – age 11 onwards

Fifth operation

- 16 years
- rhinoplasty
- le Fort I advancement to correct class III malocclusion if required

Bilateral much the same – add in:

- Presurgical orthopaedics for the protruding premaxilla
- Millard bilateral lip repair banking forked flaps
- Lengthen the columella with forked flaps at the time of pharyngoplasty ~5 years

Arm restraints in children with cleft lip/palate

Sommerlad. *Plastic Reconstruc Surg* 2003

No benefit in using any form of arm restraint demonstrated by randomized trial

The use of the operating microscope for cleft palate repair and pharyngoplasty

Sommerlad. *Plastic Reconstruc Surg* 2003

Operating microscope used for all palate and pharyngeal operations since 1991 ($n = 1000$)

- more comfortable position with reliable lighting and variable magnification
- Same view for operating surgeon, trainees and operating room staff (teaching arm or video screen)
- Anatomy more clearly displayed so potentially more accurately reconstructed

Pharyngoplasty

Site of phonation (lips, tongue, palate, pharynx, etc.) – moves backwards

Only the sounds M, N and NG normally allow nasal escape in the English language

During normal speech the soft palate ascends to close off the nasopharynx

Inadequate closure requires either lengthening/reconstruction of the soft palate or narrowing of the velopharyngeal space

Where the palate is intact, pharyngoplasty begins with a palatal split

~20% of patients post-palatoplasty require pharyngoplasty, independent of the type of palatoplasty

VPI may result from anatomic, neuromuscular, behavioural or combination disorders

VPI overcome by either lengthening the palate (push-back procedures), improving palatal movement (intravelar veloplasty) or narrowing the nasopharyngeal isthmus (pharyngoplasty)

Normal speech

24 consonants, 15 short vowel sounds and nine long vowel sounds in the English language

Classification of consonants:

- voicing of sounds
  - vocal folds vibrating – all vowels and B G D Z
  - vocal folds held apart – mainly plosive sounds P T K S
- place of articulation
  - lips – M P B
  - labiodental – F V (lower lip and upper incisors)
  - dental – TH (tongue plus teeth)
  - alveolar – T D (tongue plus alveolar ridge)
  - palato-alveolar – SH (air passes beneath the palate)
  - palatal – Y
  - velar
  - glottal

Symptoms of VPI

Hypernasality (rhinolalia)

Audible nasal escape

Lack of voice projection and articulation

Secondary symptoms of VPI

Inability to generate enough air pressure to pronounce explosive sounds such as P, T, K, B, D and G which are substituted for **glottal stop sounds**

Consonants such as S, Z, SH and occasionally CH are substituted by **pharyngeal fricative sounds**

Unintelligible vocalization, nasal grimacing, snorts and breathlessness

Investigation of VPI

Allows definition of the site and size of the gap

Speech and hearing assessment

Videofluoroscopy (pronouncing 'EE')

Nasendoscopy

MRI

Indications for surgery

Nasal escape a prominent feature and hampering the development of normal speech

VPI despite adequate correction of a palatal cleft

Conditions for surgery

Intelligence and speech development are not unduly retarded

An accurate speech assessment has been possible

Timing of surgery

After 5 years but before 12 years

After 12 years there is a decline in the rate of learning of new speech sounds

Options for correction of velopharyngeal insufficiency

Sphincteroplasty

Wardill. *BJS* 1928

First attempt at sphincteroplasty – Wardill (1928)

Muscle sphincteroplasty originally described by Hynes (1951)

Modified by Orticochea (1968) and Jackson (1985)

Indicated when there is **poor medial excursion of the lateral pharyngeal walls and a short anteroposterior diameter**

Pyloroplasty technique: horizontal incision in the posterior pharyngeal wall at the level of Passavant's ridge sutured vertically

Ledge of tissue created to act as a 'valve seating for the upper surface of the soft palate'

Pharyngoplasty by muscle transplantation

Hynes. *BJPS* 1951

Drawbacks using Wardill's technique:

- pharyngeal wall sutured under tension
- ridge of tissue on the posterior pharyngeal wall may be placed too low for velopharyngeal closure if the repaired palate is short because the palate will then approach the posterior wall at a level higher than Passavant's ridge (hypertrophy of palatopharyngeus and lower part of superior constrictor)

To be effective, pharyngoplasty must:

- reduce transverse diameter of the pharynx
- reduce the AP diameter of the pharynx at a level higher than Passavant's ridge
- maintain functional muscle around the nasopharyngeal isthmus rather than inert scar
- allow normal superior constrictor function
- minimize tension on suture lines

Superiorly based mucosal flaps from posterior tonsillar pillars including the underlying palatopharyngeus

Branch of the ascending pharyngeal A may cause some bleeding during elevation of the flaps

Preserve branches of the vagus nerve entering palatopharyngeus at the level of the soft palate

Flaps should be 3–4 cm long and ~1.5 cm wide

Close donor defect directly

Inset flaps in the midline into **a horizontal incision in the posterior pharyngeal wall, one above the other** to form a bulky ridge

Static and dynamic closure of the velopharynx

Dynamic muscle sphincter

Orticochea. *PRS* 1968

Transposition of palatopharyngeus myomucosal flaps towards the midline

Inset into an **inferiorly based posterior pharyngeal flap**

Donor defects heal by secondary intention with cicatrization which gradually closes off the lateral pharyngeal apertures

In adults or where there is a very short palate (anteroposteriorly), there is increased risk of dehiscence of the palatopharyngeus flaps – hence perform in two stages, one flap at a time

Sphincter pharyngoplasty

Jackson. *Clin Plast Surg* 1985

Similar to the Hynes pharyngoplasty except palatopharyngeus flaps are sutured **end–end** and inset into a transverse incision on the posterior pharyngeal wall

Transverse incision is placed level with the upper margin of the tonsillar fossa

Pharyngeal flaps

Superiorly or inferiorly based single flap

Static closure of velopharynx

Less air passes through lateral ports – aim for a diameter of ~0.5 cm

Over-correction leads to mouth breathing, hyponasality, and obstructive sleep apnoea

Flap raised in the plane of prevertebral fascia

Inset into reflected flaps from the soft palate of nasal mucosa

Partially close donor defect or allow to heal by secondary intention

Choice of procedure

Immobile soft palate: posterior flap pharyngoplasty

Mobile soft palate but inadequate lateral wall closure: sphincteroplasty

Nasal escape following adenoidectomy: implant (Teflon, cartilage)

Anaesthesia

Centrally placed south facing metal oral endotracheal tube (not compressed by Dingman gag)

Inflatable cuff (no pharyngeal packs)

Level of anaesthesia to be deep enough to prevent gagging but light enough to allow swift return of protective pharyngeal reflexes (cough and swallowing)

Preliminary infiltration with 1:200 000 adrenaline solution

Post-operative care

Clear fluids – 24 h

Liquid diet – 48 h

Soft diet – 2 weeks

Velocardiofacial (Shprintzen's) syndrome (including the original paper by Shprintzen)
Cleft Plate J 1978

VCF is the most common syndrome associated with clefts:

- 22q11.2 deletion using TUPLE 1 probe
- diagnosed by FISH test (fluorescent *in situ* hybridization for the gene)
- generally do badly as a group
- inadequate development of the facial neural crest tissues, resulting in defective organogenesis of pharyngeal pouch derivatives

Associated abnormalities:

- CATCH 22:
  - cardiac anomalies
  - abnormal facies (flat expressionless face)
  - thymic aplasia (overlaps with Di George syndrome)
  - cleft palate (submucous)
  - hypocalcaemia

Velo-

8% of all cases of cleft palate without cleft lip

Velopharyngeal dysfunction – poor movement in lateral pharyngeal wall

Cleft or, more commonly, submucous cleft palate

Cardio-

Medially displaced anomalous carotid As (pre-operative MRI angiography)

Bad heart problems, e.g. tetralogy of Fallot

Also VSD (most commonly), coarctation of the aorta, pulmonary stenosis

25% have median carotid artery

Facial

Vertical maxillary excess

Epicanthic folds

Anti-Mongoloid slant

Malar flattening

Class II malocclusion

Abundant scalp hair

Long face (vertical maxillary excess)

Also

Small stature

Abnormal dermatoglyphics

Mild hypotonia in early childhood

Spindling fingers

Learning difficulties

Psychotic illness in adult life

Surgical management of VPI in velocardiofacial syndrome

Mehendale. *Cleft palate-craniofacial J* 2004

42 patients with 22q11 deletion

Pre- surgical assessment:

- Intraoral examination
- Lateral videofluoroscopy $+/-$ nasendoscopy
- Intraoperative assessment of velar muscular anatomy

Surgical options (based upon assessment above)

- Radical dissection and retropositioning of velar muscles (submucous cleft palate repair)
- Hynes pharyngoplasty
- Palate repair followed by Hynes pharyngoplasty
  - Staged approach
  - Maximize palatal function first

Outcome assessment

- Evaluation of resonance and nasal airflow
- Lateral videofluoroscopy and nasendoscopy assessment of velopharyngeal function

Results

- Improvement in hypernasality in all groups
  - Staged approach showed significant improvement in nasal emission
  - SMCP repair resulted in increased velar length and increased velocity of closure

Approach to repair should be determined by assessment of velopharyngeal anatomy and function

Sphincter pharyngoplasty in VPI

Losken. *Plastic Reconstruc Surg* 2003

Review of 250 patients who underwent sphincter pharyngoplasty for VPI

- Mean age 7.6 years
- VPI alone ($n = 63$)
- VPI plus cleft palate ($n = 127$)
- 22q11 deletion ($n = 32$)

- Submucous cleft ($n = 15$)
- Other ($n = 13$)

Revision of pharyngoplasty required in 12.8%

- Most common in 22q11 deletion group
- Lowest in patients with VPI alone
- Predicted by:
  - Severe preoperative hypernasal resonance
  - Larger velopharyngeal aperture
- Favourable outcome in 94%

Randomized study of pharyngeal flap vs. sphincter pharyngoplasty

Ysunza. *Plastic Reconstruc Surg* 2002

Residual VPI following palatal repair commonly between 10–20%

50 patients with residual VPI were evaluated by videonasendoscopy and multi-view videofluoroscopy

- 25 patients underwent 'customized' pharyngeal flap repair
- 25 patients underwent 'customized' sphincter pharyngoplasty

Residual VPI following secondary surgery was similar in each group

Cleft nose

Unilateral cleft nose deformity:

- mild – wide alar base, normal alar contour, normal dome projection
- moderate – wide alar base, depressed dome or alar crease (minimal alar hypoplasia)
- severe – wide alar base, deep alar crease, under-projecting alar dome (alar hypoplasia) with **caudal rotation** (downwards) of the alar cartilage so that the dome is **retroposed** and the nose is **lengthened** on the cleft side – normal columellar angle ~60°: cleft nose is caudally rotated (>60°)
- septum is deviated away from the cleft side – pull of normal muscles not counterbalanced

Bilateral cleft nose deformity:

- short columella
- broad, depressed nasal tip

Aetiology of the cleft nose:

- extrinsic – malposition of the nose due to developmental traction (Moss' functional matrix theory)
- intrinsic – inherited tissue defect in the cleft side traced to an ectodermal deficiency

Nasal correction carried out aged 5–6 years

Rhinoplasty at ~16–17 years

Primary repair of the *unilateral* cleft lip nose
McComb. *PRS* 1975 and 1985

Surgery aims to correct caudal rotation of the alar cartilage at the time of lip repair and shorten the nose on the cleft side

Skin mobilized off cartilage framework

Alar lift achieved with mattress sutures passing from within the vestibule of the cleft nostril and tied over a bolster at the level of the nasion

Primary repair of the *bilateral* cleft lip nose
McComb. *PRS* 1990

Following primary correction of the bilateral cleft nose by elevation of the alar cartilages and columellar lengthening using forked flaps, three undesirable features become apparent at adolescence:
- nostrils are larger than normal
- broadening of the nasal tip (persistent separation of alar domes)
- downward drift of the columella base

Embryologically the columella should be reconstructed from nasal tissue rather than from the prolabium that belongs to the lip – hence the use of forked flaps questioned

Nose repaired at a first stage with repair of the lip at a second stage 1 month later – the blood supply to the prolabium, when elevated off the premaxilla, is thus not compromised by concurrent nasal tip dissection and undermining

Presurgical orthopaedics helps reduce the soft tissue cleft before operation

Stage 1:
- repair of nostril floor
- lip adhesion of prolabial segment to adjacent lip

Stage 2:
- incisions above each alar rim meeting in the midline and wide undermining to mobilize alar domes (open rhinoplasty approach)
- lip adhesions taken down and a formal lip repair performed using lateral mucomuscular flaps to the undermined prolabium
- suture together the displaced alar domes, now under less tension
- close skin incisions as a V–Y to a length of 5 mm as the vertical limb in the columella

Reverse 'U' incision for cleft lip nose
Tajima. *PRS* 1977

Makes use of an inverted 'U'-shaped incision in the nasal vestibule to mobilize up the dorsal nasal skin and allow suturing of the displaced alar cartilage (cleft side) to the normal side

As the normal anatomical correction of the alar cartilage is achieved, the mobilized dorsal skin is in slight excess and closure gives rise to a natural in-rolling effect

Much greater undermining required

Orthodontics

Tooth development and cleft orthodontics

Alveolar cleft is usually located between the lateral incisor and the canine

Lateral incisor tooth bud may develop two incisors on either side of the cleft, may erupt into the cleft space or may be absent

Permanent lateral incisors are absent in 10–40% of patients

Adjacent teeth have poorly formed enamel

Permanent lateral incisor normally erupts at 7–8 years of age

The canine erupts at 11–12 years of age

Permanent teeth are generally slower to erupt around a cleft than non-cleft teeth

Orthodontics relies upon bone resorption along the pressure side of a tooth and growth on the tension side

Stages of orthodontic treatment

Presurgical orthopaedics (see above)

- assist in closure of the wide alveolar cleft
- use while awaiting lip repair
- prosthetic plate assists feeding

Early dental management

- extraction of troublesome displaced deciduous teeth
- correction of malocclusion of erupting permanent teeth
- begin at the time of eruption of the upper central incisors, age 6 onwards

Management of permanent dentition

- orthodontic treatment aimed at realigning teeth and correcting cross-bite, age 11 onwards
- Le Fort I osteotomy and maxillary advancement or distraction

Occlusion (angle classification)

Class I – lower incisor contacts the middle part of the upper incisor (normal)

Class II – lower incisor contacts posterior to class I

Class III – lower incisor contacts anterior to class I

Essentially each upper molar tooth should sit half a tooth in front of the corresponding lower tooth

Bone–base relationship

Class I – maxilla slightly overprojects mandible (normal)

Class II – maxilla excessively overprojects

Class III – mandible overprojects maxilla

In cleft patients occlusion may be normal but there is often a class III occlusion

There are also variable degrees of cross-bite in the posterior teeth, some uppers biting inside the lowers

Unilateral clefts tend to be associated with unilateral areas of cross-bite, bilateral clefts with bilateral cross-bite

Some teeth may be significantly displaced and need to be extracted

Aims of alveolar cleft closure

Stabilize the maxillary arch (especially bilateral clefts)

Close oronasal fistulas and anterior palatal cleft

Provide periodontal support for teeth to the cleft

Provide a matrix into which permanent teeth may erupt

Gingivoperiosteoplasty (closure of the alveolar cleft using periosteal flaps – Skoog) fails to achieve all of these aims

Alveolar deformity in complete clefts

- Narrow, no collapse
- Narrow, plus collapse
- Wide, no collapse
- Wide, plus collapse

Bone grafting

Orthodontic treatment, i.e. movement of the premaxilla and maxillary segments, is impossible after bone grafting

Hence, need to establish good arch alignment before grafting

Debate regarding timing – early (5–6 years) vs. late (9–11 years)

Alternatively when 25–50% of the canine tooth is visible on the OPT

Early grafting may reduce maxillary growth and the bone graft resorbs in the absence of an erupting tooth

Late grafting deprives erupting permanent dentition of periodontal support

May require the eruption of permanent dentition to facilitate orthodontic treatment before bone grafting – bilateral clefts in particular

Conditions for surgery – must have

Robust repair of the palatal cleft

Watertight closure of nasal lining

Secure lip repair

Technique

Raise flaps of gingiva in the cleft itself and superiorly based on the alveolus to cover bone graft

Keep incisions further away from the gingivodental junction when raising flaps around permanent compared with deciduous teeth

Cancellous autograft from iliac crest

Closure of gingival flaps over the bone graft packed into the cleft

Complications

Separation of gingival flaps and graft exposure

Resorption of graft

Ear disease

Eustachian tube dysfunction – links nasopharynx with middle ear

Tensor palati and levator palati both attach to the auditory tube

Failure of opening during swallowing

Generation of negative pressure within the middle ear

Collection of serous or mucoid (glue ear) effusion in middle ear

Infected mucoid effusions = otitis media

Palatoplasty often but not always corrects dysfunction

Conductive hearing loss

Worsens speech problems

Treat by myringotomy and insertion of grommets before or at the time of palate repair

Adenoidectomy may also improve Eustachian tube patency

Hearing:

- repair of the palate alone does not improve otitis media
- natural history is to improve ~8 years of age: as mid-face grows the Eustachian tube begins to drain by gravity
- previous adenoidectomy may be due to palatal malfunction
- glue ear → 40 dB hearing loss
- insertion of grommets treats glue ear but hearing decreases by a further 15 dB
- test by evoked response audiometry

5 Hand surgery (trauma, degenerative and inflammatory disease, nerve compression, congenital abnormalities)

Examination
Injury
Dupuytren's and joint contracture
Nerve compression and CTS
Arthritis and inflammatory disorders
Congenital hand
Spastic disorders of the upper limb

Examination

Look

Start with the dorsum of hand

skin	– sudomotor changes, skin lesions benign (Garrod's pads, Heberden's nodes) or malignant (AKs, SCCs), pigment changes, scars, etc. – anything obvious
swellings	– dorsal wrist ganglia, bony exostoses
wasting	– dorsal interosseii
position of the hand	– ulnar claw, rheumatoid deformities of metacarpophalangeal joints and fingers and measure angles with goniometer

Turn the hand over to look at the volar surface

Skin	– sudomotor changes, palmar scars, palmar nodules of DD
Swellings	– volar wrist ganglion, palmar lipomata, etc.
Wasting	– interosseus, thenar muscle, hypothenar muscle

Feel

Test for **sensation** in each of the nerve territories. Need to check nerves before operating on any part of the hand, e.g. Dupuytren's where a digital nerve may be injured. Better to check sensation prior to manipulating the hand.

Feel the **relevant feature** to complete examination of texture, tenderness, mobility, etc. If a joint is the relevant feature then feel stability. Do not elicite pain!

Move

Passive range of movement

Active range of movement

- movement in an **area of special interest**
  - flexor tendon division – test FDP and FDS tendons
  - basal joint OA – ask patient to circumduct
  - RA – look at active pronation/supination at the wrist, ask patient to flex and extend at metacarpophalangeal joints
- **test the motor nerves to the whole hand** by testing the muscles innervated by each

Examination for specific nerves

Median nerve

Observe:

- wasting of the thenar musculature
- sudomotor changes in the median nerve distribution

Tests:

- motor/power
  - **median nerve at the elbow**:
    - palpable tendon of FCR with resisted wrist flexion
  - **anterior interosseus nerve sign**:
    - inability to make an 'O' sign – denervation of FDP to the index finger and FPL
    - pronation of the forearm, elbow extended to neutralize pronator teres (pronator quadratus)
  - **motor branch of median nerve**:
    - weakness in abduction of the thumb (APB)
    - opposition to the little finger (true pulp to pulp – opponens pollicis)
- sensory:
  - **moving** two-point discrimination
  - sharp/blunt sensation

Ulnar nerve

Observe:

- interosseus guttering and first dorsal interosseus wasting
- hypothenar wasting
- ulnar claw hand
- sudomotor skin changes

Tests:

- motor/power:
  - Froment's test – adductor pollicis
  - individual Froment's tests to the fingers – palmar interosseii
  - resisted abduction of the index finger (first dorsal interosseus) and little finger (ADM)
  - flex the metacarpophalangeal joint of the little finger with the proximal interphalangeal straight – FDM

- absent flexion at the distal interphalangeal joint of the ulnar two fingers (ulnar-innervated FDPs)
- sensory:
  - **moving** two-point discrimination
  - sharp/blunt sensation

Radial nerve

Observe

- sudomotor changes in the superficial branch of radial nerve distribution
- wasting of triceps, brachioradialis and extensor compartment
- wrist drop

Tests:

- motor/power:
  - above the elbow:
    - elbow extension (triceps)
  - at the elbow:
    - elbow flexion, arm in mid-pronation to neutralize biceps (brachioradialis)
    - wrist extension and radial deviation, fist clenched (ECRL and ECRB)
  - below the elbow: **posterior interosseus nerve**:
    - supination with the elbow extended to neutralize biceps (supinator)
    - thumb extension with the palm flat (EPL)
- sensory:
  - **moving** two point discrimination
  - sharp/blunt sensation

Specific provocation tests for nerve compression

In addition to the above tests

Provocation tests reproduce the symptoms of the compression neuropathy

Median nerve

Pronator syndrome: pain with resisted pronation of the flexed forearm. Pinches the median nerve between the two heads of pronator teres

Anterior interosseus syndrome – resisted FDS flexion of the middle finger

Carpal tunnel syndrome – **paraesthesia** with Tinel's and Phalen's tests

Ulnar nerve

Cubital tunnel syndrome

- **paraesthesia** with Phalen's test (flexion of the elbow)
  - Tinel's test unreliable
  - note lack of clawing due to denervation of ulnar FDPs

Ulnar tunnel syndrome (Guyon's canal) – **paraesthesia** with pressure over Guyon's canal

Radial nerve

Radial tunnel syndrome

- **pain** with middle finger test (resisted extension of the middle finger)

- ECRB inserts into the base of the third metacarpal
- tendinous medial edge compresses radial nerve in radial tunnel

Wartenberg's syndrome – dysaesthesia with compression of the superficial branch of radial nerve beneath the tendon of brachioradialis. Frinkelstein test (positive in de Quervain's) misleadingly positive

Examination for thoracic outlet syndrome

Roos' test
- abduct the arms to 90° with the elbows flexed to 90° and externally rotated, then open and close hands for 3 min
- listen for a bruit indicating subclavian artery aneurysm (most sensitive in the position of Roos' test)

Wright's test – abduct arms to 90°, hyper-extension and palpate the radial pulse as the flexed forearm is externally rotated to adopt the position of Roos' test

Addson's test
- brace shoulders backwards, turn head towards the affected side, lift chin and take a deep breath in – look for diminution of the radial pulse
- positive in 20–25% of normal subjects

reverse Addson's, head away and chin down

Falconer's, brace and pull down on arms behind the patient checking for decrease in pulse

Brachial plexus compression test – pressure applied to the brachial plexus in the posterior triangle

Costoclavicular compression test – allow shoulders to relax, supinate forearms and apply downwards and backwards traction to both arms while palpating the radial pulse

Also check for Horner's syndrome (involvement of the stellate ganglion) phrenic nerve (raised hemi-diaphragm CXR) and Brown–Sequard syndrome

Examination for cervical root compression

Spurling's test – head turned to the affected side and downwards pressure is applied to the top of the head, closes the intervertebral foramens

Sensory changes
- C5 – lateral upper arm
- C6 – lateral forearm
- C7 – central posterior arm and forearm
- C8 – medial forearm
- T1 – medial upper arm

Motor loss
- elbow flexion – C5,6
- elbow extension – C7,8
- hand intrinsics – C8,T1

Reflexes
- biceps – C5,6
- brachioradialis – C6,7
- triceps – C7,8

Injury

Hand infections

Commonest hand infection is paronychial infection due to *Staphylococcus aureus*

- highest density of dermal lymphatics in the body is in the hyponychium

Felon – abscess of the pulp space

Herpetic whitlow – HSV vesicular eruption in the fingertip

- incise only if a secondary bacterial abscess has developed
- if not then bacterial superinfection may be caused by incision

Collar stud abscess – infection in the subfascial palmar space pointing dorsally

Kanavel's four cardinal signs of flexor sheath infection:

- fusiform digital swelling
- stiffness in a semiflexed position
- tenderness along the flexor sheath into the palm
- pain with passive extension

Two bursae in the hand:

- synovial sheaths
- radial – encloses the FPL tendon
- ulnar – encloses the long tendons to the little–index fingers (and is continuous with the flexor sheath to little finger)
- most people have connections between these two bursae in the palm which extend into the wrist to form the space of Parona in front of pronator quadratus which can allow infection to spread between these two spaces

Palmar spaces in the hand:

- thenar

  hypothenar

  adductor policis

- mid-palm
- separated by fascia arising from the metacarpal of the middle finger (mid-palmar ligament)

Organisms in bites:

- human – *Staphylococcus, Streptobacillus, Eikenella corrodens*, anaerobes
- dog – *Pasteurella multocida, Streptobacillus, Staphylococcus*, anaerobes
- cat – mainly *Pasteurella multocida*

All respond to augmentin

Necrotizing fasciitis of the upper extremity

Gonzalez. *J Hand Surg* 1996

First described by Wilson 1952

Insidious onset with rapid spread along tissue planes

12 cases reviewed, all associated with IV substance abuse or diabetes

HIV positivity in three of five patients tested

β-haemolytic *Streptobacillus* or a mixed aerobic/anaerobic infection or both

Zone of fascial involvement spreads beyond zone of skin involvement

Myonecrosis in five patients

Average of three debridements including shoulder disarticulation

If debridement has been effective it should be followed by a rapid clinical response

Flexor tendon injuries

Fingers extended at time of injury – distal ends lie in the wound

Fingers flexed at time of injury – distal ends distal to the skin wound

Anatomy

All flexor tendons, the ulnar and median nerves and the ulnar artery lie in the ulnar half of the wrist, medial to PL

Dorsal branch of the ulnar nerve is at risk during excision of the ulnar head

Deep branch of the ulnar nerve dives down at the level of the pisiform into the hypothenar musculature

Palmar cutaneous branch of the median nerve arises 5–6 cm proximal to the distal wrist crease between PL and FCR

Last muscle to be supplied by the ulnar nerve is the first dorsal interosseus – and hence shows the earliest sign of wasting

FDS divides level with the distal palmar crease

Verdan's zones

Zone of tendon injury must be described as that when the fingers and thumb are extended, rather than the site of the surface laceration

Finger

zone 1: Insertion of the FDP to the insertion of FDS

zone 2: Between the insertion of FDS and the A1 pulley (distal palmar crease) 'No man's land' (Bunnell); 'critical zone' (Boyes)

zone 3: From the A1 pulley to the distal border of the carpal tunnel

zone 4: Carpal tunnel

zone 5: Carpal tunnel to musculotendinous junctions muscle bellies

Thumb

zone 1: From the A2 pulley to the insertion of FPL

zone 2: A1–2 pulley

zone 3: A1 pulley to carpal tunnel; then as above

Pulleys

Finger

Five annular pulleys, four cruciate pulleys

- A1 – overlying metacarpophalangeal joint, attached to base of PP
- A2 – overlying shaft of PP
- A3 – overlying proximal interphalangeal joint, attached to base of MP
- A4 – overlying shaft of MP
- A5 – overlying distal interphalangeal joint, attached to base of distal interphalangeal joint
- C1–4 – between annular pulleys

Thumb

Two annular pulleys, one oblique pulley

- A1 – overlying metacarpophalangeal joint, attached to volar plate
- A2 – overlying interphalangeal joint, attached to head of PP
- oblique – overlying shaft of PP (analogous to A2 in finger)
- tendon of adductor pollicis attached to A1 and oblique pulleys

Vinculae

Short vinculum attaches FDP to neck of MP

Long vinculum attaches FDP to neck of PP

FDS also has long and short vinculae both attaching to the PP

Closed avulsion of FDP

Leddy and Packer classification

I – FDP ruptures along with both vinculae but no fracture, hence tendon retracts into the palm – tender lump

II – FDP ruptures but long vinculum remains intact. Distal tendon end held by long vinculum at proximal interphalangeal joint level. May have small fracture fragment

III – Large fracture fragment caught in A4 pulley. Tendon unable to retract further hence both vinculae protected

Boyes Classification flexor tendon injuries

I Injury to tendon only

II Tendon and soft tissue

III Associated with joint contracture

IV Associated with neurovascular damage

V multiple digits or combinations of II–IV

Flexor tendon repair

Two or four strand techniques

Non-absorbable monofilament (prolene) or braided (ticron)

Absorbable sutures (PDS, maxon) also satisfactory since metabolic rate of tendon tissue is low and suture material is retained long enough to maintain tensile strength during healing

Modified Kessler plus epitendinous superior to most other techniques – epitendinous suture contributes 20% to the strength of the repair

Preserve vinculae

Keep sutures volar to preserve tendon blood supply

Zone 1 repairs may demand a reinsertion technique (Mitek anchors)

Up to 60% tendon division will have greater strength with an epitendinous stitch alone than if a core stitch is inserted

Failure of proximal interphalangeal joint flexion when considering FDS injury of the little finger:

- 15% do not have FDS to little finger
- 15% have a non-functioning FDS to little finger
- some have adhesions between FDS to ring finger and little finger preventing independent movement

Linburg's sign:

- FPL action accompanied by flexion at the distal interphalangeal joint of the index
- due to adhesions between FPL and FDP index in the carpal tunnel

Effect of partial excisions of the A2 and A4 pulleys,

Tomaino. *J Hand Surg* 1998

Fresh cadaver study quantifying angular rotation and energy required for digital flexion

Venting may be performed without compromising pulley function up to:

- 25% A2 pulley (most reduction of angular rotation at the distal interphalangeal joint)
- 75% A4 pulley
- 25% of the A2 **and** 25% of the A4 pulleys (most reduction of angular rotation at the meta-carpophalangeal joint)
- decreases in angular rotation at the proximal interphalangeal joint were negligible
- but decreases in range of movement were small even where 50% of the A2 pulley was divided in combination with A4 venting

Venting pulleys facilitates repair in zones 1 and 2 and reduces tendon impingement on intact pulleys without significant functional sequelae

Quadriga syndrome

Results from tethering of the FDP tendon to an amputation stump

Active flexion deficit in uninjured fingers

Normal passive range of movement

Due to a failure of full excursion of the tethered tendon

Lumbrical plus

Opposite of quadriga

FDP tendon left too loose and acts via its lumbrical insertion

Metacarpophalangeal flexion and interphalangeal extension

Positive Bouviere's test

Flexor tendon grafting

Indications

- primary repair not possible (tendon loss)
- failed primary repair
- need good soft tissue cover

Tendon grafting in zone 2 – one stage

For example, tendon avulsion injury, good soft tissue cover, tendon sheath and pulleys preserved

Preparation

- leave 1 cm of FDP distally
- select best flexor (FDS or FDP) as motor
- resect FDP to level of lumbrical insertion
- trim FDS proximally (unless motor) but leave insertion

Graft options

- palmaris, plantaris
- toe extensors
- FDS
- extensor indicis and extensor digiti minimi
- tendon allografts

Technique

- insert distally before proximally, options:
  - into bone – Bunnell
  - to FDP stump
  - to pulp/nail bed – Pulvetaft
- insert proximally after consideration of appropriate tension by tenodesis effect:
  - Pulvetaft weave
  - Bunnell criss-cross
  - Kessler suture

Complications

- tendon adhesion
- rupture of graft
- lumbrical plus if tendon graft too long

Tendon grafting zone 2 – two-stage

Indications

- late tendon reconstruction
- fracture or overlying skin loss
- nerve injury requiring nerve grafting
- loss of pulley system
- perceived benefit over arthrodesis or amputation

Stage 1

- insertion of Hunter rod, fixed distally
- pulley reconstruction

Stage 2

- 6 months later
- remove rod
- harvest and insert tendon graft

Complications

- intra-operative – neurovascular injury
- early
  - synovitis, infection and buckling of implant
  - implant extrusion or migration
  - pulley breakdown
  - skin flap necrosis
- late
  - chronic flexion deformity
  - CRPS type 1

FDP tendon grafting in digits where FDS is intact

Sakellarides and Papadopoulos. *J Hand Surg* 1996

Tendon grafting an alternative to distal interphalangeal joint fusion or tenodesis of the distal part of the FDP (Bunnell) in children and young patients

Must have good quality volar skin

Divided FDP >6 weeks old

Need for active distal interphalangeal joint function

Plantaris and palmaris grafts

Index and middle finger – improved pinch

Middle finger and ring finger – improved power

FPL reconstruction

For example, Mannerfeldt lesion

One-stage tendon graft

Ring FDS transfer (RA)

Consider interphalangeal joint arthrodesis – usually do well

Repair proximal to zone 2

Interposition grafts

FDS transfer

End–side with profundus

A2 and A4 pulley reconstruction

Encircling graft of extensor retinaculum of wrist (Lister)

Encircling tendon graft (two-to-four wraps if possible)

Tail of superficialis

Principles of tendon transfer

Utilizes existing motor function, none created

Power is lost during transfer at least one MRC grade therefore choose muscle with 4–5/5

Full passive ROM is required before transfer

Active control at the wrist is paramount

Transferred tendons require free passage in vascularized tissue planes

Joints must be stable

All transfers slacken

Multiple transfers may be too complicated for the patient to make them work

Complete division of recipient tendon burns bridges but attachment in-continuity compromises mechanics – concept of reversibility (baby sitting transfers in-case re-innervation of paralysed muscles occurs)

Use tenodesis effect to get the tension right

Function aimed at but not achieved cannot be restored later

Restore function only to an area which is sensate

Power must be adequate but over-powerful transfers will deform the joint

Donor muscle should be independently innervated and not act in concert with other muscles (e.g. lumbricals)

Transfers should be within synergistic muscle groups – hand opening and hand closing muscles

Requires well-motivated patient likely to be compliant with post-operative hand therapy

Opponensplasty

Camitz transfer – palmaris with extension of palmar fascia

Huber – transfer of ADM (needs intact ulnar N), mainly children, avoid ulnar N compression

Bunnell – FDS ring finger transfer

EI transfer – Burkhalter

Tenolysis

Wait ~6 months

Difficult dissection, use Beaver blade

Must free ALL adhesions

Balloon 'angioplasty' technique to expand pulleys

Adcon gel may inhibit further adhesion formation

Early post-operative movement essential, brachial plexus block helps

Tenolysed tendon is weak and may rupture at up to 2 months post-operation, avoid resisted movement

Failed tenolysis: consider two-stage tendon grafting, arthrodesis or amputation

Extensor tendon tenolysis usually easier but may need to plan for elective skin cover

> **Self-assessment: A patient is referred whom the casualty officer feels has an injury to his flexor tendon. How would you manage him?**

History
- age
- occupation (very important – complex reconstruction vs. pragmatic lesser option?)
- hobbies
- hand dominance
- state of hands before the injury – may already have had a hand problem
- mechanism of injury – laceration, crush, avulsion, etc.
- time of injury (if long-standing may need two-stage reconstruction)
- general questions relating to factors relevant to fitness for surgery and wound healing (drugs, PMSH including diabetes, smoker, etc.)
- tetanus status

Examination
- full hand examination
  - look – perfusion, old scars, swellings, sudomotor changes, wasting, hand arcade, identify zone of injury
  - feel – sensation especially distal to the injury, feel for tender mass in the palm – Leddy and Packer classification type I (both vinculae ruptured)
  - move – passive and active movement distal to the injury plus full neurological examination of the three nerves

Investigation – AP and lateral films – fractures, foreign bodies

Treatment
- anaesthesia – BPB or GA
- markings – Brunner extensions to the wound
- flexor tendon repair
  - 4/0 ticron Kessler core stitch plus 5/0 prolene epitendinous suture (even in zone 3 as epitendinous stitch adds 20% to the repair)
  - if <50–60% divided just epitendinous and protect as per flexor protocol post-operation
  - zone 1 FDP may need reinsertion technique over nail
  - tendon **loss** – consider primary graft or insertion of a Hunter rod but must have good quality soft tissue cover or be able to provide it
- post-operative protocol

- splint with wrist in neutral, metacarpophalangeals flexed to 90°, interphalangeals extended with a dorsal slab and no resisted flexion
- Belfast protocol of controlled active movement for 6 weeks under the supervision of the physiotherapists
- antibiotics of debatable value

Suppose that this is a late presentation and there is tendon loss – what are the surgical options?

Depends upon whether the FDS is intact, which digit is involved, patient factors (occupation, compliance, etc.)

Thumb with FPL loss:

- arthrodese the interphalangeal joint
- reconstruct FPL with a two-stage tendon graft
- transfer FDS from the ring finger

Digit with loss of both FDS and FDP – two-stage FDP graft – Pulvetaft insertion and Pulvetaft weave

Digit with FDS intact:

- most patients benefit from distal interphalangeal joint arthrodesis
- could consider FDP reconstruction or tenodesis of a long distal end to FDS

Zone 3 injury:

- interpositional graft
- tendonese to adjacent FDP
- FDS transfer

But all transfers/reconstruction must satisfy the following:

- full range of passive movement
- stable joints
- hospitable tissue planes
- sensation
- patient compliance

Extensor tendons

Verdan's Zones

Odd numbers overlie joints starting at zone 1 – distal interphalangeal joint
Even numbers overlie intervening segments finishing at zone 8 – distal forearm

General principles

Interrupted over–over sutures in zones 1–6
Prolene/ticron
Kessler suture as above zones 7 and 8
Tendon loss: graft if adequate skin cover or reconstruction with a distally based tendon flap
Central slip rupture/loss: reconstruct with medial portions of lateral bands
Repair sagittal band injuries in zone 4/5 or tendon will sublux into metacarpal gutter on intact side
Management of mallet – below
Gutter splint injuries in zones 2–4
Outrigger for zone 5–8 injuries plus night gutter splint

Mallet finger

Open or closed

Forced flexion of the extended digit

?Zone of relatively poor vascularity at the site of mallet ruptures

Most common type is type 1

Proximal interphalangeal joint is of utmost importance – keep active to avoid a Boutonnière deformity

Green classification

Type 1 – closed, with or without small avulsion fracture

Type 2 – open

Type 3 – open, loss of tendon substance

Type 4

- A – transepiphyseal plate fracture
- B – fracture involving 20–50% of articular surface (hyper**flexion**)
- C – hyper**extension** injury >50% of articular surface, volar subluxation

Management

Type 1

- Stack splint 6 weeks
- occupational need for early return to work or poor patient compliance – consider buried K-wire

Type 2

- suture of tendon and skin either separately or together (tenodermodesis)
- stack splint 6 weeks

Type 3

- primary tendon reconstruction (distally based EC flap) plus oblique K-wire to distal interphalangeal joint
- secondary extensor reconstruction

Type 4

- A – manipulation under anaesthetic plus Stack splint 4 weeks
- B–C – open reduction and K-wiring of distal interphalangeal joint, maintaining reduction with pull-out suture over button on pulp; miniscrew fixation
- some loss of active flexion in operated patients

Operative treatment of a mallet injury may downgrade flexion so treat conservatively if possible

Other options

Arthrodesis – comminuted intra-articular fracture, elderly

Amputation – severe soft tissue injury, devascularization

Extensor tendon: anatomy, injury, and reconstruction

Rockwell. *Plastic Reconstruc Surg* 2000

The anatomy and function of the extensor mechanism of the hand are more intricate and complex than those of the flexor system

The extensor apparatus is a linkage system created by

- radial nerve-innervated extrinsic system

- ulnar nerve and median nerve-innervated intrinsic system
- these interconnecting components can compensate for certain deficits in function

Extrinsic tendons

- the muscle bellies of the extrinsic extensors arise in the forearm and enter the hand through six compartments formed by the extensor retinaculum, a fibrous band that prevents bowstringing of the tendons
- at the wrist, tendons are covered by a synovial sheath, but not over the dorsal hand or fingers
- the extensor pollicis brevis, abductor pollicis longus, extensor pollicis longus extensor digitorum communis (EDC), extensor indicis proprius, and extensor digiti minimi have independent origins and functions
  - the extensor indicis proprius and extensor digiti minimi are usually ulnar and deep to the extensor digitorum communis at the level of the MCPJ
  - the extensor digitorum communis to the little finger is present less than 50% of the time
    - when absent, it is almost always replaced by a juncturae tendinae from the ring finger to the extensor apparatus of the little finger.
  - the four EDC tendons originate from a common muscle belly and have limited independent action
  - the extensor indicis proprius and extensor digiti minimi have independent muscle bellies and are common donor tendons for transfer
- at the wrist, the extensor tendons are more round and have sufficient bulk to hold a suture. Over the dorsum of the hand, they are thin and flat with longitudinal fibres that do not hold suture well
- The extrinsic extensor tendons have four insertions
  - the metacarpophalangeal joint palmar plate through the saggital bands
  - a tenuous insertion on the proximal phalanx
  - strong insertions on the middle and distal phalanges
  - at the metacarpophalangeal joint level, the extensor tendons are held in place by the intrinsic tendons and the sagittal band that arises from the palmar plate and the deep intermetacarpal ligament
- The extrinsic extensor tendons extend
  - the metacarpophalangeal joint primarily
  - the interphalangeal joints secondarily
  - contribute the central slip to the extensor mechanism in the finger
- The intrinsic tendons are composed of
  - four dorsal interossei (abductors)
  - three palmar interossei (adductors)
  - and four lumbrical muscles

The interossei

- originate from the lateral sides of the metacarpals
- run distally on both sides of the fingers except the ulnar side of the little finger
- the tendons enter the finger dorsal to the intermetacarpal ligament

The lumbricals

- arise from the radial side of the flexor digitorum profundus tendon
- pass palmar to the intermetacarpal ligament
- the tendons of these intrinsic muscles join to form the lateral bands, all passing palmar to the axis of the metacarpophalangeal joint

- the lateral bands join the extrinsic extensor mechanism proximal to the midportion of the proximal phalanx and continue to the distal finger dorsal to the axis of the proximal interphalangeal and distal interphalangeal joints

The intrinsic muscles

- flex the metacarpophalangeal joint
- extend the proximal and distal interphalangeal joints
- the intrinsic system contributes the lateral bands that pass palmar to the axis of the MPJ
- and dorsal to the axis at the PIPJ and DIPJ

The sagittal band

- centralizes the extensor tendon over the metacarpal head at the MCPJ

The intermetacarpal ligament

- separates the lumbrical tendon that is palmar from the interossei tendons that are dorsal

The transverse retinacular ligament

- stabilizes the extensor tendon at the PIPJ

The oblique retinacular ligament

- is a component of the linkage system
- passes palmar to the rotational axis of the PIPJ
- passes dorsal to the joint axis at the DIPJ

The triangular ligament

- helps maintain close proximity of the lateral bands over the middle phalanx

The extensor tendon has four insertions

- on the metacarpophalangeal palmar plate through the sagittal band
- the tendon then inserts on the base of the proximal, middle and distal phalanges
- over the distal portion of the proximal phalanx, the central slip trifurcates as the central slip and lateral bands share fibres
  - the central slip inserts on the base of the middle phalanx
  - the lateral band component continues to insert on the base of the distal phalanx
- at the midportion of the proximal phalanx, the central slip of the extensor mechanism trifurcates.
  - distal to this level, there is an exchange of fibres from the central slip to the lateral bands and from the lateral bands to the central slip
  - the central slip primarily attaches to the base of the middle phalanx
  - both components are capable of proximal and distal interphalangeal extension
- at the proximal interphalangeal joint, the transverse retinacular ligament maintains the position of the extensor mechanism and creates limits on its dorsal–palmar excursion

The oblique retinacular ligament

- arises proximally from the middle third of the proximal phalanx and the A2 pulley and inserts into the lateral portion of the extensor tendon along the middle phalanx
- coursing palmar to the proximal interphalangeal joint, it helps stabilize the lateral bands
  - Its previously described role of mechanically linking simultaneous PIPJ and DIPJ extension has been discounted

The triangular ligament

- connects the lateral bands over the dorsum of the middle phalanx, maintaining them in close proximity

Excursion of the extensor tendons over the finger is less when compared with the flexor tendons

- at the proximal interphalangeal joint, excursion may vary from 2 to 8 mm
- preservation of relative tendon length between the central slip and lateral bands is important
- disturbance causes deformities that are progressive, and restoration of normal balance is difficult
- overlapping linkage systems also contribute to this balance
- the components of the linkage system pass palmar to one joint and dorsal to the next
  - the intrinsic tendons create the linkage at the MCPJ and PIPJ
  - the oblique retinacular ligaments function at the PIPJ and DIPJ
- deformity at one joint may cause a reciprocal deformity at an adjacent joint

The extensor mechanism of the thumb is different from that of the fingers

- each joint has an independent tendon for extension
- the extensor pollicis longus extends the interphalangeal joint
- the extensor pollicis brevis extends the MCPJ
- abductor pollicis longus extends the carpometacarpal joint
- the abductor pollicis longus almost always has multiple tendon slips, whereas extensor pollicis brevis usually has one

The intrinsic muscles of the thumb primarily provide rotational control

- contribute to MCPJ flexion and IPJ extension
- on the radial side, the abductor pollicis brevis tendon continues to insert on the extensor pollicis longus
- on the ulnar side, fibers of the adductor pollicis also insert on the extensor pollicis longus
  - these two muscles can extend the interphalangeal joint to neutral, significantly masking an extensor pollicis longus laceration

Zone 1 Injury (mallet finger)

- disruption of continuity of the extensor tendon over the distal interphalangeal joint
- when left untreated for a prolonged time, hyperextension of the proximal interphalangeal joint (swan-neck deformity) may develop because of proximal retraction of the central band
- mallet finger injuries are classified into four types:
  - Type I: closed, with or without avulsion fracture
  - Type II: laceration at or proximal to the distal interphalangeal joint with loss of tendon continuity
  - Type III: deep abrasion with loss of skin, subcutaneous cover and tendon substance
  - Type IV:
    - (A) transepiphyseal plate fracture in children
    - (B) hyperflexion injury with fracture of the articular surface of 20 to 50%
    - (C) hyperextension injury with fracture of the articular surface usually greater than 50 per cent and with early or late palmar subluxation of the distal phalanx
- The management of mallet finger is still a topic for debate. In the vast
majority of cases, splinting alone is sufficient
- Type I injuries: continuous splinting of the distal interphalangeal joint in extension for 6 weeks, followed by 2 weeks of night splinting
  - Alternatively, and only in rare circumstances, Kirschner wire fixation of the distal interphalangeal joint in extension
- Type II injures: repaired with a simple figure-of-eight suture through the tendon alone or a roll-type suture (dermatotenodesis) incorporating the tendon and skin in the same suture. DIPJ splinted in extension for 6 weeks

- Type III injuries with loss of tendon substance require immediate soft-tissue coverage and primary grafting or late reconstruction using a free tendon graft
- Type IV-A is usually a transepiphyseal fracture of the phalanx; the extensor mechanism is attached to the basal epiphysis, so closed reduction results in correction of the deformity

Zone 2 injury (middle phalanx)

- if less than 50% of the tendon width is cut, the treatment involves routine wound care and splinting for 7 to 10 days, followed by active motion
- injuries involving more than 50% of the tendon should be repaired primarily

Zone 3 injury (boutonnière deformity)

- the boutonnière deformity is caused by disruption of the central slip at the proximal inter-phalangeal joint
- this results in loss of extension at the proximal interphalangeal joint and hyperextension at the distal interphalangeal joint
- the injury can be closed or open, and the central slip may avulse with or without a bony fragment
- usually appears 10 to 14 days after the initial injury, especially after closed rupture
- initial treatment for closed injury should be splinting of the proximal interphalangeal joint in extension
- surgical indications for closed boutonnière deformity are:
  - displaced avulsion fracture at the base of the middle phalanx
  - axial and lateral instability of the proximal interphalangeal joint associated with loss of active or passive extension of the joint
  - failed non-operative treatment

Zone 4 injuries

- usually involve the broad extensor mechanism, are usually partial, and usually spare the lateral bands
- splinting the proximal IPJ in extension for 3 to 4 weeks without repair is equivalent to repair for partial injuries
- for complete lacerations, primary repair should be performed

Zone 5 injury (metacarpophalangeal joint)

- injuries over the metacarpophalangeal joint are almost always open and human bite should be considered
- the injury more often occurs with the joint in flexion, so the tendon injury will be proximal to the level of the overlying wound
- primary tendon repair is indicated after thorough irrigation
- all involved structures should be repaired separately, including partial injuries
- early dynamic splinting has also improved outcome

Zone 6 injuries (dorsum of hand)

- may be masked by adjacent extensor tendons through the juncturae tendinae
- diagnosis made at exploration
- tendons are thicker and more oval so repair should be performed with stronger, core-type sutures

Zone 7 injuries (wrist)

- controversy exists whether excision of part of the retinaculum over the injury site is necessary to prevent post-operative adhesions
  - partial release of the retinaculum is required in most cases to gain exposure to the lacerated tendons, which retract significantly in this area

- some portion of the retinaculum should be preserved to prevent extensor bowstringing
- if early dynamic splinting is used, adhesions are less likely

Zone 8 injuries (forearm)

- multiple tendons may be injured in this area, making it difficult to identify individual tendons
- difficulty also may be encountered with injuries at the musculo-tendinous junction because the fibrous septa retract into the substance of the muscles

Thumb injuries

- terminal extensor tendon is much thicker therefore, mallet thumbs are rare
- in zones 6 and 7, the abductor pollicis longus retracts significantly when divided and usually requires that the first compartment be released for successful repair

Dynamic splinting for extensor injuries

- early controlled motion with a dynamic extensor splint has been found to decrease adhesions and subsequent contractures especially with more proximal injuries

Replantation and ring avulsion

Absolute contraindications

Head/thoraco-abdominal life-threatening injuries
Multilevel injury, widespread crush or degloving
Severe chronic illness

Relative contraindications

Single digit amputation
Avulsion of tendons, nerves and vessels
Extreme contamination
Lengthy warm ischaemia (especially macro-replants)
Elderly with micro-arterial disease
Unwilling, uncooperative or psychotic patient

Indications

Amputated thumb
Children
Multiple digits
Partial or whole hand

General principles

Resuscitate patient and exclude concomitant life-threatening injury
Keep amputated part wrapped in moist saline gauze in a polythene bag on ice
Radiographs of hand and amputated part(s)
Consent for vein, tendon and skin grafts and terminalization
Prepare amputated parts while patient is being anaesthetized, tagging Ns and vessels
Shorten the bone
Arthrodesis first
Repair extensor then flexor tendons
Digital As then dorsal vein (opens up) and Ns
Achieve good skin cover

Keep patient warm, well filled, pain free (BPB)

Elevate to 45°

White finger post-replantation:

- ensure patient is warm, well filled and pain free (prevent spasm and hypoperfusion)
- loosen dressings
- remove sutures
- re-explore

Blue finger post-replantation:

- elevate limb
- loosen dressings (venous tourniquet)
- remove sutures
- leeches
- fish mouth incision in nail bed
- heparin injections
- re-explore

Major limb replantation

Beware reperfusion injury – monitor for hyperkalaemia and myoglobinuria

Fasciotomy

Contraindicated by lengthy ischaemia time (>6 h)

Thumb reconstruction

Options:

- pollicization – mandatory if the basal carpometacarpal joint is lost
- osteoplastic reconstruction – bone graft plus neurosensory island flap
- toe–hand transfer

All metacarpal present → great toe transfer

Some metacarpal present → second toe transfer (can sacrifice metatarsal from the second toe but not from the first or will get gait disturbance)

Alternatively, replant an amputated finger on to the thumb metacarpal

> **Self-assessment: A patient arrives in casualty having cut off his thumb. What is your management?**

History

- age, occupation, hand dominance, hobbies
- pre-existing hand problems
- ischaemia time and mechanism of injury
- how the digit has been stored (ideally in a damp gauze within a plastic bag on ice)
- general health including drugs, past history, and **is the patient a smoker**?
- **tetanus** status

Examination

- amputated part:
  - level of injury
  - degree of crush/avulsion
  - skin quality
- full hand examination to identify other pathologies, e.g. crush higher up at the wrist level, etc.

Investigations – X-rays of the hand and the amputated part

Discussion

- wishes of patient for replant in view of need to return to work, complications, etc. (below)
- **absolute contraindications to replant**
  - life-threatening concomitant trauma
  - severe premorbid disease
  - severe injury to the digit – multilevel trauma, gross contamination, extensive degloving
- **relative contraindications to replant**
  - avulsion
  - lengthy warm ischaemia time
  - self-harm/psychosis
  - single finger
- **indications**
  - thumb replant
  - child
  - multiple digits or full hand

Surgery

- general anaesthesia, tourniquet, two surgeons
- dissect neurovascular bundles on amputated part and hand – tag structures
- shorten the bone and osteosynthesis
- repair extensors then flexors
- repair digital arteries and re-establish flow
- dorsal veins then open up to repair
- repair nerves
- close skin

Post-operative

- keep patient warm, well filled and pain free
- antibiotics
- elevation to 45°
- splint in a position of function
- monitor perfusion of replant

Complications:

- intra-operative – technically impossible
- early post-operative – replant loss, infection
- late post-operative – CRPS type 1, pain, stiffness, TICAS

If thumb replantation is impossible:

- toe–hand transfer (metacarpal preserved use first toe, if not preserved use second toe)
- pollicization of remaining digit

Ring avulsion

Urbaniak classification

I – Circulation adequate, circumferential laceration

II – Microvascular repair required:
- A – digital arteries only
- B – arteries plus tendon or bone
- C – digital veins only

III – Complete degloving of skin

Type III injuries are unlikely to regain adequate function and amputation is usually recommended

Ray amputation

Indication
Secondary surgery following trauma, including failed replantation

Tumours

Infections

Congenital hand reconstruction

Technique
Index finger – subperiosteal dissection of metacarpal, osteotomize at level of metacarpal flare, transpose digital nerves into interosseus space

Middle finger – two main techniques:

- **Carroll** – transposition of the index metacarpal to the base of the middle metacarpal
- alternatively suture together the intervolar plate ligaments between ring and index finger metacarpophalangeal joints (± closing wedge excision of the capitate)

Ring finger

- shares articulation to the hamate with the little finger, allowing this to slide radially after division of the carpometacarpal ligaments
- can also transpose to base of ring metacarpal as above

Little finger – preserve metacarpal base – site of insertion of FCU and ECU tendons

Digital arteries

Dominant supply:

- ulnar digital artery – thumb, index, middle finger (radial digits)
- radial digital artery – ring finger, little finger (ulnar digits)

Radial A → deep palmar arch → 1 cm proximal to the superficial arch and beneath the flexors

Ulnar A → superficial palmar arch → distal (digital vessels) and above the flexors

Also have anastomoses over the dorsal carpal arch

All digital arteries are branches of the superficial palmar arch

Artery grafts

Long revascularizations (e.g. thumb replants are best revascularized by grafts to the radial artery)

When there is a significant discrepancy between the size of proximal and distal ends

Artery grafts are harvested from the posterior interosseus or subscapular vessels

Replantation

Pederson. *Plastic Reconstruc Surg* 2001

Replantation of parts offers a result that is usually superior to any other type of reconstruction

- first successful replantation of a severed limb undertaken ~40 years ago by Malt in Boston (replanted the arm of a 12-year-old boy)
- Revascularization of incompletely severed digits by Kleinert and Kasdan in 1965
- first successful digital replantation performed by Komatsu and Tamai in Japan, in 1968

Indications

- consider status of the amputated part (sharp amputation vs. crush) and the patient (healthy vs. systemic illnesses)
- assess potential for long-term function
  - thumb replantation probably offers the best functional return
  - even with poor motion and sensation, the thumb is useful to the patient as a post for opposition
- Replantation distal to the level of the FDP tendon insertion (zone I) usually results in good function
- Multiple finger amputations present reconstructive difficulties that may be difficult to correct without replantation of one or all of the amputated digits
- Any hand amputation offers the chance of reasonable function after replantation, usually superior to available prostheses
- Although usually indicated, the replantation of any hand or arm proximal to the level of the mid-forearm must be carefully considered
- The risk of complications increases and the chance of functional return decreases with amputations above the elbow
- Replantation should be attempted with almost any part in a child including replantation and revascularization of the foot or lower leg

Contraindications

- Single-finger replantations at the level of zone II (from the A1 pulley to the distal sublimis tendon insertion) are rarely indicated, with the notable exception of the thumb
- Amputated parts that are severely crushed and those with multiple-level injuries
- Parts of fingers that have been completely degloved
- Very distal amputations at the level of the nail bed are marginally indicated, as there needs to be approximately 4 mm of intact skin proximal to the nail fold for adequate veins to be present
- Patients with:
  - severe systemic disease or trauma
  - severe mental disease
  - intractable substance abuse

Technical points

- Patient should be stabilized
- amputated part should be gently cleansed and wrapped in a moist gauze sponge, placed in a container (either sterile bag or specimen cup), and then placed in ice
- The warm ischaemic tolerance of digits is in the range of 8 hours
  - Replantation has been reported after cold ischaemia times of up to 40 hours
  - In more proximal amputations, the ischaemic tolerance is significantly shorter due to sensitivity of muscle to ischaemia
  - The absolute maximum warm ischaemic tolerance for major amputations is in the range of 4 to 6 hours, and this may be prolonged by cooling to the 10- to 12-hour range
- Examination of the part in the operating room before the patient is under anesthetic allows time for appropriate decision making
  - Vessels must be examined under the microscope
  - A corkscrew appearance of the arteries suggests that an avulsion force has been applied to them, and this segment of vessel should be excised and vein grafted

- Bruising along the course of the digit where the neurovascular bundle runs suggests a severe avulsion injury with disruption of branches of the digital artery and replantation may be unsuccessful
- There should be brisk bleeding from the veins after the digit is warmed up
- select the two veins that are bleeding the most for venous anastomosis
- The bone should be debrided minimally with a curette and managed as an open fracture
  - Distal fixation can be placed in the amputated part
  - Kirschner wires, interosseous wires or plate fixation can be used
- Tendons are repaired in standard manner
  - Where the digit has been avulsed with attached tendon the carpal tunnel should be decompressed
- If there is concerned about ischemia, then arterial repair takes precedence over nerves
- Nerve gaps should be grafted in most digital replants
- If there is volar skin loss and coverage of the neurovascular repairs will be a problem, some skin overlying the vein graft may be taken with the vein graft, and this unit used as a small flow-through venous flap
- Care must be taken to avoid compression of the veins by skin closure

Post-operative care
- Axillary infusion of marcaine may be given to provide both pain relief and a chemical sympathectomy
- systemic heparinization is widely used in replantation but it is difficult to prove its efficacy
- Chlorpromazine orally (25 mg 8 hourly) is a potent peripheral vasodilator and sedative
- Aspirin 325 mg daily useful for its anti-platelet effect (given for 3 weeks)

Fractures and dislocations

Unstable fracture – cannot be reduced closed or cannot be held reduced without fixation
Antibiotics – 30% infection rate in open DP fractures without antibiotics but 3% infection rate if treatment with antibiotics; Sloan, *Br J Hand Surg* 1987
A DP fracture underlying a subungal haematoma should be considered to be open
Healing time 4 (phalangeal fractures)–6 (metacarpal fractures) weeks
Radiological healing lags behind clinical healing

Acceptable hand fractures
Tuft of distal phalanx
AP displacement of metaphyseal fractures in children
Metacarpal neck fractures
- <15° angulation in middle finger and ring finger
- <50° angulation in index and little finger
Metacarpal base fractures
- <20° in adults
- <40° in children

Unacceptable phalangeal fractures
Rotational angulation
Severe dorsal angulation

Lateral angulation

Finger scissoring

Phalangeal fractures

Epiphyseal injuries

Salter classification:

I – Shearing through the growth plate

II – Epiphysis and growth plate separate from the metaphysis, small metaphyseal fragment attached

III – Intra-articular fracture of the epiphysis, growth plate undisturbed

IV – Fracture passes through epiphysis, growth plate and metaphysis

V – Growth plate crushed

80% of Salter–Harris fractures are type II

Indications for fixation of non-articular fractures

Angulation (except modest AP angulation in children)

Rotation

Shortening

Techniques

Lag screw fixation – spiral fractures

Screw plus miniplate (generally only metacarpal fractures)

Crossed K-wiring

Interosseus wiring/Lister loop

Bone tie (Sammut)

External fixation (S-QUATTRO) – comminuted open/closed fractures

Free and island vascularized joint transfers

Foucher. *J Hand Surg* 1994

Options for stiff and arthritic proximal interphalangeal joint:

- arthrodesis
- silicone joint replacement (reversed Swanson's)
- Skoog perichondrial arthroplasty
- non-vascularized joint transfers (in young children)

Islanded vascularized joint transfers:

- heterodigital
  - includes collateral ligaments, volar plate, extensor tendon and vascular pedicle
  - proximal interphalangeal joint from a non-functioning finger
  - distal interphalangeal joint from a non-functioning finger
- homodigital
  - islanded distal interphalangeal joint transfer (distal interphalangeal joint contributes 15° to the flexion arc whereas the proximal interphalangeal joint contributes 85°)
  - complex trauma to the proximal interphalangeal joint
  - distal interphalangeal arthrodesis
  - reinsert FDP

Free vascularized joint transfer:

- joints harvested from a non-replantable finger

- harvest of skin island and extensor tendon along with the joint
- free vascularized toe joint transfer from the second toe

Thumb fractures

Bennett's fracture
Oblique fracture of the base of the first metacarpal in the dorso-volar axis
Due to traction on the abductor pollicis longus tendon
Metacarpal base is subluxed dorsally
Anterior fragment of bone attached to ulnar collateral ligament and volar plate
Optimally treatment by screw fixation

Reversed Bennett's fracture
Same as Bennett's except occurring in the fifth metacarpal base
Due to traction on the extensor carpi ulnaris tendon
Motor branch of ulnar nerve may be injured

Rolando fracture
Same as Bennett's except that the dorsal, avulsed segment has a 'T-condylar' fracture

Metacarpal fractures
Percutaneous K-wires in parallel splinting to adjacent metacarpal ×2 intramedullary K-wires (neck fractures)
Miniplate fixation via dorsal approach

Dislocations
Open or closed
Simple (reduce easily) or complex (will not reduce due to soft tissue interposition)
In general
- complex dislocations more common in 'border' digits – thumb, index and little
- volar plate interposition between metacarpal head and base of PP
- thumb volar plate sesamoids (if present) seen separating the metacarpal and PP on X-ray
- if closed and stable begin movement as pain allows with buddy strap
Distal interphalangeal joint dislocations – usually easily reduced by longitudinal traction
Proximal interphalangeal joint dislocations
- commonly result in flexion contracture
- permanent fusiform enlargement of the joint
- mainly dorsal dislocation – volar dislocation is rare and due to central slip avulsion (need K-wire for 6 weeks to allow central slip healing)
- simple, closed dorsal dislocations (volar plate avulsion ± small volar fragment) may be treated conservatively (mobilize plus extension-block splint)
- complex dislocations require open reduction and volar plate removal and repair
Gamekeeper's thumb
- tear of the ulnar collateral ligament of the metacarpophalangeal joint
- hyperextension injury
- volar plate disruption
- **Stener lesion** – torn UCL lies superficial to the adductor expansion
- reattach ligament using an interosseus wire, suture or Mitec bone anchor

- K-wire the metacarpophalangeal joint (6 weeks)
- repair – UCL, accessory ligament, volar plate and dorsal capsule – all of these lend stability to the joint
- bony Gamekeeper's thumb may be treated conservatively if the fracture fragment involves <15–20% of the articular surface

Wrist fractures and dislocations

Wrist instability

Tearing or stretching of ligaments of the carpus

Terry Thomas sign – increased gap between scaphoid and lunate

An increase in the scapholunate angle beyond 60°

In assessing carpal height radiographically, the ratio of the distance between distal capitate and proximal lunate to the length of the third metacarpal should be 0.54 ± 0.03

Carpal ligaments

Radius and carpus rotate around the free ulna

Two types:

- interosseus
  - between adjacent bones
  - connect all four carpal bones of the distal row
  - individual carpal bones to forearm bones, e.g. **radioscapholunate ligament of Testut**
- transosseus
  - between non-adjacent bones
  - radioscaphocapitate (sling ligament)
  - radiolunate (short and long)
  - triquetrohamatocapitate

Wrist instability around the scaphoid and ligamentous laxity between proximal and distal carpal rows can be classified as dorsal or volar intercollated segment instability (VISI,DISI) and tested for by palpating the scaphoid as the wrist is put into radial and ulnar deviation

Anterior (volar) dislocation of the lunate

Signifies dorsal radiocarpal ligament failure

A cause of acute CTS

Dorsal dislocations are rare

Radiological signs

Lunate appears triangular on the AP view

Capitate does not sit in the cup of the lunate on the lateral film

In cases of perilunate dislocation, the lunate remains appropriately positioned on the radius while the rest of the carpus is displaced

Kienbock's disease

(see also Kienbock's disease. Almquist. *Clin Orth Rel Res* 1986)

Aetiology

- Avascular necrosis of the dorsal pole of the lunate (lunatomalacia) with collapse
- May be due to a primary vascular insufficiency or secondary to trauma
  - >50% have a history of wrist trauma
- Strong association with ulnar minus variant (short ulna)
  - present in 23% of normal wrists

- present in 78% of Kienbock's wrists
- ulnar minus variant subjects lunate to greater shear stress forces compromising its volar blood supply
- Fault plate hypothesis (Watson. *J Hand Surgery* – Br Vol, 1997)
  - Extrinsic factors
    - Lunate loading due to differential radii of curvature of lunate and capitate
  - Intrinsic factors
    - Cortical strength of lunate
    - Trabecular pattern
    - Vascular anatomy

Clinical features

- Male: female 4:1
- Painful, stiff, swollen wrist in young active adults
- Decreased grip strength
- Variable symptomatology and rate of progression
- Usually unilateral in the dominant wrist
- Manual workers, repetetive tasks

Investigations

- Plain radiographs
  - Radiological features
    - radiolucent line indicating compression fracture
    - demineralization surrounding a fracture line (<3 months)
    - sclerosis of the dorsal pole (~3 months)
    - fragmentation and flattening
    - wrist arthrosis
  - Lichtman staging
    1 Positive bone scan, X-ray normal – immobilization
    2 Sclerotic changes on X-ray – radial shortening to restore neutral ulnar variance
    3 Lunate collapse on X-ray (a) no scaphoid rotation (b) with scaphoid rotation – shorten radius, lunate resection, fill with tendon or capito-hamate fusion to prevent capitate subluxing into proximal carpal row in the absence of the lunate (Treatment of Kienbock's disease with capitohamate arthrodesis. Oishi. *PRS* 2002)
    4 Carpal arthritis – proximal row carpectomy or wrist fusion
  - May also see shortening of the lunate and proximal migration of the capitate
- Bone scan
- MRI
- CT (shows occult fractures)

Treatment aims:

- Prevention of deformity and restoration of normal appearance and function

Treatment options:

- splintage and analgesia (rarely effective even in the early stages)
- joint levelling procedure
  - radial shortening or ulnar lengthening
- intercarpal arthrodesis
  - scaphoid–trapezium–trapezoid fusion with excision of the radial styloid
  - scaphoid capitate fusion
  - capitate shortening and capitate–hammate intercarpal fusion

- revascularization procedures
  - pronator quadratus turnover flap
  - pedicled dorsal metacarpal artery buried in lunate
- salvage procedures
  - proximal row carpectomy
  - wrist arthrodesis
  - wrist dennervation
  - excision of the lunate and replacement with a sialastic implant, rolled tendon graft or vascularized pisiform (Saffar, 1982)

Ulnar variance

A horizontal line is drawn from the junction of the distal articular surface and sigmoid notch of the radius:

- positive variance (ulnar head above this line) – ulnar impingement syndrome
- negative variance (ulnar head below this line) – **Kienbock's disease**, SL dislocation
- neutral (ulnar head level) – normal

Scaphoid fractures

Avascular necrosis of the proximal pole

Fracture line becomes an extension of the mid-carpal joint

Movement at this mid-carpal joint promotes flexion of the distal row and extension of the proximal row, hence a loss of wrist extension

Scaphoid adopts a flexed attitude – humpback deformity

Sequence of arthritic changes in the radioscaphoid and capitolunate joints, leading to **scapholunate advanced collapse** (SLAC wrist), rotatory subluxation of the scaphoid and a decrease in the Huber index on the X-ray

Treatment

No displacement	– immobilization in a scaphoid plaster
Displacement	– open reduction and internal fixation (Herbert screw) – cancellous bone graft from radius to correct humpback deformity
Non-union without AVN	– Non vascular bone graft (Matte–Rewse)
Avascular necrosis	– Vascularized bone graft – Kuhlman procedure with bone flap from beneath PQ on a branch from radial artery excision and rolled tendon graft 4 corner fusion (Lunate to capitate to hamate to triquatral to lunate wrist arthrodesis

Arthritis

- radial styloid excision
- radioscaphoid fusion
- proximal row carpectomy
- total wrist arthrodesis (SLAC wrist)

The scaphoid is the most commonly fractured wrist bone

- avascular necrosis of the proximal pole heralded by radiological sclerosis
- scaphoid view – ulnar deviated PA
- fracture visible after 10–14 days or earlier by CT or MRI
- stable fractures managed conservatively – includes vast majority of paediatric fractures

- unstable fractures (displacement and angulation) and very proximal fractures (risk AVN) →
  open reduction and internal fixation

Primary avascular necrosis of the scaphoid: **Preiser's disease**

Hammate fracture
Open reduction and internal fixation or excise

Carpal collapse
SL ligament repair, Blatt capsulodesis

Surgical treatment of scapholunate advanced collapse
Krakauer. *J Hand Surg* 1994

Scapholunate dissociation leads to dorsiflexion intercalated segment instability (DISI),
shifting stress forces to the radioscaphoid articulation

Most cases of SLAC wrist due to scapholunate dissociation but may be caused by other
aetiologies including rheumatoid

SLAC wrist is the most common pattern of degenerative arthritis found in the wrist

Sequential degeneration of the radial styloid (stage 1), the entire scaphoid fossa of the radius
(stage 2) and the capitolunate joint (stage 3)

May have minimal symptoms

Surgical options:

- scaphoid excision and silicone implant
- scaphoid excision and intercarpal arthrodesis – capitate, lunate, triquetrum, hamate
- proximal row carpectomy
- radiocarpal arthrodesis
- total wrist arthrodesis

Non-union
Gap too large

Avascularity and infection

Soft tissue interposition

Dead bone interposition

Poor internal fixation holding ends in distraction

Excessive interfragmentary movement

Adverse systemic factors (anaemia, steroids, malnutrition, etc.)

Wrist: other points
20% of the longitudinal force applied to the wrist is transmitted through the ulnocarpal
articulation, 80% through the radiocarpal joint – positive ulnar variance increases load
through the ulna

In full supination the radius and ulna lie parallel but in full pronation they are crossed and the
radius projects less distally – hence when assessing variance the forearm must be in mid-
pronation:

- hand and wrist flat on the X-ray cassette
- shoulder abducted to 90° and elbow flexed to 90°

All axes of wrist movement pass through the capitate

Two-thirds of wrist flexion occurs at the radiocarpal joint, one-third at the mid-carpal joint

Insertion of the FCU tendon to the pisiform is the only direct insertion of extrinsic tendons to the carpus

Radiocarpal ligament connects the radius to the triquetral via the lunate

Wrist arthroscopy may be of diagnostic and therapeutic benefit to patients with wrist pathology

AP draw test – traction applied to the wrist and anteroposterior forces exerted at the mid-carpal level to test mid-carpal stability

Pivot shift test

- supinate the hand
- with a thumb behind the ulnar side of the wrist volarly sublux the ulnar carpus and move the hand from radial to ulnar deviation
- during this manoeuvre the capitate will sublux volarly if there is excessive ligamentous laxity

Examine the wrist

Look

- skin changes – scars, RSD skin changes
- generalized swelling including synovium
- masses – ganglia, prominent ulnar head, carpometacarpal boss
- position of the wrist, e.g. ulnar deviation

Feel

- masses
- areas of tenderness

Move

- flexion/extension
- supination/pronation
- radial and ulnar deviation
- AP draw test
- pivot shift test
- rotatory subluxation of the scaphoid

Scapholunate diastasis

Ligamentous laxity due to:

- OA
- RA
- AVN of the scaphoid post-number
- AVN of the lunate (Kienbock's)
- Presier's disease

Clinical signs

- RSS
- DISI – (VISI is due to lunotriquetral ligament disruption)

X-ray signs

- signet ring sign on PA radiograph due to volar tilting of the scaphoid – humpback deformity
- Terry Thomas sign of scapholunate dissociation (diastasis)
- SLAC wrist with decrease in the Huber index (disease begins at the radioscaphoid joint)

Treatment

- RSS alone:
  - triscaphe fusion – scaphoid, trapezium, trapezoid
  - provides a stable column for the radial axis
- SLAC wrist
  - excision of the scaphoid and fusion of the capitate, lunate, hamate and triquetrum

- results in significant decrease in wrist range of movement
- Kienbock's disease – ulnar lengthening, etc.

Colles' fracture – distal radius, dorsal and radial angulation

Smith's fracture – distal radius, volar angulation

Wrist dislocations:

- lunate dislocation: lunate lies dorsal or ventral to the radius on the lateral film
- perilunate dislocation: lunate is in the correct position but the capitate and the rest of the carpus are not
- mid-carpal dislocation: neither the lunate nor the capitate is in alignment with the radius

Ulnar abutment (impingement) syndrome

- positive ulnar variance
- degeneration of the TFCC
- ulnar sided wrist pain
- confirmed by MRI or arthroscopy
- treated during arthroscopy by excision of TFCC tears (as for meniscal cartilage tears in knee arthroscopy)
- salvage procedure is ulnar shortening

Self-assessment: A patient comes along with wrist pain. What is your management?

History

- age, sex, occupation, dominance, hobbies
- duration of the pain, provoking or relieving factors
- site of pain
- functional disability
- any history of trauma
- any history of rheumatoid/osteoarthritis
- drugs, allergies, PMSH, smoker

Examination

- look – swellings, scars, sudomotor changes, wasting, attitude of the hand
- feel – masses, test sensation to the hand, feel for tender areas
- move – radio-ulnar, dorsi and volar flexion, movement in fingers including power and full nerve examination
- provocation tests – pivot shift, RSS

Investigations

- AP and lateral films ($\pm$ Eaton views for basal joints)
- look for: SLAC wrist, decreased Huber index

Differential diagnoses

- radial wrist pain:
  - Bone/joint
    - basal joint OA
    - ischaemic necrosis of scaphoid
  - Soft tissues
    - de Quervain's tenosynovitis (first compartment)
    - intersection syndrome (second compartment tenosynovitis)
    - Wartenberg's syndrome (superficial branch of radial nerve entrapment)
    - synovitis

- central wrist pain:
  - Bone/joint
    - Kienbock's disease
    - ganglia/metacarpal boss
  - Soft tissues – synovitis
- ulnar wrist pain:
  - Bone/joint
    - ulnar impingement syndrome
  - Soft tissues – synovitis
    - FCU tenosynovitis

Treatment

- tailored to individual problem
  - RA, scaphoid necrosis and Kienbock's → scapholunate ligament rupture → diastasis
  - clinically manifest by DISI with rotatory subluxation of the scaphoid
  - X-rays show a SLAC wrist, decreased Huber index, Terry Thomas sign
  - primary scaphoid necrosis treatment splint, open reduction and internal fixation, excision and rolled tendon spacer
  - primary Kienbock's treatment splint, ulnar lengthening (radial shortening), capitohamate fusion, excision and rolled tendon spacer
  - early treatment, triscaphe fusion; later treatment, wrist fusion

Treatment of other basal joint OA, etc. see other sections

Nerve injury
Compartment syndrome

Volkman 1881 – paralytic contracture with tight bandages. Volkman's ischaemic contracture is the final state of ischaemic necrosis and fibrosis. Originally described in the forearm

Thomas 1909 – extrinsic compression not necessarily required

Murphy 1914 – haemorrhage and decreased venous outflow raises compartment pressure

Mubarak – compartment syndrome results from raised interstitial pressure in a closed compartment

Aetiology

Crush

Prolonged extrinsic compression

Internal bleeding

Fractures

Excessive exercise (increases muscle volume)

High tension electrical injury

Reperfusion

Symptoms and signs

Pain, especially on passive stretching, out of proportion to the injury

Weakness of compartment muscles (late), tendon contracture (very late)

Tense swelling in the compartment

Paraesthesia/hyperaesthesia

Loss of pulses (late)

Capillary refill >2 s

Pallor

Disappearance of pain may herald necrosis rather than recovery

Compartment syndrome may develop late (>3 days) after injury

Pressure >40 mmHg (perfusion pressure) >2 h causes irreversible necrosis

Classification

Acute – recognized symptoms and signs

Subacute – without easily recognizable symptoms and signs but may progress to acute

Recurrent – athletes

Chronic – unrelieved acute, ischaemia progressing to fibrosis and Volkman's

Pathophysiology

Injury is proportional to the degree of pressure elevation and the duration

Local blood flow $= P_a - P_v$/resistance (Ohm's law: $I = V/R$)

reduced P_a

- high elevation
- premorbid limb ischaemia

increased P_v

- high interstitial pressure, e.g. muscle oedema, haemorrhage, external compression
- limb dependency

increased resistance – peripheral vascular disease

Investigations

Compartment pressure measurement

- tissue $P > 20$ mmHg in a hypotensive patient
- tissue $P > 30$ mmHg in a normotensive patient

Doppler/arteriography

MRI

Clinical suspicion must be followed by operative exploration of all the compartments in the area concerned

Management

Release extrinsic compression

Limb at heart level

Fasciotomy then elevation

Splint in a position of function

Treat haemochromogenuria

Definitive wound closure

Classification of nerve injury

Wallerian degeneration

Orthograde degeneration in the nerve distal to the site of division, ultimately to the end receptor

Occurs for $\sim$6 weeks

Axonal degeneration

Retrograde degeneration in the nerve proximal to the site of division

Axons die back to the next most proximal branch

Cell body undergoes changes that include chromatolysis

Regenerative sprouting proceeds down the original Schwann cell myelin sheath but through new endoneural tubules

Classification

Seddon	Sunderland	Insult	Prognosis
Neuropraxia	First degree	Segmental demyelination	Full recovery 1–4 months
Axonotmesis	Second degree	Axon severed	Full recovery 4–18 months
Neurotmesis	Third degree	Endoneurium disrupted	Incomplete recovery
Neurotmesis	Fourth degree	Perineurium disrupted	Incomplete recovery
Neurotmesis	Fifth degree	Epineurium disrupted[†]	No recovery

[†]Loss of continuity.

Prognosis

Younger age and more distal transections do better

Sharp transection preferable to avulsion

Division close to motor end plates better than proximal division

Regeneration occurs at between 1 and 3 mm per day

Muscles can regain ~100% of function even after 1 year of denervation providing enough axons reach the motor end plates

Sensory recovery – MRC grading

S0 – no recovery

S1 – deep **pain**

S1+ – superficial pain

S2– light **touch**

S2+ – hyperaesthesia to light touch

S3 – 2pd >15 mm

S3+ – 2pd 7–15 mm

S4 – complete recovery

Motor recovery – MRC grading

M0 – no contraction

M1 – perceptible contraction

M2 – contraction with gravity eliminated

M3 – contraction against gravity

M4 – contraction against resistance

M5 – full contraction

Nerve conduction studies

Neuropraxia →   absent conduction over the site of the block, normal above and below

Incomplete lesion →   prolonged **latency**, reduced **amplitude**

Complete lesion →   no conduction

Principles of repair

Primary repair within 10 days

Good fascicular alignment

Inverting epineural suture in purely sensory or motor nerves

Fascicular (perineural) repair in mixed nerves

Avoid excessive tension and mobilization

- >20% increase in length of the nerve sutured under tension causes conduction impairment
- gaps >2–2.5 cm should be grafted

Nerve graft significant defects

Transfers for specific nerve lesions

High median nerve palsy

FCU split to restore balanced **wrist flexion**

Re-route biceps to restore **pronation**

Brachioradialis → FPL for **thumb flexion**

Opponensplasty using EI or ADM → **thumb abduction and opposition**

Suture together ulnar FDPs to median FDPs to achieve a **finger flexion** (mass action)

Low ulnar nerve palsy (claw hand)

FDS transfer to the radial lateral band (or A1 pulley) or a slip of FDS (Zancolli Lasso) to **correct metacarpophalangeal hyperextension and lack of interphalangeal extension**

Brachioradialis and graft or ECRL → adductor pollicis to **improve pinch** (Boyes)

High ulnar nerve palsy

Suture together ulnar FDPs to median FDPs to achieve a **finger flexion** (mass action)

Brachioradialis or ECRL → adductor pollicis to **improve pinch** (Boyes)

Radial nerve palsy

PT   →   ECRB to restore **wrist extension**

            Maintains some useful pronation from PT to the most central wrist extensor ECRB

FCU →   EDC to restore **finger extension**

PL   →   EPL to restore **thumb extension**

Injured nerve	Active deficit	Tendon missing	Tendon available
Median nerve (elbow)	Forearm pronation	Pronator teres	Biceps
	Wrist flexion	FCR, PL	FCU split
	Finger flexion	FDS (all), FDP (median)	Tenodese to ulnar FDPs
	Thumb IP flexion	FPL	Brachioradialis
	Thumb abduction	Thenar muscles	Opponensplasty using ADM or EI

Ulnar nerve (elbow)	Wrist flexion	FCU	Split FCR
	Finger flexion	FDP (ulnar)	Tenodesis to median FDPs
	Thumb adduction	AP	Brachioradialis
Ulnar nerve (wrist – ulnar claw)	Metacarpophalangeal flexion (hyper-extended)	Lumbricals (ulnar)	FDS to radial sagittal band
Radial nerve (elbow)	Elbow flexion	Brachioradialis	Flexor mass resited higher on humerus
	Radial wrist extension	ECRB, ECRL	Pronator teres
	Finger extension	EC, EI, EDM	FCU
	Thumb extension	EPL	Palmaris longus

Nerve conduits

Nerve grafts (autograft, allograft, xenograft)

Denatured skeletal muscle

Fibronectin

Bone

Arteries and veins

Pseudosynovial sheaths

Silicone and PTFE tubes

Human NGF and glial growth factor (GGF) may augment regeneration

Autologous nerve transplantation is nearly always possible

Neuroma

Presentation

Pain and exquisite tenderness

Pain when moving adjacent joints

Pressure pain

Dysaethesia in the distribution of the nerve

Types

Neuroma-in-continuity

- spindle – chronic irritation in an intact nerve (lateral cutaneous N of thigh entrapment)
- lateral – develops at a site of partial nerve division
- following N repair – generally smaller

End-neuroma

- following traumatic nerve division
- following amputation

Common upper limb neuromas

Palmar cutaneous branch of the median N

Superficial branches of radial nerve

Radial digital nerves

Dorsal branch of the ulnar N

Palliation

Desensitization exercises

TENS

Drugs – carbamazepine, etc.

Surgical management

Resection and coagulation – bipolar, cryotherapy, chemical (alcohol, formaldehyde), laser

Crushing

Capping (silicone, vein, histoacryl glue)

Multiple sectioning (but may form multiple smaller neuromas)

Ligation

Epineural repair over the cut end

Bury cut end in bone or muscle

- palm and digits – bury into PP or metacarpal
- wrist – bury into pronator quadratus
- forearm – bury into brachioradialis

Implantation into nerve

- centro-central implantation into another nerve
- implantation into the same nerve
- experimentally in animal models use of nerve agents to destroy cell bodies of affected nerves

Lateral neuromas treated by resection and repair of the disrupted perineurium of the involved fascicles only

Loss of sensation in a critical area of the hand → consider importing innervated tissue (e.g. Littler flap to the index pulp) – sensory integration of neurovascular island flaps occurs in up to 40% of adults, greater percentage in children

Trauma-induced cold-associated symptoms (TICAS)

What is cold intolerance?

Campbell and Kay. *J Hand Surg* 1998

A collection of acquired symptoms resulting in an abnormal aversion to cold:

- pain/discomfort (93%, most troublesome)
- stiffness
- altered sensibility
- colour change (least troublesome)
- around half of all patients experience these symptoms from the time of injury
- around half experience symptoms after a lag period of ~4 months, mostly coinciding with the first cold day of winter

Patients may experience TICAS for the two winters following injury but symptoms generally improve thereafter

Brachial plexus injuries

Main anatomy of the brachial plexus

Roots –   lie behind scalenus anterior (C5,6,7,8,T1)

Trunks –   cross the lower part of the posterior triangle

Divisions – behind the clavicle

Cords – embrace the axillary artery

- lateral cord – musculocutaneous N
- posterior cord – radial and axillary Ns
- medial cord – median, ulnar Ns and thoracodorsal N

Dorsal root: contains sensory afferents with cell bodies (but no synapses) in the dorsal root ganglion

Ventral root: contains motor efferents (relay in anterior horn cells)

Dorsal and ventral roots combine to form the spinal nerve

Spinal nerve splits into anterior and posterior rami

Anterior rami form the major plexuses – including the brachial plexus

- **hence, the 'roots' of the brachial plexus are the anterior rami of C5–T1**
- anterior ramus of T1 also contains sympathetic fibres

Posterior rami become the posterior intercostal nerves and supply the erector spinae muscles

Serratus is innervated by the long thoracic nerve – branch from the nerve roots of C5,6,7: if there is no wing scapula then the injury is in the nerve trunks

A supraganglionic lesion is where the disruption occurs at the level of the dorsal root ganglion.

- within the spinal canal hence not amenable to grafting
- hence do not waste graft on nerves where there is no central connection

This may be tested for by eliciting sensory nerve action potentials as sensory nerves remain in continuity with their cell bodies in the dorsal root ganglion however motor repair is not possible as the nerves have been separated from the spinal cord ventrally and dorsally proximal to the dorsal root ganglion.

An infraganglionic lesion is where the disruption occurs in the spinal nerve itself

Millesi classification

I – Supraganglionic

II – Infraganglionic

III – Trunk

IV – Cord

Obstetric palsies

Wait at least 3 months for recovery of elbow flexion before exploring

C5,6 Erb's palsy

Traction downwards (obstetric), lateral flexion of the cervical spine, blow to the neck

Affects lateral and posterior cords (musculocutaneous, radial and axillary Ns)

Waiter's tip position – wrist drop

Most obstetric palsies recover but if there is no return of biceps function by 3 months of age then exploration is warranted

C7,8, T1 Klumpke paralysis

Less common

- Traction upwards (breech delivery)
- Affects medial cord (ulnar and median Ns)
- Intrinsic muscle wasting

General

Open injuries – exclude concomitant axillary artery trauma → life or limb-threatening haemorrhage

Low velocity bullet injury → concussive effect on the plexus, rarely transection: explore after 3 months if no recovery

Lower trunk and long thoracic N at risk during first rib resection in thoracic outlet syndrome

Infraclavicular injuries have a better prognosis than supraclavicular injuries and if closed can wait 3–6 months for recovery before exploring

Post-anaesthetic brachial plexus palsy

- closed traction injury
- excellent prognosis → recovery within 6 weeks
- avoid hyperabduction of the arms or excessive lateral neck flexion in the unconscious patient
- nerve injury in the course of administering a brachial plexus block is rare

Investigations

- thorough clinical examination
- EMG and nerve conduction studies – must wait at least 3 weeks before fibrillation potentials as a result of denervation are produced
- MRI scan or CT myelography to demonstrate root avulsion

Non-surgical treatment

- physio to maintain joint mobility
- functional bracing
- nerve stimulation to maintain motor end plates while awaiting recovery

Surgical treatment

- external neurolysis
- primary repair or cable grafting with sural nerve or medial cutaneous nerve of the forearm – intra-operative cortical evoked potentials help determine whether there is supraganglionic injury
- arthrodeses to stabilize joints
- tendon transfers (must have good passive ROM)
- free functioning muscle transfers
  - gracilis
  - latissimus dorsi
  - must have an appropriate motor nerve for coaptation
  - can include a skin paddle for soft tissue cover
- direct neurotization of distal stumps using spinal accessory, intercostal nerves and the long thoracic nerve or crossed nerve grafts from the opposite brachial plexus
  - consider donor site morbidity
  - used for supraganglionic avulsion injuries

Shoulder

- trapezius transfer to restore abduction
- advance the origins of biceps and triceps to the acromion (flexion/extension)
- alternatively shoulder fusion to provide a stable platform for elbow transfers to work against – 30° abduction, flexion and internal rotation

Elbow

- **pectoralis major transfer** – pedicled on clavicular head into the forearm
- **latissimus dorsi transfer** (if thoracodorsal N spared)

- **triceps transfer** to the biceps insertion to provide flexion (flexion is more important than extension) when radial N (posterior cord) available but musculocutaneous nerve (lateral cord) is not
- transfer the **forearm flexor mass** (medial epicondyle) higher up on the humerus

Post-radiotherapy palsies
- gloomy prognosis
- intraneural ischaemia and fibrosis
- pain and paraesthesia
- difficult to distinguish from tumour invasion – tumour → more pain and involvement of the lower roots → Horner's syndrome
- grafts should be wrapped in vascularized tissue – omentum has been reported

Complete traumatic brachial plexus palsy

Bentolila. *Am J Hand Surg* 1999

Priorities (in order) are restoration of:
- elbow flexion (most important) → musculocutaneous N (lateral cord)
- elbow and wrist extension → radial N (posterior cord)
- finger flexion → median N (medial cord)
- shoulder abduction → axillary N (posterior cord)

If no central connection:
- accessory nerve transfer → lateral cord or musculocutaneous N itself
- grafts from intercostal, accessory and thoracodorsal nerves (if spared) to distal stumps

Access to the plexus via a lymphadenectomy approach in the posterior triangle (supraclavicular area) extended via the deltopectoral groove to the infraclavicular area; may need to split the clavicle

Patients may have a Horner's syndrome due to interruption of sympathetic outflow via the stellate ganglion

Delay between accident and operation was prognostic for return of function but need proper investigation rather than emergency surgery

>6 months → muscular atrophy, fibrosis and joint stiffness

Minimum of four cables to each cord

Pain is not alleviated by amputation

Obstetrical brachial palsy

Kay, *BJPS* 1998

About one per 1000 live births

Associated with:
- shoulder dystocia
- high birthweight
- assisted delivery – breech presentation
- prolonged labour
- multiparity
- very rare after caesarean section

Prognostic factors
- 96% → full recovery
- poor recovery with:

- lower root lesions
- associated fractures of clavicle, ribs, humerus
- avulsion injuries
- Horner's syndrome

Diagnosis

- passive but no active movement
- look for Horner's syndrome
- CXR to check for elevation of the hemidiaphragm
- EMG used to select muscles for transfer
- in ~20% of patients EMG → prolonged conduction block → good recovery
- imaging is difficult:
  - myelography in children (need GA) → high false-positive rate for root avulsion
  - MRI unreliable

Classification

- C5–6 – waiter's tip position – Erb's palsy
- C5–7 – as above, elbow slightly flexed
- C5–T1 – flail limb, claw hand, marbled appearance due to vasomotor changes, ± Horner's syndrome

Early management

- physiotherapy to maintain passive ROM awaiting recovery – also allows spheroidal moulding of the humeral head and glenoid cavity
- indications for primary plexus exploration (repair, grafting):
  - complete palsy with a flail arm
  - C5–6 palsy with no biceps contraction at 3 months
  - Horner's syndrome
  - phrenic nerve involvement

Late management – tendon transfers, etc.

Self-assessment: A patient is admitted through casualty having been knocked off his motorbike. His left arm appears to be frail. How would you manage this patient?

Emergency management

ABC – particular attention to the C-spine, etc.

Definitive management of the arm itself

History

- age, occupation, hand dominance, hobbies
- mechanism of injury: arm hyperabducted or neck laterally flexed?
- immediate or delayed weakness in the arm?
- any concomitant injuries?
- general health – drugs, PMSH, smoker, etc.

Examination

- look – attitude of the limb, wasting of muscles (if presentation delayed), sudomotor changes, scars, swellings (might have subclavian A aneurysm), look for Horner's syndrome in lower root lesions
- feel – sensation C5–T1

Move – shoulder, elbow, wrist, fingers and thumb testing individual neuromotor units and **reflexes**

Investigation

- MRI, EMG/NCS, myelography
- classify level – Millesi

Treatment

- physio, splints
- surgery after ~3 months (immediately if sharp injury)
  - nerve grafts
  - nerve transfers if supraganglionic
  - muscle transfers – local or free
  - address shoulder, elbow, wrist, fingers in sequence
- arthrodeses

The surgical treatment of brachial plexus injuries in adults

Terzis. *Plastic Reconstruc Surg* 2000

High-velocity motor vehicle accidents account for the majority of the cases of brachial plexus injury

Nature of injury

- Crush
  - direct blunt trauma to the neck and upper extremity
  - plexus is crushed between the clavicle and the first rib
- Traction
- Compression of the plexus by haematoma or adjacent tissue elements that have been injured

History

- Mechanism of injury
- Pre-existing neurologic status
- occupation and handedness

Examination

- Horner syndrome
- Use preprinted brachial plexus diagrams that include all muscle groups of the upper extremity, sensory mapping, and pain threshold to document observations
- Passive and active range of motion of all
- Evaluation of the vascularity of the arm
- Function of the phrenic nerve

Investigations

- complete radiological study of the cervical spine and the involved shoulder with special attention to the clavicle and scapula
- Fractures of the transverse processes might indicate avulsions of the corresponding roots, due to the attachments of the deep cervical fascia between the cervical roots and the transverse processes.
- CT/myelography
  - Positive predictive value of combined CT myelography more than 95% per cent
  - Avulsed roots can exist despite a normal myelogram
- MRI
  - good visualization of the brachial plexus beyond the spinal foramen

- High field strength MRI with multi planar views can easily distinguish the nerves at the distal plexus
- Electrophysiologic studies
  - Wallerian degeneration results in the emergence of spontaneous electrical discharges or fibrillations
  - Needle electromyogram of the paraspinal muscles, innervated by the dorsal rami of the spinal roots, should also be routinely performed
    - denervation of these muscles provides strong evidence of avulsion of the corresponding roots
    - if these muscles are electrically intact, then the injury is most likely infra-ganglionic and the root is most likely ruptured

Surgical exploration

- Avoidance of any kind of paralytics
- The incision for the exploration of the brachial plexus parallel to the posterior border sternocleidomastoid
- Open clavicular osteotomies have the tendency to create malunions and nonunions and should be avoided
- The omohyoid muscle and the transverse cervical vessels are identified and retracted
- The phrenic nerve is identified
- Neuromas are identified and can extend between the upper roots and the trunks
  - May also be present distally at the cord or peripheral nerve level
  - Neuromas can be in continuity or at the end of a ruptured plexus segment
  - The proximal stump of the neuroma may be used as an intra-plexus motor donor for the reconstruction of the distal plexus
- Signs of avulsion of spinal nerves:
  - feel empty to palpation
  - pale in appearance
  - negative to electrical stimulation
- Identify the level, type, and extent of the lesion
- Motor and sensory donors are matched to their corresponding distal targets
  - Intra-plexus motor donors
  - Proximal stumps of ruptured roots
  - Extra-plexus donors used in multiple-root avulsions
    - intercostal nerves
    - accessory nerve
    - contralateral C7 root
- Microneurolysis
- Longitudinal epineuriotomies
- Excision of the neuroma to healthy fascicles
- Interposition nerve grafting
  - Sural nerves

Specific aims of reconstruction

- Stability of the shoulder is a very important goal
  - The return of function in the supraspinatus and deltoid muscles is considered of prime importance
- Restore biceps mediated elbow flexion for hand–mouth function
  - Re-innervate the musculocutaneous nerve with the best motor donors

- Avoid contractures at the elbow level that might hinder its full range of motion
- One or two of the upper intercostal nerves are dedicated to neurotize the ipsilateral latissimus dorsi muscle as a reserve muscle unit to eventually enhance the power of a weakened recovering biceps
  - If the biceps restoration is complete, then the reinnervated latissimus can be used as a pedicled muscle flap to strengthen the function of the ipsilateral triceps muscle
- Reinnervation of the triceps is also of prime importance because it can give stability to the elbow joint
- Sensory protection of the hand is of prime importance in global brachial plexus injuries and can be achieved by neurotisation of the median nerve from sensory intercostal nerves or from supraclavicular sensory nerves
- Functioning free-muscle transplantation has become a reconstructive option in cases of delayed patient presentation with long denervation time, or in cases with multiple-root avulsions, especially when the lower roots of the plexus that innervate the hand are involved
- Tendon transfers
  - transfer of the clavicular and acromial insertion of the trapezius with or without fascia lata to the deltoid insertion on the humerus to enhance abduction and reverse subluxation
  - Transfer of the sternoclavicular part of the pectoralis major to the anterior deltoid for anterior flexion
  - The pectoralis minor can also be transferred to the biceps muscle to strengthen elbow flexion
  - A classic manoeuvre is also the rerouting of the latissimus dorsi tendon around the humerus to restore dynamic external rotation
- Rotational osteotomies of the humerus help improve external rotation by 30 degrees

Skin loss

Nail bed injuries
Replace lost germinal matrix with a split nail bed graft from the big toe
Severe germinal matrix injury may require nail bed ablation
Consider homodigital advancement pulp flaps (e.g. Atasoy) or heterodigital flaps with nail bed grafts from distal amputations

Pulp reconstruction
Requirements
- freedom from pain
- adequate padding
- sensation
Options
- neurovascular island flap – pedicled (**Foucher** flap – first dorsal metacarpal artery flap, may be of insufficient length to cover thumb pulp), **Littler** (1960) – from radial border of ring finger
- free neurovascular island flap from the big toe (toe–pulp transfer)
- sensory cross finger flap

Dorsal skin defects
Reversed or free radial forearm flap (see Chapter 2)

Foucher flap (1979)

- first DMCA flap
- skin paddle from the dorso-radial aspect of the proximal phalanx of the index finger is a random pattern extension from the dorso-radial aspect over the distal second metacarpal which must be raised with the flap
- raise pedicle 1–2 cm in width with fascia and epimysium
- dorsal lazy-S incision
- 20% may not have a definitive vessel – several branches
- 'sink' branch at the level of the metacarpal head needs to be ligated
- leave paratenon for graft take
- nerves are deep to veins but superficial to arteries
- originally described for dorsal thumb defects, not really for thumb pulp
- may also be rotated to reconstitute dorsal ulnar defects

Second DMCA flap

Earley and Milner 1987

- same technical principles as Foucher flap
- large anastomosing vessel between dorsal and palmar metacarpal arteries in the second web space which needs ligating (vessel for Quaba flap)
- second DMA is larger than first DMCA in one-third of hands
- but vein and artery lie either side of EC tendon, limiting arc of rotation
- may be used as a free flap

Quaba flap (1990)

- distally based flap based on communicating vessel between second DMCA and palmar vessel which runs in second web space
- no need to raise second DMCA beneath the skin paddle
- raise at level of paratenon
- useful for full-length defects of the dorsum of the finger

Posterior interosseus artery flap

Zancolli 1986

- ulnar artery gives off a common interosseus artery at the level of the neck of the radius which divides into anterior and posterior interosseus arteries
- long axis of flap on a line joining the ulnar head with the lateral epicondyle when the arm is pronated
- posterior interosseus vessels lie in the vertical septum radial to ECU and ulnar to EDM – fasciocutaneous flap
- distally pedicled, ulna head is pivot point
- include around three perforators in the tail of the flap (distally)
- dorsal skin loss

Additional flaps for dorsal digital defects

Cross-finger flap

- based upon dorsal branches of digital As
- mainly used for volar defects
- volar thumb defect – use cross-finger flap from middle finger
- de-epithelialized and reversed for dorsal defects

Flag flap

Vilain 1977

Fingertip injuries

Classification (Allen)

I – Skin and pulp distal to the nail bed – dress/SSG/hyphecan cap

II – Pulp and nail bed distal to bone – dress/SSG/flap/composite graft/hyphecan cap

III – Loss of part of terminal phalanx – flap/terminalization/hyphecan cap

IV – Amputation proximal to nail bed – flap/terminalization/replant

Homodigital flaps – fingertip injuries

Kutler. *JAMA* 1947 – lateral V–Y, distal skin

Hueston. *PRS* 1966 – volar skin transposition/advancement ± V–Y modification (*Elliot*) at base

Ataso. *J Bone Joint Surg* 1970 – volar V–Y, distal skin

Macht. *J Hand Surg* 1980 – **Moberg** flap: volar digit V–Y skin advancement

Venkataswami. *PRS* 1980 – half digit oblique volar skin advancement V–Y based on one neurovascular bundle

Step-advancement

Evans. *J Hand Surg* 1988

Exploits tissue laxity at the base of the finger

Avoids flexion contracture occasionally seen following Venkataswami flap

Skin flap angles get smaller proximally

Beneath the skin incisions fat is incised vertically in a straight line to flexor sheath

Raise at level of flexor sheath and under neurovascular bundle

Commence proximal interphalangeal extension within 1 week

Reverse digital artery island flap

Wilson. *Injury* 2004

Technique for volar pulp and fingertip reconstruction using an island of skin from the non-dominant border of the digit

Flap based upon reverse flow in the ipsilateral digital artery via volar communicating vessels from the other side at a level 5 mm proximal to the DIP joint crease

- Digital artery ligated proximal to the flap
- Can include a segment of dorsal nerve within the flap for coaption to the distal stump of the digital nerve other side to render the flap sensate

Success with this technique and good functional outcome possible even in elderly patients

Complex regional pain syndromes

Stanton–Hicks definition

'A variety of painful conditions following injury ... exceeding both in magnitude and duration the expected clinical course of the inciting event.'

CRPS type 1

- no predisposing event ('primary' CRPS) – RSD, algodystrophy
- increased uptake on the bone scan especially around the joints
- can be cited as an early and late complication of any hand surgery

CRPS type 2

- identifiable primary **nerve** insult ('secondary' CRPS) – causalgia plus vasomotor, sudomotor (sweat gland) and trophic changes
- differential diagnosis may include **Secretan's** disease: brawny swelling and induration in the hand as a result of factitious tapping/rubbing of the hand

Pathogenesis

Calder, Holten and McAllister. *J Hand Surg* 1998

Sensitization of the central nervous system following peripheral injury

Initiating stimulus → ↑ rate of firing of nociceptors and ↓ threshold

Increased numbers of Langerhans cells release IL-1 and TNF-α

IL-1 and TNF-α cause skin fibroblasts to release NGF

NGF is transported retrogradely to the neuronal cell body causing the release of substance P and calcitonin growth-related peptide (CGRP)

SP and CGRP are transported to the periphery to produce oedema and inflammation and centrally to increase the excitability of CNS NMDA receptors

Cytokine-mediated feedback (from the site of injury via spinothalamic tracts) to hypothalamus → sensitization of the CNS

Secondary effects mediated by SNS outflow from the sensitized hypothalamus

Symptoms

Pain

- **allodynia** – pain due to a stimulus which does not normally provoke pain (e.g. emotion, noise)
- **hyperalgesia** – increased pain to a normally painful stimulus
- **hyperaesthesia** – increased sensitivity to a stimulus, e.g. light touch
- **hyperpathia** – excessive perception of a painful stimulus
- **dysaesthesia** – abnormally perceived unpleasant sensation, spontaneous or provoked
- **causalgia** – burning pain, allodynia and hyperpathia after traumatic nerve injury

Swelling/oedema

Discoloration – **dermographia** – triple response to a light object drawn across the skin

Stiffness

- increased hair growth
- shiny skin
- hyperhidrosis
- atrophy of bone (osteoporosis) with reduced radiographic bone density

Predisposing factors

Increased sympathetic activity

Smokers

Surgery or trauma to hand (common after Colles fracture)

Tight dressings

Immediate

Inappropriate pain within 48 h of trauma or surgery

Early (1 week–6 months)

Pain – hyperpathia, hyperalgesia

Vasodilatation – red, sweaty, oedematous

Reduced bone density

Intermediate (6–12 months)

Pain – constant

Organized oedema ('brawny')

Discoloration and sudomotor changes – blue, cool, dry

Trophic changes – shiny skin, brittle nails

Stiffness – joint contractures

Late (>12 months – Sudek's atrophy)

Dry

Intractable pain (or may decrease)

Joint stiffness/contracture

Atrophic changes as above

Lack of shoulder movement (**shoulder–hand syndrome**)

Increased uptake on bone scan (osteoclastic resorption)

Treatment

Early

- treat primary insult
- physiotherapy (splintage and mobilization) ± BPB
- drugs (amitriptyline, carbamazepine)
- guanethidine block

Intermediate

- steroids
- stellate ganglion block

Late – sympathectomy

> **Self-assessment:** A patient returns to clinic 1 week after carpal tunnel release with a painful, red, hot, shiny, stiff hand. What would be your thoughts in this situation?

History

- what were the immediate postoperative symptoms – excessive pain?
- are the current symptoms getting worse or better?
- were there any symptoms like this pre-operatively?
- what is the nature of the pain (allodynia, hyperpathia, dysaesthesia)?
- how has the hand been splinted (?tight bandages) and has there been post-operative physiotherapy?
- smoker?

Examination

- look – observe the above features plus any other scars, swellings, sudomotor changes, wasting. Also look at the attitude of the hand, hyperhidrosis

- feel – hot skin, sweaty, tender
- move – passive and active ROM in fingers, full examination of the three nerves

Diagnosis – a presumptive diagnosis of CRPS type 1 (RSD, algodystrophy) is reached: a set of painful conditions, the extent and duration of which exceeds the expected clinical course of the stimulus which initiated them (Stanton–Hicks)

Investigations – plain X-ray → may see osteopenia

Treatment

- hand therapy team approach:
  - splint
  - physiotherapy – under BPB if necessary
  - analgesia – including carbamazepine and amitriptyline
- regular review

What is the cause of RSD and how might the patient's symptoms progress?

Cause is due to sensitization of the CNS to a painful stimulus:

- nociceptive firing stimulates Langerhans cells
- Langerhans cells → IL-2 + TNF-α
- IL-2 + TNF-α → chemo-attract fibroblasts
- fibroblasts → NGF
- NGF → neurone cell body
- neurone cell body → substance P and CRGP
- substance P and CRGP →
  - **centrally** → sensitizes CNS (hypothalamus)
  - **peripherally** → pain, oedema, skin changes, etc.

Intermediate stage 6–12 months

- development of brawny oedema
- constant pain
- stiffness with early joint contracture
- atrophic changes
- fingers blue

Last stage >6 months

- decreased pain
- permanent stiffness
- loss of bone density – Sudek's atrophy
- joint contractures
- stiff shoulder

Dupuytren's and joint contracture

Causes of flexion contracture

Skin – scar contracture

Fascia – Dupuytren's

Flexor tendon sheath – fibrous contracture

Flexor tendon – Volkman's contracture, adhesions

Capsular structures – volar plate shortening

Block to extension – osteophytes, loose bodies, etc.

Collateral ligament shortening NEVER a cause because these are held taught in all ranges of movement at the IP joints

Extension contracture

Skin – scar contracture

Extensor tendon – shortening, adhesions

Intrinsic muscles – ischaemic contracture, intrinsic plus

Capsular structures – collateral ligament shortening (lax in extension at metacarpophalangeal joint), volar plate adhesions, dorsal capsule contracture

Joint surfaces – fixed extension in post-burn contracture, bony block, loose body, OA

Flexor tendon – bulky tendon preventing excursion

Bouviere's test to confirm intrinsic tightness – flexion is impossible at proximal interphalangeal and distal interphalangeal joints when the metacarpophalangeal joints are extended; shorten intrinsics by passively flexing metacarpophalangeal joints – flexion at proximal interphalangeal and distal interphalangeal joints is now possible

Ligaments

Positions of greatest ligamentous laxity are assumed in the injured hand:

- wrist – extension
- MPjs – extension
- IPs – flexion
- thumb – adduction

The collateral ligament of the metacarpophalangeal joint and the volar plate of the IP joints will then shorten to create a contracture

Dupuytren's disease

General/anatomy

First described by Sir Astley Cooper, then by Dupuytren in 1831

'Band' is normal, 'cord' is diseased

Anatomy of the palmar fascia:

- horizontal fibres – insertion:
  - skin of palm just beyond distal palmar crease
  - spiral band of Gosset passing to lateral digital sheet
  - flexor tendon sheath just beyond proximal interphalangeal joint
- transverse fibres
- vertical fibres (of Skoog) binding to metacarpals

Involvement of **pretendinous bands** of superficial palmar fascia and the **natatory ligament** which spans the web spaces

Transverse fibres of palmar aponeurosis are usually uninvolved

Natatory ligament bifurcates at each digit to form the **lateral** band (lateral to the neurovascular bundle, intimately adherent to skin) and to attach to the pretendinous band

A further spiral band passes from the pretendinous band at the base of the finger, beneath the neurovascular bundle (displaced to the midline) and reattaches to the continuation of the pretendinous band, the central band, which itself attaches distally to the flexor sheath

A spiral cord is formed by the pre-tendinous cord, spiral cord, lateral digital sheet and Grayson's ligament. This is important operatively as a spiral cord can displace the neurovascular structures proximally medially and superficially placing them at risk of injury

Retrovascular band 'of Tomine' lies just superficial to Cleland's ligament and attaches to the periosteum of the proximal phalanx, extending to insert into the periosteum of the distal phalanx (often a cause of inadequate release)

In the little finger the spiral cord also arises from the ADM tendon

It is unusual to have diseased cords on both sides of the finger

Grayson's ligament, on the volar surface of the finger, is involved while Cleland's ligament is spared

Oblique retinacular ligament (Landsmeer)

- spirals from the volar side of the proximal interphalangeal joint to the dorsal side of the distal interphalangeal joint
- coordinates flexion and extension between these two joints
- cannot voluntarily flex distal interphalangeal joint with proximal interphalangeal joint extended
- shortens in Boutonnière deformity

Epidemiology

Disease of the Celtic race

Common in northern Europe, North America, Australasia

Oriental races and diabetics tend to have palmar disease but not joint contracture

Uncommon in pigmented races

Male:female ratio $= \sim14:1$

Both hands usually involved

Unilateral disease is more commonly a sporadic finding without a family history and is usually less severe

In females DD is seen later and is usually less severe

Aetiology

Molecular factors

- myofibroblasts; Gabiani. *Am J Pathol* 1972
- abnormality of expression of matrix metalloproteins
- fibrogenic cytokines (including IL-1), free radicals (via xanthine oxidase) and growth factors including β-FGF, GM-CSF and TGF-β3
- modulation of TGF-β receptor expression: DD fibroblasts express high-affinity type 2 receptors vs. low affinity type 1
- low levels of -interferon in DD patients (also low in black patients with keloids)
- expression of type VI collagen during the proliferative phase acts as a scaffold for DD fibroblasts
- disturbed regulation of fibroblastic terminal differentiation (apoptosis)

Genetic factors

- strong family history in some patients points to a single gene defect

- other fibroproliferative conditions (Peyronie's, Lederhosen's) may be pleiotropic effects of the same gene
- possible link with trisomy 8

Pathophysiology

Intrinsic theory (McFarlane) perivascular fibroblasts within normal fascia are source of disease

Extrinsic theory (Heuston) disease starts with proliferation of fibrous tissue de-novo as nodules appear superficial to palmar fascia

Synthesis theory (Gosset) combines both theories with nodules arising de-novo and cords from pre-existing fascia

Murrell's hypothesis : age environmental and genetic factors cause micro-vessel narrowing leading to ischaemia, free radical formation which stimulates fibroblasts.

The disease is characterized by three phases

Proliferative

Involutional

Residual

Dupuytren's diathesis (Hueston)

Aggressive DD

Young age of onset

Early recurrence

Strong family history

Other areas of involvement

Associated clinical features

Garrod's knuckle pads (proximal interphalangeal joint) – ~20% of patients, lie between skin and extensor tendon, attached to paratenon

Plantar fibromatosis (Lederhosen) but no flexion contracture

Penile curvature (Peyronie)

Frozen shoulder

Associated clinical conditions

Diabetes (30% with diabetes <5 years, 80% with diabetes >20 years), not related to the need for insulin, possible link is a micro-angiopathy

Epilepsy (2% of patients with DD are epileptic), possible aetiological factor is phenobarbitone

Alcoholics have a slightly increased incidence

Hand trauma, may be related to occupation

Common sites for palmar nodules

Base of little finger (ADM tendon)

Fourth ray

Base of thumb and first web space

Collagen

Early stage	– type III
Active stage	– type III and type V
Advanced stage	– type I

Non-operative treatment

Splintage

Steroid injections to nodules and pads

Indications for surgery

Painful palmar nodules

Painful Garrod's pads

Contracture of 30° at the metacarpophalangeal joint

Any contracture at the proximal interphalangeal joint

Contractures of the first web space

Surgical options

Fasciotomy (Sir Astley Cooper)

Regional fasciectomy

Extensive fasciectomy (McIndoe, single transverse palmar incision)

Dermofasciectomy and FTSG (Hueston) – recurrent disease, skin involved

Joint release

- incision of the flexor sheath
- incision of the accessory collateral ligaments
- incision of the check rein ligaments (proximal attachment of the volar plate)

Joint replacement

Arthrodesis is a salvage procedure for severe recurrence (>70° at proximal interphalangeal joint)

Amputation

Variety of incisions, Brunner incisions or multiple Z-plasty

Transverse wounds may be left open if short of skin and to prevent haematoma (McCash, Dupuytren)

Most extension is gained from release of metacarpophalangeal contracture rather than IP contracture

Post-operative management

Apply volar splint

Change for thermoplastic splint at ~4 days, hand exercises 1–2 hourly

Keep splint on for 2 weeks, until removal of sutures

Use splint at night only for 6 months

Complications of surgery

Intra-operative

- division of neurovascular bundles (check pre-operatively especially in 'recurrent' disease)
- over-stretch and spasm in digital arteries leading to ischaemia

Early post-operative

- haematoma

- skin flap necrosis or graft loss
- infection

Late post-operative

- loss of flexion
- inadequate release
- CRPS type 1 (4% of males, 8% of females)
- recurrent contracture
- scar-related problems

Poor prognostic factors

Early age of onset

Presence of Garrod's knuckle pads

Multiple rays involved

Epilepsy or alcoholism

Dupuytren's diathesis

Dupuytren's disease in children

Urban, Feldberg, Janssen and Elliot. *J Hand Surg* 1996

DD very rare in children

Two children with DD <13 years of age are presented

Only seven other histologically confirmed cases of DD in this age group have ever been reported

DD in children should be treated aggressively, early dermofasciectomy

Self-assessment: A patient presents to you with Dupytren's disease. What is Dupuytren's disease and how would you manage this patient?

Dupuytren's disease is abnormal thickening and contracture of the palmar fascia, affecting predominantly the longitudinal fibres and vertical fibres (of Skoog) resulting in palmar nodules and contractures of the fingers

Commonest affected digit is IV

May be associated with other fibromatoses such as Lederhosen's and Peyronie's, also retroperitoneal fibrosis

Disease affecting mainly Caucasian men of Celtic decent (male:female ratio $= \sim14:1$) in middle to late life

Strong family history points to a single gene defect, possibly affecting the expression of γ-interferon or high-affinity TGF-β receptors on fibroblasts

In other patients environmental factors seem to play a role including diabetes, alcohol intake, anti-epilepsy drugs and occupations involving the use of vibrating hand tools – possibly via an effect on the small vessels of the hand (micro-angiopathy)

History

- age, hand dominance, occupation or hobbies
- Dupuytren's diathesis:
  - age of onset of disease
  - family history
  - rate of progression of disease
  - other affected areas

- functional deficit
- drugs – aspirin/warfarin, oral hypoglycaemics, anti-epileptics
- smoking history (effects graft take and skin flap viability)
- lives alone? (implications for postoperative discharge plans)
- previous hand surgery

Examination

- Look
  - Garrod's pads (dorsum proximal interphalangeal joints)
  - dorsal scars, swellings, sudomotor changes, skin lesions, wasting, attitude of the hand
  - volar signs as above
- Feel – palmar nodules, thickening, degree of skin involvement, sensation distal to any site of proposed surgery
- Move
  - active and passive ROM of the affected digits to quantify degree of contracture
  - examination of each of the three nerves of the hand

Investigations – plain X-rays to determine degree of joint changes if long-standing to predict expected release

Treatment

- fit with a thermoplastic night splint pending any surgery
- nodules can be simply injected with hydrocortisone
- surgery indicated for:
  - painful palmar nodules or Garrod's pads
  - thumb adduction
  - metacarpophalangeal flexion $> 30°$
  - any proximal interphalangeal joint contracture
- preferred technique:
  - brachial plexus anaesthesia
  - markings then inflate tourniquet
  - regional fasciectomy via Brunner incisions $\pm$ joint release
  - open palm (McCash) technique if significant release expected or risk of haematoma
  - dermofasciectomy for re-do's and diathesis patients
  - fasciotomy for single band to thumb
  - arthrodesis or amputation as salvage procedures
  - splint 2 weeks postoperation under the supervision of OTs and physiotherapists
  - night splint 6 months
- complications – intra-operative, early and late but all patients advised that disease will recur

Dupuytren's disease: an overview
Saar JD. *Plastic Reconstruc Surg*, 2000
Cline first proposed palmar fasciotomy as a surgical cure in 1787
Dupuytren's disease is almost unique to Caucasian races, particularly those of northern European descent
Autosomal dominant condition with incomplete penetrance
The major collagen type of normal palmar fascia is predominantly type I, although small levels of type III are present. There is an increase in the ratio of type III to type I collagen in Dupuytren's disease

Increased levels of growth factors in the diseased palmar fascia of Dupuytren's disease

- basic fibroblast growth factor
- platelet-derived growth factor
- transforming growth factor-beta
- prostaglandin-F2α and lysophosphatidic acid seem to promote myofibroblast contraction

Histology and pathogenesis

- The diseased tissue possesses the biologic features of benign neoplastic fibromatosis
- 1959, Luck classification first is the
  - *proliferative stage*
  - the second, *involutional stage*, is represented by the alignment of the myofibroblasts along lines of tension.
  - during the third, *residual stage*, the tissue becomes mostly acellular and devoid of myofibroblasts.
- Severity of functional limitation vs. importance to the patient
- The rate of progression is the best indication for surgery
- Flexion contractures of 30 degrees at the metacarpal phalangeal joint and 20 degrees at the proximal interphalangeal joint are generally considered to be indications for intervention.

Management of the fascia

- *Percutaneous fasciotomy* is intended to release the tension in the fascia
- Moermans described a *limited fasciectomy*, in which only short portions of fascia are removed
- *Regional fasciectomy* is the most commonly performed operation and entails removing all involved fascia in the palm and digit by a progressive, longitudinal dissection.
- *Extensive or radical fasciectomy* removes all involved fascia with the additional removal of uninvolved fascia to try to prevent disease progression or recurrence. This procedure is usually reserved for patients who have extensive disease or an increased diathesis.

Complications in the treatment of Dupuytren's disease is high, being reported by

- McFarlane and McGrouther to be as great as 17 to 19 per cent overall.
- Nerve and or arterial injury has been reported by McFarlane to occur in 3 per cent of patients,
- Reflex sympathetic dystrophy 5 per cent of patients
- Recurrence rates after surgery range from 26 to 80% dermofasciectomy should be considered.

Nerve compression and CTS

Nerve compression and diagnosis of level of nerve injuries can be made more difficult by the presence of the following anatomical variations

Martin–Gruber anastomosis

Taams. *J Hand Surg* 1997

Branch from the median nerve to the ulnar nerve in the forearm, which carries all the motor fibres to the ulnar nerve. Present in ~23% of subjects. Lesions to the ulnar nerve above this branch cause no motor deficit, while lesions to the median nerve cause a simian hand

Riche–Cannieu anastomosis

Similar to the Martin–Gruber anastomosis but in the palm of the hand – in up to 70% of subjects
May allow for improved prognosis in low division of the median and ulnar nerves at the wrist

Nerve of Henlé

A branch of the ulnar nerve in the forearm that travels with the ulnar artery to supply sensation to the distal medial forearm and proximal hypothenar eminence. Present in ~40% of subjects. When present, the palmar cutaneous branch of the ulnar nerve is absent

Pathogenesis of nerve compression

Anatomical – carpal tunnel
Postural – occupational
Developmental – cervical rib, palmaris profundis
Inflammatory – tennis elbow, synovitis, scleroderma, amyloid, gout
Traumatic – lunate anterior dislocation, hand trauma and swelling
Metabolic – pregnancy, myxoedema, diabetes
Tumour – ganglion
Iatrogenic – trapped by plate fixation devices, positioning on operating table
Intraneural blood flow
- 20–30 mmHg → decreased venular flow
- 40–50 mmHg → decreased arteriolar and interfascicular blood flow
- >50 mmHg → no perfusion

Long-term circulatory impairment may result from mechanical injury to these intraneural blood vessels

Compression neuropathy of the median nerve

Anatomical sites of compression
Pronator syndrome
Ligament of Struthers
Bicipital aponeurosis
Humoral and ulnar heads PT
Arch FDS
Anterior interosseus syndrome (nerve to FPL, FDS index and middle, PQ
Multiple sites distal forearm
Gantzer's muscle (accessory head FPL)
Aberant radial artery
Thrombosis ulnar collateral vessel
Carpal tunnel syndrome

Pronator syndrome

Pain in the proximal volar forearm
Increases with activity
Decreased median N territory sensation
Four sites of compression

- where the nerve passes between humeral and ulnar heads of pronator teres
- beneath the ligament of Struthers (attaches humeral head of pronator teres to the humerus above the elbow – supracondyloid process syndrome)
- beneath the lacertus fibrosus (bicipital aponeurosis)
- under arch of FDS

Pain with resisted forearm pronation

NCS indicate increased latency at the elbow

Dissect out the median nerve from a point 5 cm above the elbow to below the bicipital aponeurosis

Anterior interosseus syndrome

Compression neuropathy of the anterior interosseus nerve

Anterior interosseus nerve, branch of median, supplies FPL, FDP (index and middle) and pronator quadratus

Pain in the forearm

Weakness of pinch grip (make an 'O' sign between index finger and thumb – test for FPL and index FDP)

Middle finger FDS flexion test

Multiple compression sites in the proximal forearm

NCS indicate latency in the upper forearm

Dissect out the anterior interosseus N from its origin to the lower third of the forearm (may need to detach both heads of pronator teres)

Carpal tunnel syndrome

First described by Paget 1854

50% of cases in patients between 40 and 60 years of age

Females > males ratio = 6:1

40% have bilateral involvement

Weakness/clumsiness

Pain in the hand, occasionally referred proximally

Sensory disturbance (hyperaesthesia/paraesthesia)

Morning stiffness and numbness

Motor loss

Signs: thenar muscle atrophy, sudomotor signs

Provocation tests: Tinel's, Phalen's (positive if signs <40 s) or median N compression test

Electrophysiological changes: median nerve latency >4 ms is diagnostic, but a normal latency does not rule out CTS – 10% of NCS are false negatives

Anatomy

Transverse carpal ligament attaches radially to the scaphoid tubercle and to the trapezium and ulnarly to the hook of the hamate and the pisiform

Ten structures in the carpal tunnel: median nerve, FPL and eight finger flexors

Palmar cutaneous branch arises 6 cm proximal to the flexor retinaculum and passes superficial to it (occasionally this nerve may pierce it from deep to superficial and at this point suffer from an entrapment syndrome of its own)

Variations in the anatomy of the motor branch of the median nerve (Lanz 1977):

- **extraligamentous** branch, emerging distal to the carpal ligament and recurrent to thenar muscles (~50%)
- **subligamentous** branch, emerging beneath the carpal ligament and recurrent to thenar muscles (~30%)
- **transligamentous** branch, emerging beneath the carpal ligament and piercing it to reach the thenar eminence (~20%)
- other variations are very rare

Management

Non-operative – when entrapment of the nerve may be regarded as temporary, e.g. pregnancy

- steroid injections – 25 mg hydrocortisone
  - one-third have maintained relief of symptoms at 3 months
  - 11% have relief of symptoms at 18 months
  - classical indication is temporary, reversible CTS, e.g. pregnancy
- futuro splint at night and during provoking activities
- NSAID

Operative

- longitudinal release of transverse carpal ligament (Brain 1947)
- synovectomy where indicated
- external neurolysis
- endoscopic release
- complications include a sensitive volar scar (most common), nerve injury, pillar pain, flexion weakness, pisotriquetral pain syndrome, CRPS type 1 (or type 2 if there is nerve injury)

Recovery

- 'immediate' relief of pins and needles
- 2pd – 2 weeks
- sensory and motor nerve latencies – 3–6 months
- pinch and grip strength – 6–9 months
- more severe symptoms and longer duration of symptoms → longer to recover

Recurrent CTS

- cause
  - incomplete division of the transverse carpal ligament
  - median nerve compressed by scar tissue
  - flexor tenosynovitis
- exploration warranted for:
  - positive Phalen's test
  - night symptoms
  - positive NCS after 3–6 months

Neurophysiological testing may help identify level of residual or recurrent compression

Surgery:

- re-release of ligament
- external neurolysis
- synovectomy
- revascularization of the nerve – pronator quadratus turnover flap

Diagnosis of carpal tunnel syndrome
Gunnarsson. *J Hand Surg* 1997

Clinical examination by an experienced doctor is sufficient to diagnose typical CTS

Atypical symptoms or signs or a prior history of fracture in the limb may warrant NCS

- numbness in median nerve distribution is the most sensitive symptom (95%) but not very specific (26%)
- Phalen's test is more sensitive (86%) than Tinel's sign (62%) but less specific (48 vs. 57%)
- NCS are highly sensitive (85%) and specific (87%)
  - sensitivity = proportion of patients with CTS testing positive
  - specificity = proportion of patients without CTS testing negative (i.e. how effective the test is at excluding those patients without CTS)

Endoscopic vs. open carpal tunnel release

Thoma. *Plastic Reconstruc Surg* 2004

Meta-analysis of 13 randomized controlled clinical trials

- Endoscopic release comnpared with open release:
  - Improved post-operative pinch and grip strength in the early post-operative phase (12 weeks)
  - Less scar tenderness
  - Increased risk of reversible nerve injury (3× compared with open release) – but uncommon with either technique
- No difference in:
  - Post-operative pain
  - Time to return to work

Secondary carpal tunnel surgery

Tung. *Plastic Reconstruc Surg* 2001

Complications following carpal tunnel decompression include:

- Persistent symptoms
  - 7–20% reported incidence
  - due to inadequate release of the transverse carpal ligament (usually distally)
  - additional persistent and undiagnosed proximal compression ('double crush')
  - initial misdiagnosis as carpal tunnel syndrome
- Recurrent symptoms
  - Post-operative scarring compressing the median nerve
  - Reformation of the transverse carpal ligament with recurrent compression
- New symptoms:
  - Neurological
    - Tender scar due to injury to multiple small cutaneous branches
    - Entrapment neuropathy or division of the palmar cutaneous branch of the median nerve
    - Injury to the main trunk of the median nerve, its motor branch or digital nerves
    - Bowstringing of the median nerve
    - Injury to the ulnar nerve or its branches
    - Injury to communicating branches between median and ulnar nerves
  - Vascular
    - Haematoma following injury to the superficial palmar arch

- Wrist complaints
  - Carapl arch alteration causing pain
  - Pillar pain
  - Pisotriquetral syndrome
- Tendon problems
  - Increased incidence of triggering, thought to be due to transferrence of initial pulley-related forces from transverse carpal ligament to A1 pulleys
  - Bowing of flexor tendons
  - Tendon adhesions

Management
- Clinical evaluation to assess the underlying cause of symptoms
- Surgical options
  - Internal neurolysis
  - Exploration of alternative compression sites
  - Excision of neuroma of the palmar cutaneous branch
  - Interpositional nerve grafts to injured segments of the main trunk of the median nerve
  - Tissue interposition flaps
    - Used to separate the overlying scar from the median nerve
    - Flaps described include:
      - Pronator quadratus
      - Abductor digiti minimi
      - Palmaris brevis
      - Distally based radial forearm fascial flap

CTS vs. pronator syndrome

With pronator syndrome:
- no Tinel's sign at the wrist
- nerve conduction is delayed but not at the wrist
- Phalen's test is positive in 50% of patients with pronator syndrome

Compression neuropathy of the ulnar nerve

Anatomical sites of compression
Arcade of Struthers fibrous condensation of intermuscular septum
Medial intermuscular septum
Hypertrophy medial head triceps
Stretching caused by cubital valgus (e.g. post-supracondylar)
Cubital tunnel syndrome (Osborne's canal)
Tumours, lipomas, accessory muscle anconeus epitrochlearis, OA, RA
Facial band of Mardio between FCU and flexors
Guyon's canal

Cubital tunnel syndrome

Passage of ulnar nerve beneath the aponeurosis joining heads of FCU
Trauma at the elbow
Recurrent dislocation of the nerve in the ulnar groove of the medial condyle – neuritis
Humero-ulnar OA or RA
Ganglion at the humero-ulnar joint

Anconeus epitrochlearis

Symptoms

- ill-defined pain in the arm
- numbness in the ulnar digits
- pain with elbow flexion
- weakness of pinch grip (adductor pollicis)

Signs

- dysaesthesia in the distribution of the dorsal branch of ulnar nerve
- wasting of the first dorsal interosseus
- Tinel's sign at the elbow
- Phalen's sign at the elbow (flexion)
- positive Froment's sign
- lack of clawing (palsy above the branch to FDP – if at the wrist then long flexor causes IP flexion while there is a failure of lumbrical-mediated extension at the interphalangeals and flexion at metacarpophalangeals. However, FDPs are rarely affected so clawing may indeed be present.)
- Wartenberg's sign
  - abducted little finger in the presence of an ulnar nerve injury at the wrist and an ulnar claw hand
  - due to insertion of the EDM tendon into the tendon of ADM
- delayed nerve conduction at the elbow
- if the problem is in the neck, dysaesthesia is encountered in the C8/T1 dermatomes – inner aspect of forearm and elbow

X-rays

- AP and lateral
- cubital tunnel view – elbow flexed

McGowan classification

I – Mild, intermittent dysaesthesia

II – Persistent dysaesthesia, early motor loss

III – Marked atrophy and weakness

Treatment options

Splint/steroids

Division of aponeurosis connecting humeral and ulnar heads of FCU (**Osbourne**) – grade I and II neuropathy

Subcutaneous or submuscular anterior transposition (**Learmonth**)

- in patients in whom decompression has failed
- grade III neuropathy
- severe ulnar neuritis or persistent valgus deformity
- technique – split medial intermuscular septum above the elbow where the ulnar nerve passes through it (to enter the volar compartment of the forearm) and divide the fascia connecting the two heads of FCU
- transpose the nerve anteriorly over the muscle belly of FCU (subcutaneous transposition) or beneath the humeral head of FCU (submuscular transposition)
- transposition risks devascularization of the nerve

Medial epicondylectomy

Ulnar tunnel syndrome (compression within Guyon's canal)

Ulnar nerve and artery lie beneath the volar carpal ligament on top of transverse carpal ligament in Guyon's canal

These pass radial to the pisiform and beneath the hook of the hamate

Within the canal the nerve divides into the motor branch (can be rolled over the hook of the hamate) and the palmar cutaneous branch

In isolation, mainly due to ganglia, otherwise due to anomalous muscles or aneurysm of the ulnar A

Sensory, motor or mixed disturbance

Ulnar nerve signs

- altered sensation in ulnar N distribution
- positive Froment's sign
- positive Froment's sign between fingers
- intrinsic and hypothenar wasting
- ulnar claw posture
- Wartenberg's sign (abduction little finger due to unopposed action of EDM, which inserts on the ulnar side of the extensor expansion)
- test for pure intrinsic function – flex metacarpophalangeals and abduct/adduct the fingers

If the dorsal sensory branch is involved, the compression cannot be in Guyon's canal – must be proximal to it, i.e. cubital tunnel

Treatment is by release of the volar carpal ligament, isolating the ulnar N proximal to the wrist initially with a longitudinal incision radial to FCU

Volume of Guyon's canal increases after carpal tunnel release – ulnar compression symptoms improved in one-third of patients following CTR alone

Radial nerve compression

Anatomical sites of compression

Triangular space

Radial tunnel syndrome

    Fibrous band to radio-humoral joint

    Leash of Henry

    Arcade of Frohse

    Tendinous edge ECRB

Posterior interosseous syndrome

    Trauma

    Dislocation elbow

    Radial head

    Ganglions

    Lipomas

Wartenberg's syndrome

Radial tunnel syndrome

Radial nerve passes through triangular space formed by humerus laterally, triceps (long head) medially and teres major superiorly, to lie in the bicipital groove in the posterior compartment of the arm

Pierces lateral intermuscular septum

Enters the radial tunnel and becomes compressed between supinator and the head of the radius

Within the radial tunnel, the nerve gives off the motor branch (posterior interosseus N, third extensor compartment) and continues as a purely sensory nerve

All forearm extensors supplied by posterior interosseus nerve (C7,8) apart from:

- ECRL and ECRB (radial nerve above the elbow)
- brachioradialis (radial nerve above the elbow)

Three constriction points within the radial tunnel

Sharp tendinous medial border of extensor carpi radialis brevis

Fan of vessels from the radial recurrent artery (**leash of Henry**)

Arcade of Frohse – free aponeurotic margin of supinator: posterior interosseus N passes beneath this (posterior interosseus nerve syndrome)

Symptoms and signs

Pain in the radial tunnel

Sensory disturbance radiating to the distribution of the superficial branch of radial nerve

Positive **middle finger test** – pain upon extension against resistance (ECRB inserts into middle finger metacarpal)

Tenderness over the supinator mass

Distinguish from tennis elbow – tenderness over the lateral epicondyle (golfer's elbow = medial epicondylitis)

Management

Decompression

Brachioradialis muscle-splitting or anterolateral approaches

Good prognosis if symptoms are relieved pre-operatively by nerve block

Wartenberg's syndrome

Neuritis of the superficial branches of the radial N

Entrapped beneath the tendinous insertion of brachioradialis, anomalous fascial bands, tight jewellery and watch bands

Tenderness 4 cm proximal to the wrist

Numbness or pain in the distribution of the superficial branch of radial nerve

Treated by surgical exploration and release of constricting tissues

Thoracic outlet syndrome

Thoracic outlet
- first rib – inferiorly
- scalenus anterior – anteriorly
- scalenus medius – behind

Aetiology
- cervical rib or ligamentous band
- trauma – clavicular fractures
- posture – holding the shoulders excessively backwards or forwards
- swellings – aneurysms of subclavian artery

Neuropathy	Congenital/anatomical	Acquired
Pronator syndrome	Between heads of PT Ligament of Struthers Lacertus fibrosus (biceps)	Swellings: lipoma, ganglion
Anterior interosseus syndrome	All the above plus: fibrous bands of FDS and Ganzer's muscle (Acc, FPL)	Swellings: lipoma, ganglion
Carpal tunnel syndrome	High insertion of lumbricals Persistent median artery	Swellings: lipoma, ganglion, bony exostoses Inflammatory: RA, OA Metabolic: pregnancy, hypothyroidism, renal failure Traumatic: lunate dislocation
Cubital tunnel syndrome	Anconeus epitrochlearis Two heads of FCU	Swellings: lipoma, ganglion Inflammatory: RA, OA Traumatic: cubitus valgus, supracondylar fracture
Ulnar tunnel syndrome	Accessory PL tendon High insertion of hypothenar muscles	Swellings: lipoma, ganglion Inflammatory: RA, OA Traumatic: fracture hook of hamate
Radial tunnel syndrome	Arcade of Frohse (supinator) Leash of Henry	Swellings: lipoma, ganglion Inflammatory: RA, OA Traumatic: elbow dislocation,
	Tendinous border of ECRB	Monteggia fracture
Posterior inter-osseus syndrome	As for radial tunnel syndrome	As for radial tunnel syndrome
Wartenberg's syndrome	Free edge of brachioradialis	Extrinsic compression by watchbands, etc.

Symptoms and signs

Often bilateral

Pain, sensory disturbance, motor loss, vascular changes (including Raynaud's phenomenon)

Affects T1 and the lower trunk of the brachial plexus

Dysaesthesia of the ulnar nerve + medial cutaneous N of arm + medial cutaneous N of forearm = thoracic outlet syndrome

Symptoms on lateral neck flexion towards the affected side = root compression

Symptoms on lateral flexion away from the affected side = thoracic outlet syndrome

If there is ulnar and median wasting in the hand a thoracic outlet syndrome should be suspected

Vascular observations

Colour and temperature difference – often more obvious on the radial side of the hand

Diminished pulses

Lower blood pressure

Thrill and bruit

Provocation tests

See above – examination section

Management

First rib resection (plus cervical rib if present)

Scalene release

Polyneuropathy

Drugs, metabolic and vitamin deficiencies

Connective tissue diseases including RA

Malignancies

Post-infective (Guillain–Barré)

Hereditary (e.g. peroneal muscular atrophy = Charcot–Marie–Tooth: champagne bottle legs)

Multiple mononeuropathy

Diabetes

Leprosy, sarcoid, amyloid

Connective tissue diseases including SLE

Malignancies

Neurofibromatosis

> **Self-assessment: A patient is sent along by the GP who feels he/she may have a carpal tunnel syndrome. What is carpal tunnel syndrome, what causes it and how would you manage it?**

CTS is compression of the median nerve within the carpal canal

Causes are either congenital or acquired but in the majority of cases it is idiopathic

Congenital:

- persistent median artery
- high origin of lumbrical muscles

Acquired:

- inflammatory – synovitis, RA, gout
- traumatic – perilunate dislocation, Colles fracture
- fluid retention – pregnancy, renal failure, CCF, myxoedema, diabetes, steroid medication
- space occupying lesions – lipoma, ganglion

Management:

- history:
  - age, occupation, hand dominance, hobbies

- numbness
- pins and needles
- clumsiness
- morning stiffness
- general questioning to exclude the above aetiologies including drug treatment
- live alone – need to be able to manage post-operation
- examination – routine hand examination with attention focused particularly on:
  - median nerve sudomotor changes, wasting, sensory deficit and motor deficit
  - resisted pronation to exclude compression higher up
  - ulnar nerve signs – may be also compressed in Guyon's canal
  - exclude first carpometacarpal joint tenderness – differential diagnosis basal joint OA
  - provocation tests – median nerve compression test and Phalen's test
- investigations:
  - NCS only if unsure – 10% false negative
  - Eaton views of basal joint
- treatment – conservative or surgical or treat the underlying cause
  - conservative
    - futura splint, rest and elevation
    - NSAID
    - steroid injections – temporary causes, temporary relief
  - surgical
    - carpal tunnel release
      - LA plus tourniquet
      - incision in line with radial border fourth ray and ulnar back-cut
      - spread superficial palmar fascia preserving transversely orientated nerves
      - divide transverse carpal ligament to fat pad preserving median nerve under direct vision
      - if concerned about motor branch look for this specifically – 50% divide extraligamentous, 30% subligamentous, 20% transligamentous
      - if concerned about ulnar nerve release this also
      - wash out and 5/0 prolene
      - post-operative splint 3–4 days then futura
      - removal of sutures 2 weeks
      - keep elevated
  - complications:
    - intra-operative – injury to median N or deep palmar arch
    - early – infection, haematoma, dehiscence
    - late – inadequate release, pillar pain, flexion weakness, tender scar, CRPS type 1

Arthritis and inflammatory disorders

Pigmentedvillonodular synovitis (giant cell tumour of tendon sheath)

Benign tumour

Bossellated swelling volar surface of finger or around a joint

Treatment by excision

High rate of recurrence, possibly reduced by electron treatment

Types of arthroplasty

Perichondrial arthroplasty – young patients, restore cartilage

Resection arthroplasty, e.g. basal joint of the thumb

Silicone joint replacement – metacarpophalangeals and interphalangeals

Interpositional arthroplasty – poor bone stock: volar plate arthroplasty

Non-vascularized bone transfer, e.g. replace metacarpal with metatarsal

Vascularized joint transfer – in children, epiphysis allows continued growth

Arthrodesis – mainly distal interphalangeal disease, intra-articular fractures

Arthrodesis angles at proximal interphalangeal joint:

- index – 20°
- middle – 30°
- ring – 40°
- little – 50°

Ganglions

Mucin-filled cyst continuous with the underlying joint capsule

Three times more common in women

70% occur in the <40 s

Uncommon associations: metacarpal boss, de Quervain's disease (first extensor compartment ganglion), Heberden's nodes (mucous cysts)

Differential diagnoses over the dorsum of the hand include lipoma and extensor tenosynovitis

Present due to cosmesis, pain, wrist weakness

History of trauma in up to 10%

No correlation with occupation

No reported case of malignancy

Subside with rest, enlarge with activity

Spontaneous rupture and resolution

50% recurrence if inadequately excised

Pathogenesis poorly understood (Angelini and Wallis. *J Hand Surg* 1985)

Ball valve effect

Metaplasia produces microcysts and fibrous metaplasia forms mucoid cells

Embryonic rests (ganglions may arise away from synovial joints)

Test for rotatory subluxation of the scaphoid – if present (clunking) then the ganglion is likely to recur following excision

Recurrence may also be related to the presence of occult intra-osseous ganglions

Management

Non-operative

- aspiration and injection of steroid (small or occult dorsal ganglions)
- extrinsic rupture

Operative treatment

- excision without closing the joint capsule
- closure of joint capsule leads to prolonged immobilization and stiffness
- avoid injury to superficial branch of radial nerve

Common ganglions of the wrist and hand

Dorsal wrist ganglion

70% of all ganglions

Directly over scapholunate ligament (midline) or connected to it by a pedicle

Occult ganglions may only be identified by volar wrist flexion and may be associated with underlying scapholunate diastasis (e.g. RA)

Transverse incision and exposure of the ganglion between thumb and index finger extensors (ECRL, ECRB and EPL radially and EC and EI ulnarly)

Note: the rare **extensor tendon ganglions** are located more distally over the back of the hand

No treatment unless there is pain, functional disability, a long history (>4 years) or RSS: **60% of dorsal wrist ganglions will resolve**

Volar wrist ganglion

Second most common ganglion (20%)

Arise mainly from the radiocarpal ligament

Lie under the volar wrist crease between FCR and APL

Care to preserve the radial artery during surgery – often intimately attached to, or encircled by, the ganglion (hence perform Allen's test before surgery – lack of ulnar perfusion may contra-indicate surgery)

Flexor sheath (seed) ganglions

- ~10% of ganglions
- Arise from the A1 pulley or occasionally more distally
- Small, firm, tender mass in the palm or base of the finger
- Excise with a small portion of the flexor sheath

Mucous cyst

Ganglion of the distal interphalangeal joint

Older patients

Dorsum of the finger lying to one side of the central slip insertion

Overlying taught skin and may necrose

Associated with OA (and osteophytes of DIPJ which need to be removed)

Carpometacarpal boss

Second/third carpometacarpal joints

Twice as common in women

Twice as common on the right hand

20–30s

Pain and decreased extension at the wrist

Palpable bony lump (exostosis) confirmed by X-ray

30% associated with wrist ganglion

Excision may lead to recurrence – rongeur bone after excision

Cast for up to 6 weeks post-operation

Recurrence may require fusion

Bone tumours

Benign:

- enchondromas commonest
- multiple enchondromas = Ollier's disease
- multiple enchondromas + vascular malformations = Maffucci syndrome
- both can → chondrosarcoma (>25% before 40 years)
- differential diagnoses:
  - fibrous dysplasia
  - infection
  - myeloma
  - hyperparathyroidism
  - gout – peri-articular erosions

Osteoid osteoma

Characterised by pain relieved by NSAIDS

Hot spot bone scan

Radiolucent nidus with surrounding sclerosis

Usually in young adults

Surgery involves curettage plus/minus bone grafting

May be treated with radiofrequency ablation

Malignant – commonest are metastases, especially bronchial Ca

Most common tumour of the upper limb is SCC

Rhabdomyosarcoma is the commonest sarcoma of childhood

Dorsal compartments of the wrist/forearm

1 APL, EPB
2 ECRB, ECRL
3 EPL
4 EDC, EI
5 EDM
6 ECU

Radial wrist pain

- De Quervain's
- Intersection syndrome
- Radial nerve entrapment (Wartenberg's syndrome)

De Quervain's disease (1895)

Musculotendinous units become inflamed either where they pass through tunnels or at a bony attachment

Stenosing tenovaginitis of APL within the first dorsal compartment at the radial styloid

APL and EPB become constricted in a synovially lined compartment under the extensor retinaculum before forming the inferior border to the snuffbox

In 20–30% of patients there may be two separate tunnels for each tendon

EPB is absent in ∼5% of people

History
- several months of pain at the radial side of the wrist aggravated by movement
- overuse of the wrist and hand
- commonly middle-aged women

Signs
- positive **Frinkelstein** test (pain on ulnar deviation with the thumb clasped in the fist)
- may have a small ganglion in the first dorsal compartment
- may co-exist with basal joint OA
- differentiated from the intersection syndrome (pain more proximally located)

Management
- non-operative
  - steroid injections
  - wrist immobilization
  - local heat
  - NSAID
- operative
  - 2 cm transverse incision over first dorsal compartment just above the level of the radial styloid
  - preserve superficial branch of radial nerve
  - longitudinal release of the first compartment by incising extensor retinaculum
  - synovectomy may be required where there is RA

Intersection syndrome

Pain and swelling of **muscle bellies** of APL and EPB at the site at which they cross the tendons of the second dorsal compartment, ECRL and ECRB, 4 cm proximal to the wrist
Basic pathology relates to a tenosynovitis of the second dorsal compartment
Operative treatment is by release of the second compartment

Trigger finger

Stenosing tenosynovitis of the flexor tendon
Primary (including congenital) or secondary
Secondary due to RA, gout, diabetes
May co-exist with de Quervain's disease or with CTS
Ring and middle fingers mostly affected in adults (index rarely)
Steroid injections of benefit only to triggering of short duration but recurs frequently
Release of A1 pulley offers operative cure
In general beware releasing the pulley in RA – A1 pulley attaches to the head of the metacarpal, release may exacerbate tendency towards volar subluxation

Tennis elbow

Lateral epicondylitis
Distinguish from radial tunnel syndrome by the middle finger test (no pain in tennis elbow)
May be due to partial tears of the extensor origin

Treatment options

Rest, splints, anaesthetic steroid injections

Surgery – repair of tears, release of the extensor origin, partial excision of the annular ligament – all fairly unsuccessful

Differential diagnoses of arthritides

Juvenile RA – poly-/mono-/pauci-articular; 80% seronegative; splint

Ankylosing spondylitis – sacroiliac joints; HLA B27; 20% have RA features; 10% seropositive

SLE – antinuclear antibody; ligamentous joint deformity; Raynaud's

Scleroderma – fibrous deformity; calcinosis circumscripta; digital ischaemia; 40% seropositive; CREST

Psoriatic arthritis – seronegative; distal interphalangeal joints; phalangeal erosions; periosteal new bone

Ulcerative colitis – transient arthritis; related to UC disease activity; seronegative

Behçet's syndrome – oral and genital ulcers; iritis; elbow and wrist arthritis

Reiter's syndrome – polyarthritis; urethritis; conjunctivitis; HLA B27

Disease in the distal interphalangeal joint more likely to be psoriatic arthritis than RA – in RA is usually secondary to proximal interphalangeal deformity

RA – non-articular problems:

- uveitis
- anaemia
- polyneuropathy
- lung changes
- vasculitic skin ulcers

Extra-articular manifestations of SLE:

- commonest of the connective tissue diseases (but RA 20× more common)
- especially prevalent in pigmented races – 1 in 250
- women 20–40 years
- antinuclear antibody
- 90% get joint involvement although SLE arthritis affects mainly the soft tissues rather than joint surfaces
- **butterfly rash on face**
- liver palms, purpuric rash in fingers, Raynaud's phenomenon
- vasculitis affecting heart, lungs and kidneys
- may also have neurological and GI manifestations

Felty's syndrome

RA

Lymphadenopathy

Splenomegaly, granulocytopenia, anaemia, thrombocytopenia

Sjögren's syndrome

Keratoconjunctivitis sicca

Xerostomia

Basal joint OA

Commonest-affected OA joint

Usual symptoms and X-ray changes (narrowed joint space, sclerosis, cysts, osteophytes, etc.)

Pain staging (Arnot and Saint Laurent):

- 0 – no pain
- 1 – pain during particular activities
- 2 – pain during daily activities
- 3 – episodes of spontaneous pain
- 4 – constant pain

High density of oestrogen receptors in the basal joint of the thumb (and in the hip) which mediate in degenerative changes (hence higher incidence in post-menopausal women)

Treatment includes:

- splinting
- intra-articular steroids
- basal osteotomy (wedge osteotomy, removing radial cortex to change the vector of stress forces acting on the joint)
- trapeziectomy with FCR sling (Burton Pellegrini)
- joint replacement
- arthrodesis

Radiological staging

Ask for Eaton views: thumbs against each other in resisted abduction, palms flat

  I   – < one-third subluxation at carpometacarpal joint

  II   – > one-third subluxation, osteophytes

  III   – Sclerosis, joint space narrowing and osteophytes > 2 mm

  IV   – Advanced degenerative changes, also involving scaphotrapezial joint

Heberden's nodes – osteophytes at the distal interphalangeal joint

Bouchard's nodes – osteophytes at the proximal interphalangeal joint

OA of the metacarpophalangeal joint of the thumb is best treated by arthrodesis

Rheumatoid arthritis

Rheumatoid factor – macroglobulin present in >70% of patients with RA

Obliterative arteritis

Radial deviation of the wrist

Ulnar deviation at metacarpophalangeal joints

Synovial disease

Stages

Proliferative – synovial swelling, pain, restricted movement, nerve compression

Destructive – tendon rupture, capsular disruption, joint subluxation, bone erosion

Reparative – fibrosis, tendon adhesions, fibrous ankylosis, fixed deformity

Pattern

Moncyclic – one episode, spontaneous remission, 10%

Polycyclic – remissions and relapses, 45%

Progressive – inexorable course, 45%

Surgery in RA is only indicated where there is pain and loss of function – deformity alone is not an indication:

- preventative – synovectomy

- reconstructive – tendon transfers
- salvage – joint surgery including lower end ulna excision, replacement, fusions
- address proximal joints before distal ones

Rheumatoid nodules (fibrinoid necrosis) are a poor prognostic factor

Most commonly found on the subcutaneous border of the ulna

Palmar erythema

First dorsal interosseus wasting, masked by an adduction deformity of the thumb

Extensor tendon ruptures due to:
- synovitis
- attrition on prominent ulna head or Lister's tubercle
- devascularization due to rheumatoid arteritis

Failure of digital extension in RA:
- attrition rupture of tendons
- subluxation of extensor tendons into metacarpal gutters
- radial tunnel syndrome with posterior interosseus nerve palsy
- metacarpophalangeal joint disruption

Neck

Atlanto-axial subluxation

Superior migration of the odontoid peg into the foramen magnum

Anterior subluxation of vertebral bodies

Wrist

Ulnar styloid and head become involved earliest

Ulna caput (head) syndrome:
- **dorsal dislocation of the ulna head**, becomes prominent and DRUJ instability
- **supination of the carpus** on the hand, limiting wrist dorsiflexion and supination on the forearm
- **volar subluxation of ECU** allowing radial deviation of the wrist and promoting attrition rupture of ulnar extensors over the prominent ulna head
- seen in up to one-third of RA patients undergoing surgery

Radial carpal rotation (increase in Shapiro angle, normally ~112°) due to erosion of the sling ligament (radioscaphocapitate)

This causes scaphoid to adopt volar-flexed position with secondary loss of carpal height

Synovitis around the ulnar head causes erosion of the triangular fibrocartilage and the ligamentous supports to the wrist

Radial scalloping

Anterior subluxation of the wrist renders flexor tendons less effective and promotes intrinsic plus, hence fingers adopt a swan neck deformity

Ulnar head (DRUJ) instability detected by the *piano key test* – depress head and release – will spring back

Options

Tenosynovectomy, tendon transfers (ECRL to ECU to reduce radial carpal rotation) and joint synovectomy

Ulnar head surgery

- resection
  - dorsal approach, preserve ECU and dorsal branches of ulnar nerve
  - limited **excision of head** (distal 2 cm) and burr edges
  - **synovectomy** of DRUJ
  - **stabilize the distal end of ulna** – distally based slip of ECU passed through a hole in the dorsal cortex of the distal end of ulna and sutured back on to itself
  - turnover flap of extensor retinaculum to pass under ECU and back on itself to **stabilize ECU radial and dorsal**
- Sauve–Kapandji procedure
  - fuse distal ulna to radial head
  - remove a segment of ulna proximal to this to allow forearm rotation
  - suited to younger patients with painful DRUJ

Limited wrist fusion

- early collapse
- destruction limited to radiocarpal joints
  - synovectomy and removal of articular cartilage from affected joints
  - proximal row fusion – radius, scaphoid and lunate
  - mid-carpal fusion – all joints surrounding the capitate
- cancellous bone graft from distal radius or excised ulna head
- K-wires, removed at 6 weeks

Total wrist fusion

- young patients, high, long-term stresses on joint
- significant wrist deformity/instability
- poor wrist extensor function
- poor bone stock
  - ulna head excision
  - cartilage removed from distal radius and proximal carpal row
  - Steinman pin introduced through third metacarpal and passed via carpus into medullary canal of radius, wrist in neutral
  - alternatively two pins exiting via second and third interosseus spaces, but these need removing after ~**4–6 months**
  - cancellous bone graft
  - arthrodesis using a plate allows for 50° dorsal angulation to be created
- complications
  - pseudo-arthrosis
  - pin migration
  - nerve injury
  - fracture of healed fusion at ends of pin

Tenosynovitis

Extensor tenosynovitis and tendon rupture (Vaughn–Jackson lesion)

Pain and swelling dorsum of the hand

May be accompanied by radiocarpal or radio-ulnar instability

Fibrinoid 'rice bodies' within the tendon sheath

Hypertrophic synovium erodes tendon

Attrition rupture
- radial tubercle (Lister) – EPL
- ulnar head – EDM, EDC

Management
NSAID

Steroid injections

Splints

Dorsal tenosynovectomy ± wrist joint synovectomy
- complications:
  - skin necrosis exposing tendons
  - haematoma
  - bowstringing if strip of extensor retinaculum not preserved

EPL rupture – EI transfer, APL slip transfer or interphalangeal joint arthrodesis

Rupture of finger extensor
- single – suture to an adjacent intact extensor tendon
- multiple – ring finger FDS transfer (Boyes) to motor several tendons

Differential diagnosis of extensor tendon rupture
- volar dislocation of the metacarpophalangeal joint
- dislocation of the extensor tendon into the ulnar metacarpal valley
- paralysis of extensor musculature – posterior interosseus N compression (e.g. radial tunnel syndrome, see above)

Flexor tenosynovitis and tendon rupture
Symptoms and signs as above

May also get triggering

Attrition rupture
- ridge of the trapezium – FCR
- hook of the hamate – FCU
- scaphoid bone – FPL (Mannerfelat lesion)

Management
Conservative treatment as above

Flexor tenosynovectomy plus CTR

FPL rupture – PL tendon graft or FDS transfer

FDP rupture – distal interphalangeal arthrodesis – often the best option

FDS and FDP rupture – adjacent FDS transfer to ruptured FDP

Normal 'rules' regarding tendon transfers do not always apply in RA patients:
- hostile territory
- motor tendons may be weak
- full range of passive movement may not be available

Metacarpophalangeal joints and joint arthroplasty

To look at metacarpophalangeal joints ask for Brewerton views: metacarpophalangeals flexed to 60° with the extensor surfaces of the fingers flat on the X-ray plate

Sequence of events destabilizing the metacarpophalangeal joint in RA

Ulnar drift (ulnar rotation + ulnar shift of the phalangeal base at the metacarpophalangeal joints) in the fingers due to:

- synovial erosion of the radial sagittal bands of the extensor tendons causing extensors to dislocate in an ulnar direction
- synovitis erodes the thin radial collateral ligaments but not the thicker ulnar ligaments

Volar subluxation due to:

- weakening of dorsal capsule and volar subluxation of extensor tendons
- synovial erosion and loosening of the collateral and accessory collateral ligaments weakens the attachment of the volar plate to the metacarpal and allows the pull of the flexor tendon on the A1 pulley to be transmitted to the base of the PP (instead of to the head of the metacarpal)

Palmar subluxation leads to telescoping

Metacarpophalangeal joint synovectomy

Persistent metacarpophalangeal joint synovitis

Minimal radiological changes

Little or no joint deformity

Adequate trial of conservative treatment including splints and steroids

Often combined with soft tissue reconstruction, e.g. relocation of extensor tendons and intrinsic release

High incidence of recurrence

Intrinsic muscle procedures

Anatomy of the intrinsics:

- **interosseus muscles**
  - palmar interosseii adduct towards the axis of the middle finger (PAD)
    - three small muscles (adductor pollicis to the thumb) serving index, ring and little fingers
    - arise from the middle finger side of their own metacarpal and insert into the same side of the extensor expansion and PP
  - dorsal interosseii abduct away from the axis of the middle finger (DAB)
    - four muscles (ADM to the little finger and APB to the thumb) serving index, middle and ring fingers
    - arise by two heads, one from each metacarpal bordering the interosseus space and into extensor expansion and PP on the side away from the middle finger
    - the middle finger has a dorsal interosseus on each side
  - all supplied by ulnar N; occasional variant is for first dorsal interosseus to be supplied by the median N
- **lumbricals**
  - arise from each of the four FDP tendons
  - pass radial to the metacarpophalangeal joint and insert into the dorsum of the extensor expansion at the sagittal bands, distal to the insertion of the interosseii
  - no bony insertion
  - lumbricals to index and middle finger are innervated by the median N, those to ring finger and little finger by the ulnar N
  - ulnar-innervated lumbricals are bicipital – arise by two heads from adjacent FDP tendons

- median-innervated lumbricals are unicipital
- metacarpophalangeal flexion, IP extension

Intrinsic release

Intrinsic tightness contributing to swan neck deformity

Division of the insertion of intrinsics into the ulnar sagittal band ± bony attachment

Hence intrinsics inserting ulnarly include dorsal interosseii ring and middle fingers, ADM, palmar interosseus to index

Crossed intrinsic transfer

Restores finger alignment, long-term correction of ulnar drift

Release of intrinsic insertions on the ulnar side of the ring, middle and index fingers

Usually combined with other soft tissue or joint procedures

Insertion cut and tendon mobilized up to musculotendinous junction

Insertion relocated and sutured to the RCL of the metacarpophalangeal joint (rather than the radial sagittal band as this may promote swan necking)

Swanson arthroplasty long-term follow-up
Wilson, Sykes and Niranjan. *BJHS* 1993

'A spacing device for the joint which guides encapsulation' (Swanson 1972).

Metacarpophalangeal joint is the key joint for finger function

Metacarpophalangeal joint is the joint most commonly involved in RA

Aims of surgery:

- painless joint
- functional range of movement
- joint stability
- produce a more cosmetic hand

Indications for surgery:

- pain
- loss of function

Swanson's prosthesis:

- dynamic joint spacer
- maintains alignment
- fibrous encapsulation stabilizes the joint
- relies upon a telescoping effect

Results at long-term follow-up:

- deterioration in range of motion with time
- majority of patients had sustained improvement in pain and range of movement

Complications:

- infection (1.3%)
- recurrence of deformity
- fracture or dislocation of the implant requiring revision (3.2%) – some fractures do not impair movement and do not require revision
- giant cell reactive synovitis (no patients in this study)
- bone resorption (14%)

Operative steps

Dorsal longitudinal (Swanson) or transverse incision across metacarpophalangeal joints preserving dorsal Ns and Vs

Release ulnar sagittal band (intrinsic release)

Longitudinal capsulotomy

Excision of metacarpal head preserving RCL on its distal attachment to the base of the PP

Broach and ream proximally and distally

Drill hole in dorsal cortex of metacarpal for reattachment of RCL

Swanson silicone joint replacement inserted

Reattachment of RCL

Close capsule

Plication of radial sagittal band

Irrigation, Swanson's drain and skin closure

Optional extras include division of abductor digiti minimi tendon and the ulnar intrinsics and crossed intrinsic transfer

Volar plate arthroplasty
Tupper. *J Hand Surg* 1989

Overview of the anatomy of the metacarpophalangeal joint

Collateral ligaments have two main parts:

- metacarpophalangeal part – between these two bones
- metacarpoglenoid part – from the M/C head to the volar plate – the accessory collateral ligament

Volar plate at the metacarpophalangeal joint is continuous with the transverse metacarpal ligament

Volar plate has a strong attachment to the PP but is attached to the metacarpal head by only a membranous insertion and the two lateral check rein ligaments

Accessory collateral ligament thus effectively anchors the volar plate to the metacarpal head

At the point of insertion of the accessory collateral ligament to the volar plate two other structures attach:

- the sagittal bands of the extensor tendon – keep the extensor tendon in a central position and stabilize the joint
- the proximal attachment of the flexor sheath – the A1 pulley

Intrinsic muscles pass volar to the axis of the metacarpophalangeal joint

Aims of volar plate arthrodesis

Remove the cause of the joint disorganization – synovectomy

Restore joint stability – tighten ligaments

Correct the deforming forces – realignment of long flexors and interosseii

Useful in the patient with poor bone stock

Resection arthroplasty

Transverse incision, ulnar release, capsulotomy, division of collateral ligaments (preserving RCL for later repair), synovectomy, excision of metacarpal head

Then:

- Vainio's method
  - cut the extensor tendon proximal to the metacarpophalangeal joint

- attach the distal end to the volar plate – providing an interpositional tissue
- reinsert the cut proximal end to the dorsal surface of the extensor at the proximal edge of the PP
- Tupper's criticism of Vainio's method:
  - interpositional substance not robust enough
  - impairs functioning of the extensor
  - does not correct the volar pull of the flexor on the base of the PP via the A1 pulley
- Tupper's method:
  - incise the volar plate at the proximal end – junction between fibrocartilaginous and membranous areas
  - separate the attachment of the A1 pulley from the volar plate
  - reflect the proximal end of the volar plate into the joint and attach to the dorsal edge of the cut metacarpal
- Advantages:
  - thick interpositional substance
  - elevates base of PP
  - re-establishes anchorage of the volar plate to the metacarpal

Small joint arthrodesis

Operative steps:
- dorsal incision
- split extensor tendon longitudinally
- capsulotomy and excision of joint surfaces at appropriate angles
- Lister loop (0.45 interosseus wire) and oblique K-wire
- repair extensor mechanism
- irrigation and skin closure

Fingers and thumb

Swan neck and Boutonnière deformities

	Thumb	Fingers
Swan neck	Flexion deformity at CMC joint	Intrinsic tightness or mallet
Boutonniere	Rupture of EPB	Rupture of central slip of EDC

RA – Nalebuff classification of thumb deformity
- I – Boutonnière
- II – Boutonnière plus metacarpal adduction
- III – Swan neck deformity
- IV – Gamekeeper's thumb

Boutonnière deformity
- metacarpophalangeal extension, proximal interphalangeal flexion, distal interphalangeal hyperextension
- originates at the proximal interphalangeal joint only – central slip attenuation and lengthening or rupture
- Capner splint – dynamic extension splint

- reconstruction of the extensor apparatus: dorsalize lateral bands
- Fowler tenotomy (releases distal interphalangeal joint hyperextension)

Swan neck deformity

- proximal interphalangeal hyperextension, distal interphalangeal flexion
- may originate at proximal interphalangeal joint (intrinsic tightness) or distal interphalangeal joint (lateral band ruptures cause mallet)
- management:
  - (passively correctable) proximal interphalangeal joint extension-block splint and later proximal interphalangeal silver ring splint – dynamic flexion splint
  - lateral band mobilization to bring intrinsic insertion volar to the axis of the proximal interphalangeal joint: split extensor tendon and plicating lateral and volar to proximal interphalangeal joint (± distal interphalangeal joint fusion)
  - Littler procedure
    - intrinsic tenodesis technique
    - distally based lateral band passed through a drill hole in the neck of the PP volar to Cleland's ligament and secured to a button on the other side
  - proximal interphalangeal joint fusion
  - proximal interphalangeal joint arthroplasty

For both:

- synovectomy
- arthrodesis or replacement arthroplasty (joint disruption)

Boutonnière deformity of the thumb (Nalebuff 1 and 2)

Metacarpophalangeal flexion and IP extension

Disease at the metacarpophalangeal joint

Attrition of EPB causes loss of metacarpophalangeal extension

Ulnar subluxation of EPL, extension at IP joint

Intrinsics (AP and APB) exacerbate flexion at metacarpophalangeal and extension at IP joint

Surgical treatment concentrated at the interphalangeal joint – may need to consider interphalangeal joint fusion

Try to maintain metacarpophalangeal joint mobility by dorsalizing EPL ± silicone arthroplasty

Swan neck deformity of the thumb (Nalebuff 3)

Metacarpophalangeal extension and interphalangeal joint flexion

Disease at the trapeziometacarpal joint leading to subluxation and metacarpal adduction contracture

Patient is unable to extend at the carpometacarpal – instead extension forces are transmitted to the metacarpophalangeal joint

Surgical treatment concentrated at the carpometacarpal – trapeziectomy or arthrodesis

Self assessment: Describe the various abnormalities of soft tissues and joint which may be seen in a rheumatoid wrist and hand and how they arise

Soft tissues
Synovitis

Autoimmune phenomenon – RF is a circulating macroglobulin present in 70% of RA patients

Synovial inflammation, formation of pannus, erosive enzymes

Tender boggy swelling dorsum of wrist and around flexor tendons in the carpal canal leading to tendon ruptures and disruption of the stabilizing structures around joints

Tenosynovitis of flexor tendons and triggering (A1 release worsens volar subluxation of proximal phalanges – held by pulley to volar plate and to the head of the metacarpal)

Rheumatoid nodules
Foci of fibrinoid necrosis
Ulnar border of forearm
Poor prognostic sign

Tendon ruptures
May be due to synovitis, e.g. extensor communis, horn sign
Attrition ruptures – ulnar head (EDM, EDC), scaphoid tubercle (FPL, Mannerfeldt lesion), Lister's tubercle (EPL)
Rupture of juncturae allowing ulnar subluxation into metacarpal gutters

Nerve compression
e.g. Carpal tunnel syndrome

Joints
Ulnar head syndrome
Prominent ulnar head due to disruption of radio-ulnar ligament and DRUJ instability
Supination of the carpus
Volar subluxation of ECU (permits radial wrist deviation)

Wrist joint
Supinated, radially deviated, volarly subluxed
Scapholunate diastasis with DISI
Unstable due to ligamentous and capsular erosion
Joints grossly deranged

Metacarpophalangeals
Ulnar drift = ulnar displacement and ulnar rotation due to erosion of radial sagittal bands and radial collateral ligaments
Volar subluxation of base of proximal phalanx due to erosion of dorsal capsule and attachment of membranous part of volar plate to head of metacarpal
Telescoping

Fingers
Swan neck deformity – volar subluxation of wrist renders flexor tendons ineffective; these adopt intrinsic plus deformity, intrinsics hyperextend proximal interphalangeal joints via lateral bands
Boutonnière deformity – erosion of central slip at proximal interphalangeal joint, lateral bands fall into flexion

Thumb

Nalebuff classification:

1 Boutonnière deformity, IP joint hyperextended, rupture of EPB at the level of the metacarpophalangeal joint
2 Boutonnière deformity with adduction contracture – rare
3 Swan neck deformity – volar subluxation of the thumb at the level of the carpometacarpal joint
4 Ulnar collateral ligament rupture with radial deviation of the thumb at the metacarpophalangeal joint

Congenital hand

Overview of limb development in relation to congenital hand anomalies
Tickle. *Ann Rev Cell Biol* 1994; Cohn. *Cell* 1995; Tabin. *Cell* 1995; Tickle. *BJPS* 1997
Occurs between weeks 6–8 in the human embryo

Formation of the chick limb bud

A morphogenetic field is a cluster of cells in the embryo which undergo similar development because they lie within the same set of boundaries

- Limb bud fields are related to *Hox* gene expression which makes the limb field competent to respond to initiating factors such as FGF

Limb bud mesoderm induces overlying ectodermal cells (slightly ventral) to elongate, become pseudostratified and form the apical ectodermal ridge (AER) – both the AER and the underlying mesoderm are thus required for limb development

- removal of the AER or loss of contact of the AER with limb bud mesoderm prevents limb development
- grafting AERs on to an existing limb bud generates additional digits
- grafting leg mesoderm beneath wing AER produces toes at the end of a wing

Hence cells in the limb bud mesoderm instruct the AER to develop a certain type of limb while AER cells are responsible for sustained growth and development of that limb

Development in a proximo-distal axis

AER is required for proximo-distal outgrowth and patterning
Mesenchymal cells beneath the AER proliferate rapidly to form the progress zone (PZ)

- AER prevents cells in the PZ from differentiating by releasing a factor which promotes proliferation, but once they have left the PZ and are no longer exposed to the factor they differentiate in a regionally specific manner
  - Potential morphogens include FGF-2, FGF-4 and FGF-8
- FGF-1, -2 and -4 soaked beads can replace the AER and when applied to flank somitic mesoderm result in:
  - outgrowth of limb bud and PD patterning
  - *Shh* expression and AP patterning (flank zone of polarizing activity (ZPA))
  - ectopic expression of *Hoxd-13* indicating formation of AER
  - new AER takes over to maintain new ZPA
  - wings grow from anterior somites while legs grow from posterior somites and nearly all limbs have *reversed AP polarity*

- FGF-4 expressed mainly posteriorly within the AER (hence interaction with ZPA) while FGF-8 is expressed uniformly

Effect of removing AER

- Cells leaving the progress zone early become proximal structures while those leaving later, having undergone numerous mitotic divisions, form distal structures
- Hence removing the AER early results in a severely truncated limb (e.g. formation of a humerus only), while later removal allows formation of more distal structures (e.g. radius and ulna, etc.)
- Truncation that results from removing the AER at a given stage of development is two segments behind the number of segments which have already been specified by that stage
  - For example, if all eight limb segments have been specified in the limb bud – cells having left the progress zone and beginning to differentiate into humerus (1), radius and ulna (2), first row carpals (3), second row carpals (4), metacarpals (5), proximal phalanges (6), mid-phalanges (7), and distal phalanges (8) – the resulting truncation would be a loss of middle and distal phalanges
- Can graft a young AER on to an old limb bud, which has already specified most limb segments, and cause a second limb to grow from it

Progress zone

- Undifferentiated mesenchymal cells
- *Msx-1* gene (homologue of muscle segment homeobox in *Drosophila*) is expressed in the PZ, which encodes a transcription factor promoting proliferation
- *Msx-1* expression is stimulated by FGF from the AER
- Hox genes are expressed within the progress zone
  - Contain a DNA binding site to directly regulate gene expression
  - Series of overlapping expression domains: the *Hox* code
    - Spacial and temporal co-linearity between *Hox* gene expression in the limb
    - Coordinate model for PD patterning in the PZ
  - *Hox* gene expression is dependent upon FGF and a polarizing signal (retinoic acid and/ or *Shh*)
  - Disruption of the *Hox* code results in homeotic transformations

A–P axis specification

ZPA is a small block of mesoderm at the junction of the posterior part of the limb bud and the body wall

Programmed cell death in the anterior necrotic zone results in loss of digit 1 (chick)

Diffusable morphogen model (Wolpert 1969)

- a soluble morphogen is released from the ZPA creating a P–A concentration gradient (insertion of a non-permeable barrier in the mid-line of the A–P axis prevents development of anterior structures)
- cells exposed to high concentration of the morphogen form digit 4 and those exposed to low concentration (furthest away) form digit 2

Grafting a ZPA to the anterior necrotic zone of another limb bud produces a mirror image duplication of those limb bud segments remaining to be specified (e.g. grafting late in development results in digit duplications)

- Retinoic acid-soaked beads have the same dose-dependent effect – RA expression co-localizes with the ZPA by *in situ* hybridization and when extracted from anterior and posterior halves of the limb bud confirms a higher concentration in the posterior half

- RA activates downstream expression of *Shh* expression

A feedback loop exists between *Shh* expression and FGF-4 expression by the AER

- remove AER from limb bud → decreased *Shh* expression
- add FGF bead to same bud → *Shh* expression re-instated
- a gradient of ZPA exists along flank mesoderm (somites 21–25), peaking at the site of anterior and posterior limb buds but with an addition peak in between, i.e. can respond to FGF bead by expression of *Shh*

Shh (and hence RA) also activates *BMP-2* expression and *BMP-2* activates FGF-4 expression, hence part of feedback loop

- Talpid mutant: polydactylous chick as a result of ectopic *BMP-2* expression throughout the limb bud (i.e. not posteriorly restricted by *Shh* induction)
- But *BMP-2* cannot induce digit duplications alone (therefore not the ZPA morphogen)

D–V specification

Homeobox-containing gene *engrailed-1* is only expressed by ventral ectoderm, BMPs may also be ventralizing

- *wnt-7a* only expressed by dorsal ectoderm: inactivation → double ventral phenotype
- *wnt-7a* is a transcription factor acting through *Lmx-1*

Removal of ectoderm and replacement with reversed DV polarity results in a similar reversal in the orientation of the foot

Summary

In the developing vertebrate limb, antero-posterior patterning (defined embryologically by the thumb-to-little finger axis) is dependent upon a gradient of morphogen emanating from the zone of polarizing activity (ZPA) in the posterior mesoderm of the limb bud. The ZPA also maintains the apical ectodermal ridge (AER), an ectodermal thickening capping the limb bud that, in turn, is responsible for initiating and maintaining growth and development of the limb

The ZPA co-localizes with the expression domain of sonic hedgehog (*Shh*), the vertebrate equivalent of the *Drosophila* patterning gene hedgehog. *Shh* encodes a secreted factor that may act directly as the limb morphogen or, perhaps more likely, leads to transcriptional activation of the true morphogen. Downstream of *Shh* is *BMP-2*, which interacts with another group of patterning genes, the *Hox* genes

Hox genes are expressed in an overlapping series of domains in the limb bud to generate a combinatorial code in the mesenchyme. This code specifies the developmental fate of groups of cells throughout the limb, and bud if disrupted, results in a homeotic transformation. For example, ectopic expression of *Shh* in anterior mesenchyme (inducing ectopic expression of downstream *BMP-2* and *Hox* genes) causes the outgrowth of a mirror image duplicated limb. *BMP-2* also appears to inhibit proximo-distal limb growth by antagonizing fibroblast growth factor-4 (FGF-4), the mitogenic signal from the AER

Congenital limb abnormalities, involving either absence or duplication of parts, may thus be attributed to:

Disruptions of antero-posterior patterning

- mediated by ZPA
- *Shh* → *BMP-2* →*Hox* genes

- 'longitudinal disorders'
- syndactyly – failure of apoptosis in web zones
- polydactyly – homeotic transformation – anterior ectopic *Shh* expression and disruption of *Hox* gene combinatorial code

Proximo-distal limb outgrowth disorders

- failure of AER signalling
- transverse deficiencies secondary to premature failure of specification of parts by the AER via FGF
- symbrachydactyly
- amelia

Combination of AP and PD patterning

- intercalated deficiencies
- phocomelia

Swanson classification of congenital hand deformities

About one in 600 children is born with a congenital upper limb deformity

Failure of formation of parts

Transverse – amelia, brachymetacarpia

Longitudinal –radial club hand, cleft hand

Mixed –phocomelia, symbrachydactyly (terminal differentiation)

Failure of differentiation of parts

Camptodactyly, clinodactyly, symphalangism, syndactyly, arthrogryposis

Duplication

Polydactyly

Mirror hand

Overgrowth

Macrodactyly

Undergrowth

Madelung's deformity

Constriction ring syndrome
Symbrachydactyly

Four types:

- peromelic type – digits are nubbins
- short finger type – short fingers, telescoped due to the action of rudimentary long tendons
- cleft hand type (**ulnar** side more affected)
- monodactylous type

Ulnar side more affected

Association with Poland's syndrome

Surgical options

Distraction manoplasty – 4–6 weeks, pull the digits out to length with wires, then: phalangeal transfer – before 15 months, transplant a toe proximal phalanx, problems with growth

Toe–hand transfer

Phocomelia

Complete   – hand attaches to trunk

Proximal   – forearm attaches to trunk

Distal   – hand attaches to humerus

Types:

- pre-axial
- postaxial
- central
- intercalated defect

Palmar plate prosthesis

Myoelectric prosthesis

Radial club hand

Hypoplasia or absence of the radius

Radial deviation of the hand

Bilateral in up to 75%

In unilateral cases, the opposite thumb is hypoplastic

25% have a duplicated median nerve which replaces an absent radial nerve

Fixed extension at the elbow

Impaired movement in the radial digits – index and middle

Almost all muscles are abnormal in the limb

Ulna is bowed and thickened and only 60% of its normal length

Humerus also shorter

Carpal fusion

Cardiac lesions and blood dyscrasias (**Fanconi's anaemia**)

Fanconi syndrome: pancytopenia, predisposition to malignancies

Bayne classification:

- I – Deficient radial epiphysis
- II – Hypoplastic radius
- III – Partial absence distally
- IV – Total absence distally

Syndromic radial club hand:

- Holt–Oram syndrome – association between radial club hand and cardiac septal defects
- Vater syndrome:
  - vertebral abnormalities
  - anal atresia
  - tracheo-oesophageal fistula
  - renal abnormalities

Management

Manipulation

Restore elbow flexion (physio) then centralization:

ulnar carpal excision

ulnar transfer of radial wrist motors
wedge osteotomy of ulna
Pollicization

Ulnar club hand
Less common than radial club hand
Shows the reverse skeletal abnormalities
Bayne's classification
- hypoplastic ulna
- partial aplasia
- total aplasia
- radiohumeral synostosis

Cleft hand
Bones are absent or malpositioned, but never rudimentary
Radial side more affected – hence can distinguish from symbrachydactyly-type of cleft hand (ulnar)
In severe forms only remaining digit is the little finger (in severe symbrachydactyly only remaining digit is the thumb)
Range of deformity from absence of middle ray to monodactyly
Lobster claw hand – syndactyly – care during separation, tenuous blood supply

Options
Separate syndactyly
Tendon transfers
Toe–hand transfers
Pollicization
Snow Littler procedure
- palmar-based flap from the cleft
- correction of syndactyly between thumb and index
- index metacarpal transposed ulnarly
- palmar flap inset into first web space
Radio-ulnar synostosis
Fusion of the proximal radio-ulnar joint
Primary – radial head is absent
Secondary – radial head is dislocated
Fixed pronation deformity
Compensatory hypermobility at the wrist
Radius thickened and bowed
Ulnar straight and narrow
Bilateral in 60%

Options
Minor – no treatment
Severe – rotational osteotomy through the synostosis
Synostosis can occur at a number of sites in the hand, e.g. metacarpal synostosis
Hereditary symphalangism

Congenital stiffness of the phalanges at IP joints, mainly proximal interphalangeal

Autosomal dominant trait

Affects mainly ulnar digits

Also commonly have symbrachydactyly of the middle finger

May be associated with hearing defects

Non-hereditary symphalangism associated with Apert's and Poland's syndromes

Camptodactyly

Congenital flexion deformity of the digit, usually little finger, usually at the proximal interphalangeal joint

Commonly bilateral

Occasionally inherited as an autosomal dominant trait

May present in adolescence, in females

Abnormal insertion of lumbrical or FDS

Secondary changes in proximal interphalangeal joint

Distal interphalangeal joint never involved, unless as a result of a secondary Boutonnière deformity

Options

Splintage rarely successful – <15° contracture, passively correctable

Normal joint, passively correctable

- release of anomalous intrinsic insertion
- correction of soft tissue contracture (see below)
- (Phillipe) Saffar procedure – subperiosteal lift, division of collateral and accessory collateral ligaments and check rein ligaments

Deranged joint

dorsal angulation osteotomy

arthrodesis if severely contracted

Camptodactyly: a unifying theory

Grobbelar and Smith. *J Hand Surg* 1998

Camptodactyly first described by Tamplin in 1846

- Affects <1% of the population
- No functional significance in the majority
- Static or progressive
- Surgery should be reserved for patients with a flexion contracture of >60°
- Release skin, fascia, tendon sheaths, intrinsics, collateral ligaments and volar plate
- Lengthen FDS tendon
- Plicate central slip
- All are implicated in the pathogenesis of camptodactyly but to varying degrees

Clinodactyly

Curvature of a digit in a radio-ulnar plane

Usually radial deviation at the proximal interphalangeal joint

Most commonly due to a 'δ-' phalanx (Blundell Jones, 1964) with a 'J'-shaped epiphysis – **longitudinally bracketed epiphysis**

Occasionally due to a fibrous band on the ulnar side of the digit

Phalanx may also be shortened (brachyphalangia)

Marked clinodactyly may be associated with mental retardation including trisomy 21

Many other associations including Poland's, Treacher Collins and Klinefelter's syndromes

Incidence in Down's patients up to 80%

Incidence in normal population 1–20%

Less common in Caucasians ($\sim$1%)

More common in males

Usually bilateral

Autosomal dominant inheritance with variable penetrance

Options

Surgery is essentially cosmetic

- closing wedge osteotomy (phalanx normal length)
- opening wedge osteotomy plus bone graft (phalanx short)
- reversed wedge osteotomy (wedge from long cortex turned over and inserted into shorter side)
- Vickers' procedure – rongeur of δ-phalanx epiphysis and free fat graft, useful before 6 years of age

Kirner's deformity

- May be mistaken for clinodactyly
- Volar and radial curvature at distal interphalangeal joint level
- Not congenital
- Females 7–14 years
- Starts as a painless swelling
- Arthrogryposis
- 'Windblown' hand
- Curved joints
- Disturbance in the neuromuscular control of joint movement
- Hence neurogenic – constitutes >90% of cases
- Myogenic
- Immobility leading to contractures (non-progressive)
- Includes clasped thumb deformity
- Treatment:
    - splints (may need to be continued until school age)
    - soft tissue releases
        - skin – FTSG
        - capsulotomy
        - tendon lengthening/transfers

Differential diagnoses of a flexed thumb

Fixed flexion at interphalangeal joint due to triggering (Notta's nodule) – may resolve spontaneously <2 years of age

Clasped thumb involving interphalangeal joint and metacarpophalangeal joint

- weak or absent EPL tendon
- may have UCL instability

Syndactyly

General

Incidence: 1 in 2000 live births

Family history in 10–40% (highest incidence in a small cluster in Iowa)

50% bilaterality

Twice as common in males

In order of decreasing frequency, most affected web space is third web space, then fourth, second, first

May be complicated by central polydactyly

Commonly associated with almost any other congenital abnormality

Second commonest congenital limb abnormality after polydactyly

Pathology

Always short of skin

Fascial interconnections

Shared flexor and extensor tendons

May share anomalous digital nerve and artery

Degrees of bone abnormalities varying in complexity

Individual joints commonly preserved unless there is symphalangism – joints remain incompletely differentiated and progress to ankylosis

Classification

Complete – digits united as far as distal phalanx

Incomplete – digits united beyond mid-point of proximal phalanx but not as far as the distal phalanx

Complex – metacarpal or phalangeal synostosis

Simple – no synostosis

Acrosyndactyly

- shortened digits united distally but with proximal fenestration
- association with constriction ring syndrome

Contraindications to surgery

Minor degree of webbing, not cosmetically or functionally significant

Severe complex syndactyly, digits share common structures including digital N and A

Hypoplastic digits where one digit functions better than would two

Adjacent webs should not be released simultaneously

Feet? (hypertrophic scars)

Timing of surgery

Most hand movements are learned between 6 and 24 months so argument made for operating before 2 years of age

Indications for early surgery in syndactyly:

- border digits
- length discrepancy

Surgical technique

Dorsal and palmar zigzag incisions (or lazy-S)

- to midline of digits
- to lateral borders (Zachariae)

Dorsal and volar inverted V flaps at the base of the web or

Larger rectangular dorsal flap inset into a horizontal incision on the palmar surface

FTSG from groin

Map flaps from the dorsal to the volar surface markings

Zigzags should make ~60° angles

Buck–Gramcko technique for division of the syndactyly nail: use matching tongue flaps at the tip of the finger curled around the raw edge of the ipsilateral nail bed

Visualization of neurovascular structures is easier from the volar surface

Tie in grafts without tension

Deepening of web spaces achieved by four-flap Z-plasty (120° Z-plasty) or jumping man flap

Postoperative complications

Intra-operative and early

- division of nerve or tendon
- circulatory deficit (grafts too tight or digital A injury/shared)
- haematoma
- infection
- graft loss

Late

- destabilization of joints
- deformity of the digit or web
- creeping of the web during growth spurt

Polydactyly

Commonest congenital limb abnormality

Stelling classification

I – Skin only

II – Part of a digit articulating with a phalanx or bifid metacarpal

III – Complete ray, including metacarpal (rare)

Central duplication

Types I–II

Type II is invariably within what appears clinically to be a simple complete syndactyly

Duplicate thumb

General

0.8 per 1000 live births

Male:female ratio = 2.5:1

~50% are Wassel type IV

Wassel type VII has the strongest familial tendency

Wassel classification

I – Bifid distal phalanx

II – Duplicated distal phalanx

III – Bifid proximal phalanx

IV – Duplicated proximal phalanx

V – Bifid metacarpal

VI – Duplicated metacarpal

VII – Partially duplicated metacarpal (also hypoplastic duplicate thumb (no skeletal elements) and triphalangia)

Interconnections similar as for syndactyly

Often shorter and thinner than normal thumbs (triphalangia approaches length of fingers)

Hypoplasia of soft tissues and bone in the central portion

Eccentric insertion of tendons along central borders, pulling thumbs together

Radial duplicate receives the hypothenar musculature

Ulnar duplicate receives adductor pollicis and the first dorsal interosseus

Absence or hypoplasia of these muscles is common

Anomalous insertion of FPL into the extensor expansion (Lister) promoting abduction

Surgery

Excision (pouce flottant), combination, revision

Excision

- appropriate where the duplicate is rudimentary (hypoplastic) without skeletal elements
- also where the accessory thumb is widely separated from a normal thumb

Combination

- required for all other duplications to provide optimal function and cosmesis
- combination 1 (C1, symmetric), combination 2 (C2, asymmetric) and combination 3 (C3, on-top-plasty) procedures
  - C1 – Bilhaut–Cloquet procedure
    - excision of adjacent marginal structures
    - merger of bone and soft tissue in a side-to-side fashion
    - Wassel types I and II
  - C2
    - nearly all of one digit is retained
    - augmented with tissues from the other digit, e.g. skin only
    - tissues from the 'spare-part' duplicate which are not used are excised
    - Wassel type IV
  - C3
    - segmental digital transposition
    - brings the best distal segment of one duplicate on to the best proximal segment of the other

Revision

- secondary surgery
- intrinsic transfer
- realignment of eccentric tendon insertions

Mirror hand (ulnar dimelia)

Rare upper limb abnormality

Duplication of the ulna

Absence of the radius

Polydactyly with midline symmetry

Usually have seven fingers (5–4–3–2–3–4–5)

Six cases of multiple hand described in the literature

Macrodactyly

Congenital enlargement of a digit

Probably a form of neurofibromatosis, also vascular malformations

Tendons and blood vessels are of normal size (relative ischaemia)

Metacarpals normal size, phalanges enlarged

Little movement

Gross curvature

Static – development of the digit keeps pace with growth of the hand

Progressive – more common, more aggressive, rapid growth

Treatment

Amputation may be best option, otherwise:

Debulking of fat

Nerve stripping

Reduction and longitudinal osteotomy

Epiphyseal ablation

Hypoplasia of the thumb

Commonly requires pollicization of the index finger in the first year of life

Buck–Gramcko classification

I – Hypoplasia – normal skeleton and musculature but *all hypoplastic*

II – Hypoplasia

- reduced volume or absence of thenar muscles
- first web space **adduction contracture**
- bones narrow

III – Hypoplasia

- **absence of thenar muscles**
- severe first web space contracture
- metacarpophalangeal joint instability
- may have absence of trapezium and scaphoid

IV – Pouce flottant

- rudimentary appendage attached by small skin bridge
- no metacarpal, trapezium or scaphoid
- neurovascular pedicle within the skin bridge
- **treatment by amputation and pollicization**

V – Total aplasia

- no skeletal or soft tissue elements
- compensatory changes in index finger
- **treatment by pollicization**

Thumb reconstruction

Principles

Allow opposition

Must be sensate

Must have good circumduction at carpometacarpal joint

Joints must be stable to allow pinch grip

Distal end of a pollicized digit must reach to the proximal interphalangeal finger crease of the middle finger when the thumb is adducted

Pollicization

Pollicization used for type III–V hypoplastic thumbs

- metacarpal head assumes role of trapezium
- thumb dissected as an island flap pedicled on neurovascular bundles and long tendons
- pronation of 160° and hyperextension at the metacarpophalangeal joint
- first dorsal interosseus assumes role of APB
- first palmar interosseus assumes role of adductor pollicis
- extensor communis to the index becomes APL
- extensor indicis becomes EPL

Littler 1953

- suited to the amputated thumb
- palmar and dorsal skin flaps
- resection of the index metacarpal (and metacarpophalangeal joint) and distal half of thumb metacarpal
- base of index PP fused to base of thumb metacarpal in 120° pronation, 10° flexion
- advancement of flaps into new first web space
- transfer of first dorsal interosseus insertion to radial border of index
- transfer of EPL to EDC of index
- late transfer of FPL to FDP in the forearm
- maintain two digital As and their VCs **plus** one dorsal vein
- need to ligate the branch of the common digital A to the radial border of the middle finger to allow full mobilization of the index ray
- common digital nerve is split longitudinally

Zancoli 1960

- first pollicization technique for the congenitally absent thumb
- index metacarpal head fused to the trapezoid
- origin of 'first' dorsal interosseus transposed across the palm to the hypothenar eminence to cause adduction of the new thumb
- no shortening of long extensors and flexors

Carroll 1988

- removal of the diaphyseal segment of the index metacarpal and fusion in 120° pronation
- shortening of extensors but not flexors
- detachment of palmar and dorsal interosseii from the base of the PP and reinsertion into the base of the MP to achieve adduction and abduction

Buck–Gramcko 1971

- subcapital excision of the index metacarpal
- hyperextend the base of the PP on the metacarpal head and suture this complex to the carpus in 160° pronation
- shorten the EI tendon and use this as a permanent motor
- redirect EDC volarly to act in adduction
- distal advancement of interosseii as above

- no need to shorten flexor tendon
- may need later opponensplasty as described above (FDS ring finger, ADM transfer)

Following trauma
Thumb replantation
Finger replantation with pollicization
Toe–hand transfer/wrap-around (first or second toes)

Madelung's deformity
Autosomal dominant inheritance
Presentation ages 8–12 years
Abnormality of radial epiphysis in ulnar anterior portion
Radius: short, radial inclination >20° with the horizontal
Ulnar: dorsal subluxation, enlarged ulnar head
Carpus: wedge shaped
Pain and decreased supination at the forearm

Treatment options
Excision of ulnar head (prominent)
Wedge osteotomies of the radius

Constriction ring syndrome
Patterson classification
Simple constriction
Constriction and lymphoedema
Constriction and acrosyndactyly
Amputation
- urgent release is required to reduce lymphoedema
- multiple circumferential Z-plasty
- may have paramedian facial cleft
- may have trunk defects

Self-assessment: A newborn baby with a radial club hand deformity is referred from your paediatrician colleague. What is your approach to management?

Assessment, investigation, planning and treatment within a multidisciplinary team environment
- plastic/hand surgeon
- paediatrician
- paediatric nurse
- physiotherapist and occupational therapist
- geneticist

History
- age, sex (mostly males affected)
- one or both hands (75% are bilateral)
- events relating to pregnancy (?antenatal diagnosis)

- any other symptoms diagnosed by the paediatrician – **radial club hand a feature of**:
  - Fanconi's syndrome: pancytopenia and predisposition to malignancy
  - Holt–Oram syndrome: cardiac septal defects
  - VATER syndrome: **v**ertebral anomalies, **a**norectal atresia, **t**racheo-**e**sophageal fistula, **r**enal anomalies
- family history of congenital hand abnormalities
- how does the child use the hand and elbow?
- can the hand be put to the mouth?
- development in general

Examination

- general body habitus and morphology
- both sides:
  - degree of hypoplasia of the upper limb as a whole
  - degree of radial angulation of the hand
  - degree of hypoplasia of the thumb (Blauth)
  - shoulder movements, elbow movement (may be extended due to humeroulnar synostosis)
  - wrist and hand movements passive and active (fingers may be stiff)

Investigations

- AP and lateral plain X-rays
- determine Bayne type:
  - hypoplastic radius
  - partial aplasia distally
  - remnant/fibrous anlage
  - total aplasia
- investigations relating to syndromal anomalies

Treatment

- splints and physiotherapy to maximize elbow movements
- centralization if good elbow movement:
  - closing wedge osteotomy of ulna
  - closing wedge osteotomy of ulnar carpus
  - release/transfer of radial deviators – FCR, ECRB, ECRL
  - release of radial soft tissues – Z-plasty
  - Steinman pin through third metacarpal
- if elbow movement is less good → radialization through second metacarpal
- Buck–Gramcko pollicization

Spastic disorders of the upper limb

Aims of treatment:

- restore function
- relieve pressure areas and enable personal hygiene
- relieve pain from nerve compression
- delay rebalancing surgery until neurological recovery is maximal – distinguish between reversible brain injury and non-reversible injury – chronic spasticity disorders (including cerebral palsy)

- regional anaesthesia helps to differentiate between spasticity and established contractures

Non-operative treatment:

- maintain passive ROM
- serial splintage
- protect pressure areas
- intraneural phenol injections of motor nerves
- Botox injections

Surgical treatment:

- stabilize joints
- tendon lengthening (partial tenotomy at musculotendinous junction)
- nerve decompression (carpal tunnel and Guyon's canal)
- address three groups of muscles:
  - extrinsic wrist and digital extensors and flexors
  - intrinsics
  - thumb and first web space

In the functioning hand:

- forearm pronation – tenotomy of pronator teres
- thumb adduction – release skin contracture (four-flap Z-plasty or jumping man) and release adductor pollicis from its origin on the third metacarpal and transverse carpal ligament (avoiding injury to the ulnar nerve)
- intrinsic tightness – release

In the non-functioning hand:

- extrinsic flexor tendon contracture – superficialis to profundus transfer with tenodesis to form a single juncturae
- ulnar motor branch neurectomy at the wrist for intrinsic spasticity if passively correctable under anaesthesia and tendon lengthening achieves metacarpophalangeal extension to neutral; if, under anaesthesia, the deformity is not passively correctable then intrinsic release is indicated for established tightness
- proximal row carpectomy and wrist arthrodesis
- arthrodesis of the subluxed thumb metacarpophalangeal or interphalangeal joint
- bone block between thumb and index metacarpals

6 Burns (pathophysiology and acute and long-term management)

Epidemiology

0.5–1% of the UK population sustains burns each year

10% requires admission

Of admitted burns, 10% are life threatening

75 000 burn victims admitted to hospital each year in the USA

45% of US admissions for scalds are in children <5 years of age

Kitchen and bathroom are commonest locations for injury in the home

Flame burns are the largest group of patients admitted to a burns unit

Burns sustained during road traffic accidents have a high incidence of concomitant injury

Acid burns commonest among people working in plating or fertilizing industries

Alkali burns commonly seen following use of oven cleaners or soap manufacture

Dyes, fertilizers, plastics and explosives manufacture associated with phenol burns

HF burns – etching processes, petroleum refinement, air conditioner cleaning

1000 deaths/year in USA due to electrical injury, including 80 due to lightning

Outcome

Burn size vs. mortality shows a sigmoid distribution, 0% with low TBSA% and plateauing at 100% mortality rate with 100% burn

LD_{50} (%BSA resulting in death of half the cohort) in 1950 for 21-year olds was 45%; in 1990 increased to 85%

Improvements in mortality rate due to:

- early and effective resuscitation
- control of sepsis
- improved management of inhalation injury
- early excision
- development of alternative wound closure materials

Resuscitation of major burns

First aid at the scene:

- extinguish flame, switch off power source, remove chemical-soaked clothes, etc.
- cool the burn wound
  - reduces direct thermal trauma and stabilizes mast cells, reducing release of histamine and other inflammatory mediators
  - cooling achieves some pain relief, also hydrogel dressings
  - 15 °C running water (avoid iced water – vasospasm and further compromise of tissue perfusion)
  - keep ambient temperature high
  - worth considering even up to 2 h post-burn
  - remove molten synthetics
- dilute acids and alkali

In A&E – approach as for any multiply traumatized patient – ABC

- **A**irway with C-spine control
  - ensure C-spine control
    - sand bags and tape
    - in-line immobilization
    - hard collar
  - provide 100% oxygen at 8 litres/min
  - check airway patency – talk to patient
  - use Yankhauer sucker to remove debris from mouth
  - chin lift or jaw thrust manoeuvre
  - secure the airway
    - Guedel airway (nose to angle of mandible for approximate size)
    - nasopharyngeal airway (exclude cribriform plate fracture)
    - endotracheal tube
      - adults size 7 (female) or 8 (male)
      - children – formula: age/4 + 4 (or size of nostril/little finger nail)
    - emergency cricothyroidotomy

- **B**reathing
  - look, feel, listen
  - pneumothorax
    - large-bore cannula mid-clavicular line second intercostal space
    - chest drain
  - may need emergency chest escharotomy – including FT thoraco-abdominal injuries in children – diaphragmatic breathing
- **C**irculation with haemorrhage control
  - apply pressure to actively bleeding wounds
  - assess fluid deficit – check peripheral and central pulses and BP
  - insert and secure two large-bore cannulae preferably through unburned skin (antecubital fossae) – consider interosseus infusion in children <2 years of age
  - take blood for FBC, U&Es, glucose, Gp&S or X-match, COHb, ABGs
  - commence Hartmann's infusion

Disability
- AVPU:
  - alert
  - responding to voice
  - responding to pain
  - unresponsive
- pupils

Exposure
- remove all clothing but maintain a warm ambient temperature
- remove all jewellery
- log roll patient to check back
- estimate %BSA according to Wallace rule of nines
- estimate depth
- recognize need for escharotomy

Fluids
- calculate fluid requirement according to the Parkland formula:
  - 3–4 ml/kg body weight/%TBSA
  - give 4 ml if there is:
    - inhalational injury
    - child
    - pre-existing dehydration
      - alcohol or other drug
      - delay in transfer
    - electrocution injury with concealed tissue damage
    - concomitant injury causing loss of circulating volume (may need blood)
  - give **half** in the first 8 h, backdating to the time of the injury
  - give the remaining **half** over the next 16 h
  - children need maintenance fluid:
    - use dextrose saline
    - watch for hypoglycaemia (low hepatic glycogen stores)
    - watch for hyponatraemia (use half normal saline if transfer is delayed)
    - 100 ml/kg up to 10 kg
    - 50 ml/kg up to 20 kg

- 20 ml/kg up to 30 kg
- fluid formulae are only guides – need to monitor resuscitation

Monitoring

- continue to monitor pulse, BP, respirations and core temperature
- ECG
- pulse oximeter (beware CO poisoning)
- insert urinary catheter
  - require 0.5–1.0 ml/kg/h in adults
  - require 1.0–2.0 ml/kg/h in children
  - if urine output falls then consider:
    - fluid challenge 5–10 ml/kg
    - increase next hourly fluids by 150%
    - manage haemochromogenuria with:
      - high urine output
        - 12.5 g/litre mannitol
        - 25 mmol/litre $NaHCO_3$
  - check specific gravity (1.010–1.020)
- insert nasogastric tube (exclude basal skull fracture)
- X-rays – C-spine, chest, pelvis
- analgesia
  - slow IV infusion
  - incremental doses of morphine
  - 0.1 mg/kg morphine repeated after 5 min

Re-evaluation of primary survey

Secondary survey

- **Ample** history
  - allergies
  - medications
  - past medical or surgical history
  - last meal
  - events and environment of injury
- head-to-toe examination
- non-life-threatening injuries
- consider escharotomy (see below)

Following resuscitation:

- management of the burn wound
  - toilet with aqueous chlorhexidine
  - dress with clingfilm
  - silver sulphadiazine topically if burn wound is contaminated, transfer delayed and agreed by the receiving burns unit
    - contraindicated in pregnant or nursing mothers and children <2 months due to kernicterus – mental retardation, deafness, epilepsy, spasticity (haemolysis followed by bile pigment deposition in the basal ganglia)
    - impedes re-epithelialization (effect on keratinocyte DNA?)
- documentation
- contact burns unit
- make arrangements for transfer

- emotional support to relatives
- tetanus prophylaxis

Criteria for transfer to a burns unit

Burns at extremes of age unless minor

FT or deep PT burns >10% in children or 15% in adults

Inhalation injury

Burns of special areas:

- face
- perineum
- hands and feet

Electrical or chemical burns

Burns requiring escharotomy

Burns of the female genitalia
Burd. *Burns* 1996

Genital burns more common in females than males ratio $= \sim$3:1

Flame burns in adults, scalds in children

Also electrical and chemical injuries

Principles of treatment:

- urinary diversion (but remember that catheter is a potential portal for infection)
- prevention of infection – daily bath/shower rather than prophylactic systemic antibiotics
- burn wound managed by exposure and topical SSD
- conservative rather than surgical approach
- vaginal stents
- late release of scar contracture

Burn shock and oedema

Increased pulmonary and systemic vascular resistance and myocardial depression despite adequate volaemic resuscitation due to local and systemic inflammatory mediators

Burn wound oedema plus severe and sustained oedema in non-burned tissues

Development of burn wound oedema is biphasic:

- immediate formation of oedema within the first hour of injury
- second phase of fluid sequestration at 12–24 h post-burn
- resolution phase begins $\sim$48–72 h
- normal Starling's forces indicate a slight filtration pressure overall, with this being matched by lymphatic drainage

Oedema impairs oxygen delivery

Globulins and fibrinogens, large protein molecules, tend to be retained in the circulation while smaller proteins including albumin leak out, even though capillary pore sizes are larger than the largest proteins

May be due to the capillary basement membrane remaining intact despite injury to the endothelium

Burn wound oedema develops due to:

- increased capillary permeability (inflammatory mediators)
- increased capillary hydrostatic pressure – nearly doubled (hyperaemia, inflammatory mediators, post-capillary sludging of erythrocytes, venular constriction)
- decreased tissue hydrostatic pressure (unfolding of complex macromolecules including collagen)
- decreased plasma oncotic pressure (loss of albumin into the tissues)
- increased tissue oncotic pressure (accumulation of albumin in the tissues and breakdown of protein macromolecules into smaller and more osmotically active subunits)

Mediators of burn wound injury

Histamine

- responsible for the early phase of increased capillary permeability
- release from mast cells in heat-injured skin
- arteriolar dilatation and venular constriction
- stimulation of xanthine oxidase
- ameliorated in rats by mast cell stabilizers (cromoglycate) or H_2 antagonists (cimetidine)

Prostaglandins, leukotrienes and thromboxane

- products of the arachidonic acid pathway
- prostaglandins and leukotrienes
- released from neutrophils (arrive at 4–5 days post-burn) and macrophages (follow arrival of neutrophils)
- neutrophil-blocking antibodies given post-burn shown to reduce oedema
- PGE2 (most important prostaglandin in the pathogenesis of burn wound oedema) and LB4–LD4 all cause increased vascular permeability
- PGI2 is a vasodilator and increases capillary permeability
- TXA2 produced locally by platelets
- TXA2 less important in oedema formation but cause vasoconstriction to extend the zone of coagulative necrosis
- serum TXA2:PGI2 ratios increased in burn patients
- systemic ibuprofen in sheep reduces post-burn tissue ischaemia by blocking TXA2 production but has little effect on burn wound oedema

Kinins and serotonin

- bradykinins increase capillary permeability
- serotonin causes vasoconstriction but increases permeability

Catecholamines

- vasoconstriction
- affect vessels in non-burned skin, muscle and viscera

Oxygen radicals

- unpaired electron, strong oxidizing agents
- superoxide anion (O^{2-}), H_2O_2, hydroxyl ion (OH^-)
- hydroxyl ion is the most damaging ($Fe^{2+} + H_2O_2 \rightarrow Fe^{3+} + 2OH^-$)
- catalase neutralizes H_2O_2 while superoxide dismutase neutralizes O^{2-}
- iron chelators (desferrioxamine) may be protective against OH^- formation
- mechanism of generation of free radicals:
  - destruction of membrane phospholipids by thermal injury

- phospholipase A_2 acts on free phospholipids, converting them along arachidonic acid pathways
- products of arachidonic acid pathway are chemotactic to neutrophils
- neutrophils are a source of O_2 free radicals that injure further membrane lipids and stimulate further phospholipase A_2
- xanthine oxidase may be the pivotal mediator in free radical production
  - xanthine oxidase catalyses the conversion of hypoxanthine to xanthine in endothelial cells
  - free radicals are released as byproducts of this process
  - histamine stimulates xanthine oxidase
  - hence cromoglycate, H_2 receptor antagonists and allopurinol (inhibits xanthine oxidase) may all be beneficial
- reperfusion injury results as flow is re-established to a zone of stasis, providing oxygen to drive renewed free radical production

Angiotensin II and vasopressin (ADH)

- fall in renal perfusion pressure stimulates the release of renin from juxtaglomerular cells (afferent arteriolar cells) – monitor renal perfusion in the kidney
- renin converts a circulating α-globulin, angiotensinogen, to angiotensin I
- angiotensin I is converted in the circulation (mainly pulmonary endothelial cells) by angiotensin-converting enzyme (ACE) to angiotensin II
- angiotensin II
  - acts upon the hypothalamus to release ADH
    - ADH also released by the hypothalamus due to stimulation of osmoreceptors monitoring plasma osmolality
    - promotes water re-absorption from the collecting ducts
    - feeds back to inhibit renin secretion
  - acts at the adrenal cortex (zona glomerulosa) to release aldosterone
    - aldosterone also released due to sympathetic efferent discharge
    - aldosterone increases sodium (and water) retention at the distal convoluted tubule
  - causes vasoconstriction including the efferent renal arterioles
  - induces thirst
  - feeds back to inhibit renin secretion

Catabolic stress hormones

- glucagon
- ACTH and glucocorticoids

Macrophages and post-burn immune dysfunction

Schwacha. *Burns* 2003

Macrophages are major producers of inflammatory cytokines including:

- Prostaglandin E2
- Reactive nitrogen intermediates
  - Inducible nitric oxide synthetase within macrophages leads to the formation of nitric oxide
    - Cytotoxic and cytostatic effects
    - Lymphocyte suppression
- Interleukin-6
- Tumour necrosis factor alpha

An exccessive ('hyper-reactive') macrophage response leads to over-production of inflammatory mediators and immune dysfunction

Nitric oxide, inflammation and acute burn injury

Rawlingson. *Burns* 2003

L-arginine – oxidation by nitric oxide synthetase $\rightarrow$ nitric oxide ($NO^\bullet$)

Role of $NO^\bullet$:

- Produced by many cell types including vascular endothelium
- Important regulator of vasomotor tone (previously 'endothelium-derived relaxing factor')
  - Increased capillary permeability
- Inhibits platelet aggregation
- Systemic effects as a neurotransmitter
- Required for leukocyte-mediated killing – may contribute to resistance to infection and wound healing at later stages of inflammation
- Interacts with cyclo-oxygenase and inducible nitric oxide synthetase (to regulate its own synthesis)
- Reacts with superoxide free radicals to produce the highly reactive peroxynitrite molecule
  - Cellular dysfunction and tissue injury
- Implicated in local burn wound inflammation and the systemic inflammatory response to a major burn including pulmonary and cardiovascular dysfunction
  - Dysregulation to $NO^\bullet$ production is associated with multiple organ failure

> **Self-assessment: What do you understand by the term 'inflammatory mediators' in the context of a burn injury?**

Inflammatory mediators are those local and systemic factors that are responsible for the physiological reaction to thermal injury

Responsible for changes in the capillary microcirculation promoting oedema

- increased capillary pressure (vasodilatation)
- increased capillary permeability (vasodilatation)
- decreased capillary oncotic pressure (loss of albumin from the circulation)
- increased tissue oncotic pressure (albumin leaks out of circulation, large proteins break up into more osmotically active units)
- decreased tissue hydrostatic pressure (unfolding of macromolecules)

Local

- histamine – released by mast cells in burned skin
  - arteriolar dilatation and venular constriction
  - pain
  - increased capillary permeability $\rightarrow$ early peak of oedema (first hour)
  - stimulation of xanthine oxidase pathways
    - endothelial cell membrane hypoxanthine $\rightarrow$ xanthine
    - are a byproduct of oxygen free radicals
- prostaglandins
  - PGE2-α and prostacyclin – neutrophils – arteriolar vasodilatation
  - neutrophils also a source of oxygen free radicals
  - second peak in oedema (24 h)

- leukotrienes
- kinins
- thromboxane – platelets – thrombosis → extends zone of necrosis

Systemic

- stress response – catecholamines, glucagon, cortisol
- homeostasis response
  - decreased BP → juxtaglomerular cells → renin
  - renin → angiotensinogen → A1 → lungs (ACE) → A2 (+ osmoreceptors) → hypothalamus → ADH → collecting ducts → water resorption
  - A2 (+ SNS discharge) → adrenal → aldosterone → sodium and water retention at the distal convoluted tubule

Systemic effects of a major burn

Reduced cardiac output
- decreased venous return
- inadequate preload
- increased afterload – increased systemic vascular resistance
- decreased myocardial contractility – myocardial depressant factor?
- persists despite adequate resuscitation

Increased SVR
- catecholamines
- sympathetic activity
- neuropeptide Y
- ADH
- angiotensin II

Pulmonary oedema
- increased pulmonary vascular resistance
- increased capillary pressure
- increased capillary permeability
- left heart failure
- hypoproteinaemia
- direct vascular injury following inhalation

Protein metabolism
Increased metabolic rate
Growth inhibition

Burn wound

Jackson's burn wound model
- zone of central coagulative necrosis
- zone of stasis

- restore capillary microcirculation
- re-establish tissue perfusion
- limit the production of free radicals
- zone of hyperaemia – burns >25% BSA incorporate the whole of the body in the zone of hyperaemia

Skin

Skin area $\sim$0.2–0.3 m^2 in the newborn; 1.5–2.0 m^2 in the adult

Epidermal thickness 0.05 mm (eyelids)–1 mm (sole of the foot)

Dermis 10∞ thicker than epidermis site for site

Males have thicker skin

Children have thinner skin

Functions:
- mechanical barrier to bacterial invasion
- immunological organ
- control of fluid loss
- thermoregulation
- neurosensory
- social interaction
- vitamin D metabolism

Depth assessment
- erythema
  - epidermal burn
  - sunburn
  - not included in area estimations
  - painful
  - blanch
- superficial partial thickness
  - painful
  - blisters
  - blanch
  - hair follicles
- deep partial thickness
  - may be painless
  - small or no blisters
  - fixed staining in tissues
- full-thickness
  - waxy white or charred eschar
  - painless
  - no blisters

Blisters
- leakage of plasma from heat-damage vessels
- epidermis separates from the dermis due to damage to the dermo-epidermal junction
- osmotically active particles within blister fluid cause enlargement with time
- contain harmful inflammatory mediators

- considered as an open wound since the overlying skin has lost the normal functions of skin
- de-roof large blisters but can leave smaller blisters alone

Eschar

- an open wound
- retains none of the normal functions of skin:
  - mechanical barrier to infection
  - thermoregulation
  - control of fluid loss
- continued source of protein loss including complement
  - exacerbates immunosuppression
  - compromises wound healing
  - consumption of clotting factors, fibrinogen and platelets
- medium for bacterial growth
- source of heat-derived inflammatory mediators and toxins which may compromise distant organ function
- if circumferential may impede distal circulation
- thoracic and thoraco-abdominal eschars may compromise ventilation

Resuscitation fluids

Resuscitation must take account of obligatory burn oedema

Give the least amount of fluid required to maintain tissue perfusion avoiding both under and over-resuscitation

Replace sufficient salt (lost into burn tissue from the extracellular fluid)

Formulae are only guides

Choice of resuscitation fluids:

- crystalloid
  - recommended by the BBA
  - Parkland formula (above)
  - Hartmann's solution
- colloid
  - but may leak out of the circulation and potentiate third space losses (although non-burned tissues re-establish normal permeability shortly after injury)
  - avoids hypoproteinaemia which drops capillary oncotic pressure and worsens oedema
  - Muir and Barclay formula:
    - TBSA% × weight kg/2 = one ration
    - give one ration 4 hourly in the first 12 h
    - give one ration 6 hourly in the next 12 h
    - give remaining ration over 12 h
- hypertonic saline
  - reduces volume of resuscitation fluid required
  - causes shift of intracellular water to the extracellular space causing intracellular dehydration
  - also complicated by excessive Na^+ retention and hypernatraemia

- dextran
  - high molecular weight polysaccharide (polymerized glucose)
  - 40 000, 70 000 and 150 000 dalton molecules
  - 40% excreted in the urine, remainder slowly metabolized
  - dextran 40 improves flow by reducing red cell sludging
  - dextran 70 causes more allergic reactions and compromises blood grouping
- fresh frozen plasma
  - use in children
  - delivers passive immunity
  - risk of viral transmission
  - hypoproteinaemia develops rapidly in paediatric patients
- plasma exchange – indications
  - ongoing fluid requirements $>2\times$ that predicted by the Parkland formula
  - despite resuscitation with hypertonic saline
  - major thermal injury

Albumin debate

Report in *BMJ* (July 1998) by Cochrane injuries group
- meta-analysis of 30 studies comparing albumin with crystalloid resuscitation fluid in three groups:
  - hypovolaemia
  - burns
  - hypoproteinaemia
- risk of death higher in albumin-treated group
- relative risk for hypovolaemia was 1.46
- relative risk for burns was 2.40
- for every 17 patients treated with albumin there is one additional death (six for every 100)

Criticisms of the report:
- 80% of paediatric burns $>95\%$ TBSA in the USA given albumin survive
- only three burns studies were included (1979, 1983, 1995)
  - dissimilar studies
  - <150 patients
  - indications and regimens for giving albumin in these studies were not standard policy in burns units

Fluid replacement after 24 h
- oedema has peaked
- if hypertonic saline was used need to give free water to contain serum hyperosmolality
- if crystalloid was given need to give protein to treat hypoproteinaemia (5% albumin)
- albumin may be given according to the Brooke formula: 0.5 ml 5% albumin/kg/%TBSA
- maintenance fluid via enteral feeding
- K^+ requirements double to 120 mmol/24 h
- 24–48 h post-burn urine output is an unreliable guide to volaemic status
  - glucose intolerance (anti-insulin stress hormones) leading to osmotic diuresis

- disturbances of ADH secretion (inappropriate ADH, diabetes insipidus)
- high respiratory water loss
- patients generally require a urine output of:
  - 1500–2000 ml/24 h (adult)
  - 3–4 ml/kg/h (children)
- monitor hydration by plasma sodium and urea concentration

Self-assessment: Describe your fluid resuscitation protocol for a burns patient during the first 48 h post-burn

Use the Parkland formula, Hartmann's solution (BBA guidelines regarding 3 or 4 ml)
- 3–4 ml × weight (kg) × %TBSA
- half in the first 8 h, back to time of injury
- remainder in the next 16 h
- only a guide – monitor UO
  - adults – 0.5–1.0 ml/kg/h
  - children – 1.0–2.0 ml/kg/h
- plus maintenance in children (dextrose saline)
  - 100 ml × first 10 kg
  - 50 ml × next 10 kg
  - 20 ml × next 10 kg

Next 24 h
- urine output no longer a guide to volaemic status:
  - hyperglycaemia → glycosuria → osmotic diuresis
  - may have syndrome inappropriate ADH
  - may have diabetes insipidus
- oedema has peaked and need to restore serum albumin
- Brooke formula – 0.5 ml 5% albumin/kg/%TBSA

Alternative resuscitation fluids:
- albumin – Muir and Barclay formula
  - weight (kg) × %TBSA/2 = one ration
  - give one ration 4 hourly first 12 h
  - one ration 6 hourly next 12 h
  - one ration next 12 h
  - less total fluid given compared with Parkland formula
- Cochrane injuries group report, *BMJ* 1998
  - multivariate analysis of deaths following albumin resuscitation in
    - hypovolaemia
    - hypoproteinaemia
    - burns
  - relative risk of death in burns 2.40
  - but three dissimilar studies only, <150 patients, not using UK protocols
  - and does not equate with the US experience of >85% survival in children >95% TBSA
- other fluids:
  - dextran
  - fresh frozen plasma (albumin and passive immunity but viral risk)

Enteral feeding as maintenance – double potassium requirement

Burn wound dressings and topical agents

Protective

Reduce evaporative heat and water loss

Absorb wound exudate

Pain relief

Burn wound eschar may become infected

Organisms include *Staphylococcus aureus*, Gram-negative bacteria including *Proteus* and *Klebsiella* and mixed anaerobes including *Escherichia coli*

Eschar needs cleansing with aqueous chlorhexidine at each dressing change

Mafenide acetate may be used as a topical antiseptic but is painful to apply and, through inhibition of carbonic anhydrase, may contribute to a metabolic acidosis

Silver sulphadiazine

Broad-spectrum activity – active against all of the above

Also active against *Pseudomonas* and *Candida*

But penetrates eschar poorly – not suitable for treating invasive infection in an eschar, only for prophylaxis

Commonest toxic side-effects:
- transient neutropenia (5–15%)
  - 2–3 days after initiation
  - monitor blood counts carefully
  - recovers even if SSD is not withdrawn
  - no increase in infection rate
- maculopapular rash (5%)
- haemolytic anaemia in patients with glucose 6-PD deficiency
- methaemoglobinuria
  - rare side-effect
  - oxidation of Fe^{2+} (ferrous) to Fe^{3+} (ferric – inactive) in haemoglobin
  - 3% of all haemoglobin is methaemoglobin normally – converted back by methaemoglobin reductase – deficiency inherited
  - treat with 1 ml/kg 1% methylene blue

Do not use on face – silver deposits

Change dressing daily

Formation of a pseudo-eschar

May inactivate enzyme-debriding agents (varidase)

Can cause kernicterus in children <2 months old

0.5% silver nitrate

Active against *Staphylococcus*, *Pseudomonas* and other Gram-negatives

Insoluble limiting toxicity by systemic absorption

Leaching of electrolytes, especially sodium, from the burn wound and oral supplements are essential especially in children to avoid rapid hyponatraemia

May also rarely cause methaemoglobinaemia

Incorporated into wet gauze dressings – over-concentrating beyond 0.5% is toxic to normal cells

Prophylactic use only

Stains overlying materials brown/black

Surgical management of the burn wound

Types of burn surgery:

- immediate – escharotomy, tracheostomy
- early – tangential excision and grafting <72 h
- intermediate – tangential excision and grafting >72 h
- late – post-burn reconstruction

Rationale for early excision (days 1–2)

- improved survival rate
- decreased hospital stay (<1 day per %BSA)
- fewer metabolic complications
- reduced blood loss
- reduced expenditure
- all confirmed by a number of studies
  - Burke. *J Trauma* 1986
  - Herndon. *J Trauma* 1986
  - Pietsch. *J Paediatr Surg* 1986
  - Tompkins. *Ann Surg*
  - Herndon. *Ann Surg* 1989
  - Muller. *Lancet* 1994

Rationale for excision >3 weeks

- easier to determine which areas are non-viable
- hence, less BSA grafted

Tangential excision

- first described by Janzekovic 1975
- ungrafted deep PT burns form hypertrophic scars
- hot water scalds in children are the exception to early excision; should be excised only after 3 weeks to avoid excess blood loss and removal of viable tissue – often indeterminate depth
- inject adrenaline subcutaneously before excision and use tourniquet where possible

Fascial excision

- indicated where fat is deeply involved
- poor cosmetic appearance
- less bleeding
- good graft take
- lymphoedema

Intra-operative patient care

- monitor core temperature
  - oesophageal, rectal or bladder probes
  - keep ambient temperature high
- avoid hypo- or hypervolaemia

- urine output
- central venous pressure monitoring
- arterial lines
- estimate blood loss
  - $0.4\,\text{ml/cm}^2$ if within 24 h
  - $0.75\,\text{ml/cm}^2$ between 2 and 16 days post-burn
- ensure good haemostasis
  - tourniquets
  - topical thrombin spray
  - topical adrenaline soaks 1:10 000
  - cautery
  - temporary pressure dressings
- care of pressure areas

Wound closure

- sheet or meshed SSG
  - sheet graft hands, face, flexural creases
  - scalp, scrotum and axillae may be the only available donor areas
- cadeveric allograft
  - meshed 1:1.5 and laid over 3:1 meshed autograft
  - burns patients are immunosuppressed so rejection delayed
  - reduced water and electrolyte losses
  - reduced protein loss
  - reduction in pain and wound infection
  - must be retrieved within 24 h of death from a refrigerated cadaver under aseptic conditions
  - serology for HBV, HCV, HIV
  - skin samples for culture of bacteria, yeast and fungi
  - storage
    - in nutrient media at $4\,°\text{C}$ for up to 1 week
    - cryopreserved
      - must be performed within 72 h of retrieval
      - controlled freezing at $0.5\text{--}5\,°\text{C/min}$ to $-196\,°\text{C}$
      - liquid nitrogen and a cryoprotectant solution
      - rapidly rewarmed to $50\text{--}70\,°\text{C}$ ($\sim3\text{--}4\,°\text{C/min}$)
      - 85% viability at 1 year
  - 32 000 square feet of allograft skin used in the USA annually (equivalent to ~1500 full adult skins)
  - 30–50 skin banks in USA
  - donor exclusion criteria:
    - high-risk categories for HIV
      - homosexuals
      - drug abusers
      - tattoos
      - prostitutes
      - haemophiliacs
    - infection/sepsis
    - neoplasia

- autoimmune disease
- >3 million tissue transplants (including skin) have been carried out since the recognition of HIV with only two cases of viral transmission

Organization of skin banks in the UK
Freedlander. *Burns* 1998

Similar inclusion/exclusion criteria to the above

One-page questionnaire to GP requesting information on past medical and
social history

Preservation media comprising of 15% glycerol in PBS with penicillin, streptomycin and
amphotericin B added

Skin banked in 15% glycerol at −80 °C (viable)

Alternatively in 98% glycerol at room temperature

- non-viable but 2-year shelf life
- biological dressing
- eliminates intracellular viruses

Biological skin substitutes

Including Jones. *Br J Plastic Surg* 2002

Products available for wound *cover*:

- Biobrane
  - Silicone sheet on a nylon mesh
    - Nylon mesh coated with porcine collagen
  - Peeled away as the wound heals over 10–14 days
  - Clean superficial partial thickness burns
  - Split skin graft donor sites
  - Temporary cover of excised deeper burns
- Transcyte
  - Similar to Biobrane but collagen-coated nylon mesh is seeded with neonatal fibroblasts to improve wound healing via the synthesis of:
    - fibronectin
    - type 1 collagen
    - proteoglycans
    - growth factors
  - Cryopreservation renders fibroblasts non-viable
  - Suited to the treatment of partial thickness burns but expensive and no proven benefit compared with Biobrane
- Apligraft
  - Cultured allogeneic neonatal keratinocytes on a gel matrix of bovine type 1 collagen seeded with viable neonatal fibroblasts
    - Keratinocytes fail to express MHC type II antigen after 7 days of culture
  - Main indication is in chronic wounds (e.g. venous ulcers) but very expensive
- Dermagraft
  - cultured human fetal fibroblasts in polyglycolic acid (Dexon) or polyglactin-910 (Vicryl) mesh
  - fibroblasts remain viable despite cryopreservation

- stimulates in-growth of fibrovasular tissue from the bed and margins of the wound and migration of host keratinocytes
- main use in diabetic and chronic ulcers
- may be useful for dermal replacement beneath split skin autograft at excised burn wound sites
- AlloDerm
  - Function similar to that of Dermagraft
  - Human cadaveric skin
  - Epidermis removed
  - Cellular components extracted to remove immunocompetency
  - Functions as dermal replacement only
  - Split skin autograft required
  - Reduces contractured at reconstructed sites of deep burn wounds
- Xenograft

Products available for wound *closure*:

- Integra
  - dermal matrix composed of bovine collagen and shark proteoglycan (chondroitin 6-sulphate)
  - silicone elastomer membrane
    - removed ~3 weeks
    - covered with thin epithelial autograft
  - in-growth of fibroblasts and vascular endothelial cells
  - less hypertrophic scarring
  - remains pliable (no contracture)
  - infection risk – silver nitrate soaks
  - must have good haemostasis and a favourable bed
  - may insulate sufficiently to provoke hyperthermia if used to close massive burns
  - can be meshed
  - expensive
  - take ~80%
  - good cosmetic and functional outcomes
- Cultured epithelial autograft (CEA)
  - requires a full-thickness skin biopsy of several square centimetres
  - fragile sheet (fibrin glue delivery system)
  - $1.8\,m^2$ sheet five cells thick
  - 3 weeks' preparation time
  - separates easily from underlying dermis – bullae contain high levels of TXA2 and PGE2 suggesting on-going inflammation
  - 80% graft take, late loss
  - suspension
    - fibrin glue suspension
    - takes less time
    - cells less mature
    - less ligand-specific integrins/adhesion molecules are expressed facilitating graft take
    - may be used in combination with meshed SSG
    - donor site re-epithelialization

Growth hormone therapy and conservatively managed burns
Singh. *Burns* 1998

rhGH given subcutaneously once daily for 2 weeks

Reported benefits were:

- improved donor and burn wound healing
- preservation of serum albumin
- increased GFR
- reduction in weight loss
- shorter hospital stay

Potential problems:

- transient hypercalcaemia
- albuminuria
- hyperglycaemia

0.2 mg/kg growth hormone SC daily accelerates burn and donor site healing

- one-third of patients experience transient hyperglycaemia requiring insulin
- induces positive protein balance
- reduces hospital stay in massive burns

Inhalation injury

Above the larynx – thermal injury to the upper airways

Below the larynx – chemical injury to alveoli due to dissolved acidic products of combustion

Systemic – toxic effects of inhaled poisons

80% of fire-related deaths are due to inhalation injury

Maximum upper airway oedema and narrowing occurs $\sim$24 h post-injury

Inhalation injury in an adult worsens mortality rate by 40%

Inhalation injury plus pneumonia worsens mortality rate by 70%

Carbon monoxide toxicity

Haemoglobin (Hb) O_2 dissociation curve shifted to the left

Toxic symptoms at levels >20% (headache) and progressive deterioration until death at levels >60%

COHb >5% indicative of inhalation injury but not severity

200–250 × greater affinity for Hb than oxygen

Also binds cytochromes – sick cell syndrome – cytochrome-bound CO washed out after $\sim$24 h causing secondary rise in serum COHb and possibly post-intoxication encephalopathy

Half-life of COHb $\sim$250 min on air and 40–60 min on 100% oxygen

Hyperbaric oxygen accelerates breakdown of COHb (30 min at 3 atm)

Late neurological deterioration several months afterwards

Hydrogen cyanide toxicity

Binds to and inhibits cytochrome oxidase – uncouples oxidative phosphorylation

Rapidly fatal at inspired concentrations >20 ppm and serum levels >1 mg/l

Smokers have $\sim$0.1 mg/l

Bitter almond odour

ST elevation

Increased ventilation via stimulation of peripheral chemoreceptors makes toxicity worse

Treatment:

- amyl nitrite
  - traps cyanide on to Hb rather than the cytochromes:
    - Hb (Fe^{2+}) + amyl nitrite $\rightarrow$ Hb (Fe^{3+})
    - Hb (Fe^{3+}) + cyanide $\rightarrow$ cyanohaemoglobin
- sodium thiosulphate
  - provides the sodium substrate for conversion of cyanide (bound to Hb) to thiocyanate (SCN) by rhodanase: S + CN – **hepatic rhodanase** $\rightarrow$ SCN
  - slow action
  - SCN excreted in the urine resulting in an osmotic diuresis
- hydroxycobalamin
  - chelating agent
  - complexes with free cyanide to aid renal excretion
- 100% O_2

Other toxic gases

- HCl – alveolar injury and pulmonary oedema
- NO – pulmonary oedema, cardiovascular depression
- aldehydes

Pathophysiology of inhalation injury

- release of inflammatory mediators
- increased pulmonary artery blood flow
- bronchoconstriction (TXA2) and increased airway resistance
- hence V–Q mismatch
- decreased pulmonary compliance – predisposes to barotrauma in the ventilated patient
- interstitial oedema
- fibrin casts within the airways – acts as a culture medium to promote infection and cause distal atelectasis
- formation of a pseudomembrane during the healing phase – $\sim$18 days post-injury
- permanent airway stenosis/fibrosis

Symptoms

- shortness of breath/dyspnoea
- brassy cough
- **hoarseness**
- wheezing

Signs

- circumoral soot and burns
- soot within the mouth
- increased respiratory rate
- increased effort of ventilation
- **stridor**
- altered consciousness

Investigations

- arterial blood gases

- carboxyhaemoglobin
- chest X-ray
- fibreoptic bronchoscopy

General management

- always give supplementary humidified O_2
- elevate bed to reduce pulmonary oedema and pressure on the diaphragm by abdominal viscera
- increase the fluid resuscitation where there are concomitant cutaneous burns
- intubate early if significant inhalational injury is suspected
- physiotherapy and sputum culture
- bronchoalveloar lavage/suctioning/toilet
- mechanical ventilatory support
- avoid barotrauma, even if $PaCO_2$ is slightly high
  - high-frequency (jet) ventilation reduces tidal volume and airway pressures
  - barotrauma results in:
    - pneumothorax
    - pneumomediastinum
    - surgical emphysema
- aerosolized or systemic bronchodilators
- aerosolized acetyl cysteine – powerful mucolytic
- antibiotics predispose to over-population with opportunistic organisms
  - treat only recognized infective complications rather than prophylactically
  - source of infection either from ET tube or opportunistic from patient's GI and skin commensals
  - stress ulcer prophylaxis with either sucralfate or H_2 receptor antagonists does not affect pneumonia rates; Cioffi. *J Trauma* 1994
- avoid tracheomalacia and long-term tracheal stenosis
  - ensure cuff pressures of <20 cm H_2O
  - conversion from ET to tracheostomy if period of supported ventilation is prolonged

Extracorporeal membrane oxygenation in the treatment of inhalation injury
O'Toole. *Burns* 1998

Conventional ventilation does not always ensure adequate oxygenation

ECMO used to treat severe but reversible cardiorespiratory failure

Must tolerate limited heparinization

Right internal jugular vein via ECMO and back to right carotid artery

Two paediatric burn cases reported

Paediatric burns

Two-thirds of paediatric burns are scalds

A child with an uncomplicated 95% burn has ∼50% chance of survival

Larger surface area:volume ratio

Paediatric circulating volume is ~80 ml/kg; adult 60 ml/kg

Alteration in the rule of nines to reflect proportionately larger head and smaller lower limbs

Need a higher urine output ~1–2 ml/kg/h

Prone to hypoglycaemia (less stored glycogen) and hyponatraemia (cerebral oedema)

Interosseous infusion allows delivery of up to 100 ml/h of fluid – low marrow fat content hence fat embolus is rare

May only show signs of hypovolaemia late – when up to 25% of circulating volume has been lost

- normally have a lower BP than adults (~100 mmHg systolic)
- immature kidneys, less concentrating ability, urine output continues despite hypovolaemia
- HR poorly indicative of hypovolaemia in a child
- delayed refill, pallor, sweating, obtunded consciousness are ominous late signs
- but avoid volume overload which may easily precipitate right heart failure and also pulmonary oedema
- cardiac output, is more closely related to HR than filling pressure

Resuscitation is accompanied by a diuresis which washes out potassium – replace with potassium phosphate since hypophosphataemia may also occur

Paediatric airways develop more rapid resistance for a given degree of swelling compared with adults because they are smaller

In comparison with the adult the paediatric larynx/upper airway is:

- shorter
- more prone to laryngomalacia
- occluded by tonsils and adenoids
- larger floppy epiglottis
- more prone to bronchial irritability and thus spasm

Greater surface area:volume ratio and fewer thermoregulatory compensatory mechanisms:

- no shivering reflex in neonates
- less insulating fat
- poorly developed pilo erection
- all result in tendency towards hypothermia:
  - ventricular arrhythmias
  - oxyhaemoglobin dissociation curve shifted to the left
  - CNS and respiratory depression
  - burned patients normally have a temperature ~38 °C, hence concern if lower
  - maintain ambient temperature of ~30 °C
  - minimize evaporative water loss

Beware non-accidental injury

Longer-term problems in children:

- inhibition of growth during the 3 years post-burn without subsequent compensatory catch-up
- breast development may be unimpaired, even where there is burn to the nipple–areolar complex
- circumferential truncal burns do not cause problems during later pregnancy in adult life
- joint contractures appear to be more of a problem in children than adults, more so where excision has been to fascia rather than fat
- limitation in respiratory reserve where there has been inhalation injury up to 2.5 years post-burn
- psychosocial problems

Differences are encountered during the resuscitation phase and longer-term phase of treatment

A – airway narrower (tonsils, adenoids) and shorter, floppy epiglottis, more prone to laryngomalacia and spasm

B – rely upon diaphragmatic respiration hence thoraco-abdominal burns, even if not circumferential, may need escharotomy

C – larger circulating volume (80 vs. 60 ml/kg), HR less of an indicator of volaemic status, BP maintained well until late, may need to gain access by intra-osseus infusion, need a higher urine output

D – less able to cooperate with neurological examination

E – larger surface area:volume ratio therefore lose heat more quickly and less thermoregulation response, skin thinner hence burns deeper, different Wallace rule of nine values for head and lower limbs

F – use 4 ml/kg/%TBSA, also need maintenance, beware hypoglycaemia due to less stored glycogen

AMPLE – different premorbid conditions, e.g. more asthma less angina, may be the victim for NAI, different type of burn injury – usually scalds

Emotional response – different needs

Longer-term – different calorie requirements, growth retardation an issue in children, long-term reduction in respiratory reserve following inhalation injury

Burn complications

MRSA

MRSA vs. the burn patient

Cook. *Burns* 1998

Common cause of nosocomial infection

Combination of open wounds and immunosuppression

Burn wound colonization may lead to loss of skin grafts and systemic sepsis

MRSA carry *mec-A* gene encoding low affinity bacterial cell wall penicillin-binding proteins with reduced affinity for β-lactam

Strain typing useful to monitor spread of infection and response to treatment

Some strains produce an enterotoxin leading to toxic shock syndrome

High incidence of environmental contamination in burns units

Infection control measures may be inadequate in this setting

Around one-quarter of *Staphylococcus aureus* wound swabs in burns patients grow MRSA; Lesseva, *Burns* 1996

Burns patients should be screened and barrier nursed

Careful use of antibiotics

Treatment
- early wound closure
- topical mupirocin (resistance now being reported)

- topical silver sulphadiazine
- systemic vancomycin (resistance now being reported in Japan – very high incidence of MRSA –60–90% of all *Staphylococcus aureus* infection)

MRSA in burns patients – why all the fuss?

Reardon. *Burns* 1998

No difference in length of stay, number of operations or mortality rate between MRSA positive and age and burn-matched control MRSA-negative patients

Excessive isolation of MRSA patients compromises nurse contact, rehabilitation and patient morale

Must eradicate all *Staphylococcus aureus* infection regardless of methicillin sensitivity or resistance

Prevention and control of MRSA infections (including *Current Opinion in Infectious Disease Farr. 2004*)

MRSA first identified in 1961

Increased use of vancomycin has led to the development of vancomycin-resistant *Enterococcus*

MRSA accounts for 50% of all nosocomial infections in the US

- Increased morbidity
- Prolonged hospital stay

Close proximity to infected patients and inadequate hand washing by healthcare personnel are risk factors for spread

- Also use of quinolone antibiotics and ciprofloxacin

Detection methods:

- Culture and susceptibility testing
- Slide latex agglutination test
- Polymerase chain reaction

Prevention

- Hand hygiene
  - Hand washing
  - Alcohol hand rubs
    - Rapidly bactericidal *in vivo*
    - Slow regrowth
    - Acts by protein denaturation
- Environmental decontamination (disinfection)
- Isolation of infected patients
- Decolonisation of infected patients
  - 5-day course of:
    - nasal bactroban
    - chlorhexidine throat gargle
    - bactroban wound ointment daily
    - triclosan skin cleanser

Treatment of MRSA infection

- vancomycin alone or in combination with:
  - frusidin
  - rifampicin

- high spontaneous mutation rate and development of resistance
- no contraindication to wound closure by split skin graft or other means

What's new in burn microbiology?

Edwards-Jones. *Burns* 2003.

Infection accounts for over 50% of deaths from major burns

- immunosupression
  - especially with burns >30% TBSA
- lack of antibiotics
- warm ambient temperature
- moist environment
- most burns units advocate early wound debridement and grafting and silver sulfadiazine antimicrobial wound dressings
  - other topical atimicrobial agents include povidone iodine and cerium nitrate
    - silver sulfadiazine + cerium nitrate = Flammacerium™
- infective complications may be mistaken for the hypermetabolic response to the burn injury

Pathogens

- *Staphylococcus aureus*
  - Accounts for up to 75% of infections
  - MRSA showing increasing resistance to vancomycin
  - Collagenases and proteinases
  - Exotoxin, e.g. toxin shock syndrome toxin-1 (TSST-1)
  - Enterotoxins A, B and C
- *Pseudomonas aeruginosa*
  - Accompanies *S. aureus* mainly at large wound sites
  - Up to 25% of burn wounds
  - Produces a toxin pigment pyocyanin
  - Also produces exotoxin A
- Other pathogens
  - *Streptococcus pyogenes*
  - Coliform bacilli
  - Fungi including *Candida* and *Aspergillus*

Toxic shock syndrome

- May be associated with a genetic predisposition
- Related to the production of TSST-1
  - Causes an overstimulation of the immune system
- Symptoms:
  - Pyrexia
  - Rash
  - Diarrhoea and vomiting
  - Hypotension
- Mortality
  - May be up to 50%
  - Also reported in small burns (<10%) in children
- Treatment
  - Early targeted antibiotic therapy
  - Anti-TSST-1 immunoglobulin

Splanchnic ischaemia

Acalculous cholecystitis

- rare complication (<0.5% of burned patients)
- fever, right upper quadrant pain and tenderness, leukocytosis
- high mortality
- average burn size ~50%
- 2–4 weeks post-burn
- ultrasound diagnosis
- treat by cholecystectomy

Curling's ulceration

- occurs more frequently in the presence of sepsis
- gastric ulcer multiple, duodenal ulcer solitary
- only one-third report pain
- usually present with haematemesis
- 12% perforate
- prophylaxis:
  - effective fluid resuscitation
  - antacid therapy/mucosal protectants – sucralfate
  - enteral feeding

All have reduced incidence from 86 to 2%

Ischaemic enterocolitis

- mucosal ischaemia
- bacterial translocation
- high mortality
- selective digestive tract decontamination (SDD):
  - cefotaxime
  - tobramycin
  - polymixin
  - amphotericin B
  - but may increase Gram-positive colonization including MRSA

Hypercatabolic metabolism

Weight loss

Catabolism of protein

Impaired wound healing and immunity

Metabolic rate of patients with burns >40% TBSA is 100–150% above basal

Indirect calorimetry:

- respiratory quotient is the ratio of CO_2 production to O_2 consumption
- normal fasting ratio = 0.70–0.85
- increase = increased CO_2 production, i.e. carbohydrate metabolism
- decrease = inadequate calorie intake

Daily calorie requirements:

- two-thirds of the non-protein calorie intake is provided by carbohydrate, the rest as fat (20% protein, 28% fat, 52% carbohydrate)

- children have less body fat and a smaller muscle mass, hence need proportionately greater intake of calories
- Sutherland formulae:
  - children – 60 kcal/kg + 35 kcal/%TBSA
  - adults – 20 kcal/kg + 70 kcal/%TBSA

Protein needs:

- greatest nitrogen losses between days 5 and 10
- 20% of kcals should be provided by protein to replace that lost over the burn wound
- Davies formulae:
  - children – 3 g/kg + 1 g/% TBSA
  - adults – 1 g/kg + 3 g/% TBSA

Intragastric feeding of ventilated burns patients

Raff. *Burns* 1997

Burned patients continue to catabolize protein during the first week post-burn despite aggressive feeding

Aims of feeding are to minimize net protein loss and to protect the gut from bacterial translocation and prevent Gram-negative septicaemia

Feeding should be instituted as early as possible and may avoid gastric ileus

Where gastric ileus is established tubes may be sited in the duodenum or jejunum but hormonal stimulation of the liver and pancreas is greatly reduced by non-placement in the stomach

Metoclopramide and cisapride may be used to assist gastric emptying

Begin feeding at low infusion rates and increase after resuscitation:

- feeding increases gut blood flow
- shock decreases gut blood flow
- hence feeding in the presence of shock may make the gut even more sensitive to the effects of relative ischaemia

Complicated by inadvertent dislodgement, diarrhoea and pulmonary aspiration

Nutrition and anabolic agents in burned patients

Andel. *Burns* 2003

Enteral feedining is superior to parenteral feeding in the burned patient

- TPN is associated with impaired mucosal immunity and enhanced endotoxin translocation
- Also related to upregulated expression of TNF-alpha which adversely affects survival
- Enteral nutrition preserves mucosal integrity, protects against bactreial translocation in the gut and is associated with improved regulation of the inflammatory cytokine response

Duodenal feeding preferred over gastric feeding

- Less regurgitation of feed
- May reduce aspiration pneumonia

Support of the metabolic response to burn injury

Herndon. *The Lancet* 2004

Basal metabolic rate increases dramatically during the acute injury phase

- 180% for burn inuries more than 40% TBSA
- BMR remains higher than normal for up to 12 months post-injury

Oxygen consuption and carbon dioxide production steadily increase over the first 5 days post-injury

- Associated increase in protein, fat and glycogen catabolism
  - Negative nitrogen balance persists up to 9 months post-injury
  - Growth delay for up to 2 years in children
- Post-receptor insulin resistance
  - Enhanced glucose delivery to cells including fibroblasts, inflammatory cells and endothelial cells at the burn wound

Reducing the hypercatabolic response

- Early wound closure
  - Including biosynthetic skin substitutes and cadaveric allograft
- Prevention of infection

Supporting the catabolic response

- Nutritional support
  - Continuous enteral feeding
    - Adults: 25 kcal/kg + 40 kcal/%BSA per day
    - Children: 1800 kcal + 2200 kcal/m^2 burn area per day
  - Parenteral feeding if there is a prolonged ileus or intolerance of enteral feeding
- High carbohydrate regimen
  - 3% fat
  - 82% carbohydrate
  - 15% protein
    - stimulates protein synthesis
    - promotes insulin release
    - improves lean body mass
- Raising the ambient temperature
  - Body temperature increases to 2 °C above normal
  - Increasing the ambient temperature to 33 °C offsets energy expenditure required to maintain raised body temperature

Modulation of the hormonal response (provision of anabolic hormones)

- Growth hormone
  - rhGH (0.2 mg/kg/day) reduces wound healing time
  - rhGH (0.05 mg/kg/day) in children improves growth for up to 3 years post-burn
  - side effects include hyperglycaemia (but not seen in children)
- Other potentially useful hormones:
  - Insulin-like growth factor-1
  - Insulin
  - Oxandrolone (weak testosterone analogue)
  - β blockade – propranolol (to block the raised catecholamine response)

Physical exercise as part of post-burn rehabilitation also shown to improve muscle mass

Suppurative thrombophlebitis

Mainly at peripheral cannulation sites

Related to duration of cannula placement

Usually occult – only one-third show clinical signs – sepsis/positive cultures with unknown source

Organisms:
- non-burned patients – *Staphylococcus, Klebsiella, Candida*
- burned patients – same as those cultured from the burn wound

Heterotopic bone formation

Mainly between the olecranon and the medial supracondylar ridge of the humerus
Once matured, excision does not lead to recurrence
Calcification around joints in children gradually disappears
Calcification increases as long as wounds remain open/granulating

Heterotopic ossification after severe burns
Richards. *Burns* 1997
Different from myositis ossificans which results from direct muscle trauma
Associated with head and spinal injuries, orthopaedic surgery and polio
Overall incidence 1–3% of burns patients
More common in patients with >20% TBSA
Joints underlying areas of FT burn may be at increased risk
Associated with aggressive passive mobilization of shoulder and elbow
Onset 3 weeks–3 months
Serum calcium and phosphate remain unchanged, alkaline phosphatase may rise but unreliable indicators
Early radiographic signs (calcification) may be reversed by effective burn wound closure
Decreased activity on bone scan indicative of maturation of bone and helps guide timing of excision (>12 months post-burn)
NSAID may be of help – prevent osteoblastic differentiation of mesenchymal cells
Diphosphonates bind calcium and phosphates to prevent hydroxyapatite crystallization
Hence bone matrix not mineralized but becomes mineralized after treatment stopped

Marjolin's ulcer

Hypopigmentation

Management of post-burn hypopigmentation
Grover. *Burns* 1996
Most common in the hands and head and neck
Most obvious in pigmented races
Usually permanent
Epidermal melanin unit made up from:
- melanocyte
  - synthesizes melanin and packages it into melanosomes
  - transported via dendritic processes to keratinocyte
Post-burn scar is a barrier to melanocyte migration and melanosome transport
Vitiligo is distinct (autoimmune phenomenon) although overlaps with Koebner's phenomenon – induction of vitiligo by trauma
Treatment options:
- dermabrasion and thin SSG

- tattooing
- natural dyes – henna – especially Asian skin
- camouflage make-up

Electrical burns

Pathophysiology

Joule effect – conversion of electrical energy into heat: $J = I^2RT$, where J is heat produced, I is current, R is resistance and T is duration of current

Hence, greatest generation of heat occurs when electrical energy passes along a tissue of high resistance, e.g. bone

Nerve and blood vessels have least resistance

Ohm's law: $I = V/R$, where I is current, V is voltage and R is resistance

Classification

Low voltage
- <1000 V
- local tissue necrosis
- similar to thermal injury
- often AC power supply
  - muscle tetany
  - cardiac arrest

High voltage
- >1000 V
- deep muscle injury
- compartment syndrome
- haemochromogenuria
- exit wounds on the soles of the feet
- cardiorespiratory arrest
- may have fractures/dislocations
- perforation of bowel or paralytic ileus
- physiological spinal cord transection in up to 25%
- bone sequestration in 15%

Lightning injury
- high voltage, high current, short duration
- direct strike
- side flash
- ground splash
- stride potential
- Lichtenberg flowers are pathognomonic
- cardiorespiratory arrest – prolonged resuscitation worthwhile
- may have fractures/dislocations and corneal injury and tympanic perforation

Cardiac dysrhythmias are diagnosed in up to 30% of high voltage injuries

- RBBB
- supraventricular tachycardia
- ectopics

Burn wounds

Entry and exit points
Arcing
Thermal burns following ignition of clothing

Management

ABC
Monitor for haemochromogenuria and compartment syndrome – fasciotomy, carpal tunnel release
Debridement and definitive wound closure after 24–72 h
- salvage of devitalized tissues with emergency free flaps – bring in additional blood supply
- amputation where necessary

Free tissue transfer in burns management

Platt. *Burns* 1996
Of burns patients treated surgically over 5 years, 1.5% had a free flap
Free flap failure rate was 22% (2/9)
Emergency free flaps mainly suited to electrical burns
Consider vein grafts to ensure that anastomoses are performed outside the zone of injury

Early complications
Myocardial injury
Intra-abdominal injury
Vascular injury

Delayed complications
Cardiac dysrhythmias
Neurological problems
- central (from 6 months)
  - epilepsy
  - encephalopathy
  - brainstem dysfunction
  - cord problems including progressive muscular atrophy, amyotrophic lateral sclerosis and transverse myelitis
- peripheral (from months to up to 3 years) – progressive neural demyelination
Cataracts (from 6 months) – occur in up to 30% of patients with high voltage electrical burns involving the head and neck

Emergency reconstruction of electrical injuries

Zhu. *Burns* 2003

Review of 14 years' experience in Shen Zhen, China

- 155 patients with electrical burns
- 459 wounds
- 102 patients with high voltage injuries (2000–100 000 V)

Comprehensive urgent reconstruction alternative (CURA)

- early conservative wound debridement but preserving vital structures (nerves, tendons, bone) even where viability is in doubt
- flap cover (including vascularized transplantation of nerves etc)
  - continuous irrigation of the wound bed beneath the flap with a solution of lignocaine and chloromycetin in saline for up to 72 hours post-reconstruction

Results

- 70% of patients underwent debridement within 1 hour of admission
- reconstruction within 48 hours can lead to good results
- 398 flaps used for reconstruction
  - 8 free flaps
    - 1 flap lost
  - 23 island flaps
  - 1 greater omentum
  - 119 'ultra-thin' flaps (dermal random pattern flaps)
  - 236 random pattern flaps pedicled from the abdominal wall
  - 6 cross leg flaps and 1 cross arm flap
- reconstruction of vital structures
  - tendon transplantation in 11 patients
    - bone (2)
    - nerve (5)

Frostbite

Cold injury either local (frostbite) or systemic (hypothermia)

Predisposing factors for hypothermia:

- extremes of age
- alcohol (peripheral vascular dilatation)
- mental instability
- low ambient temperature with strong air currents (wind chill)

Frostbite:

- temperature
- duration of contact
- moisture content vs. oil content of the skin
- wind chill factor
- pre-existing hypoperfusion (atherosclerosis, etc.)
- smoking causes vascular spasm

Four phases:

- prefreeze (3–10 °C)

- before formation of ice crystals
- increased vascular permeability
- freeze–thaw (–6 to –15 °C)
  - formation of extra- and intracellular ice crystals occurs at –4 °C, i.e. when the skin is supercooled
  - must have supercooling to develop ice crystals owing to the underlying generation of metabolic heat
  - at –20 °C, 90% of all available water is frozen
- vascular stasis
  - dilatation
  - stasis and coagulation
  - shunting away from the affected part
- late ischaemic phase
  - cell death
  - gangrene

Effect of thawing:
- initial reversible vasoconstriction then hyperaemia
- restoration of the dermal circulation
- endothelial cell damage
- formation of microemboli leading to distal occlusion and thrombosis (no reflow)
- liberation of inflammatory mediators and oxygen free radicals which contribute to the frostbite injury
- oedema
- formation of blisters and later an eschar

Symptoms:
- coldness
- numbness
- pain on rewarming

Long-term sequelae:
- residual burning sensations for up to 6 weeks, precipitated by warming
- may have permanent sensory loss
- hyperhidrosis as a manifestation of altered SNS activity
- cold intolerance/Raynaud's phenomenon
- localized areas of bone resorption
- joint pain and stiffness

Management
- stages 1 and 2
- avoid vigorous rubbing
- rapid rewarming by immersion in circulating water at 40–42 °C for ~30 min
- analgesia during rewarming (NSAID)
- leave blisters
- elevation and splinting of extremities
- tetanus and antibiotic prophylaxis
- delay amputation as long as possible
  - line of demarcation may be indeterminate for many weeks
  - often achieve good recovery

Chemical burns

~3% of burns centre admissions

Acids, alkalis, organic hydrocarbons

Majority are work-related

Majority in men

Military chemical injuries mainly white phosphorus

Civilian chemical burns mainly acids and alkalis

Most commonly affect upper extremities

Continued tissue damage long after the initial injury

Severity related to

- temperature
- volume
- concentration
- duration of exposure
- site affected
- mechanism of chemical action

Emergency management

- removal of contaminated clothing
- copious lavage with running water but avoid hypothermia
- blood gas monitoring
    - correct acidosis with i.v. NaHCO$_3$
    - encourage diuresis with mannitol to prevent renal complications
- emergency debridement

Alkalis

NaOH, KOH, lime

Mechanism of injury:

- saponification of fat – liquefractive necrosis
- tissue desiccation
- protein denaturation

Capable of deep penetration

Severe pain

Severe eye injury including scarring, ulceration and opacification of the cornea

Cement

- calcium oxide
- exothemic reaction with the water of sweat to form CaOH (alkali)
- desiccation injury
- delayed symptoms and presentation

Acids

Coagulative necrosis

Formic acid

- industrial descaling and hay preservative
- absorption from the skin leads to:

- metabolic acidosis
- haemolysis and haemochromogenuria
- ARDS
- necrotizing pancreatitis
- wound has a greenish colour with blistering and oedema
- surgical excision

Hydrofluoric acid (HF)

- used in the glass industry for dissolving silica
- severe injury
- desiccation, corrosion, protein denaturation
- complexes with cations including Ca^{2+} and Mg^{2+}
- binding intracellular Ca^{2+} leads to cell death
- liquefractive necrosis and bone decalcification
- F^- binds to Na/K ATPase resulting in K^+ efflux from cells and hyperkalaemia
- concentrations:
  - <20% – injury becomes apparent after 24 h
  - 20–50% – injury becomes apparent after several hours
  - 50% – injury immediately painful
  - unrecognized injuries inevitably progress to extensive tissue destruction including bone
- hypocalcaemia leads to cardiac dysrhythmia
- refractory (fatal) VF may be induced by the action of F^- on the myocardium
- management:
  - emergency management
    - neutralization by copious irrigation
    - topical calcium gluconate gel ± injection of calcium gluconate solution into deeper tissues beneath the burn, from the periphery of the burn, with a 27-gauge needle
    - injection of calcium reduces wound pain
    - subsequent return of pain may indicate need for repeat injections
    - wound debridement
  - correct hypocalcaemia and hypomagnesaemia – i.v. calcium chloride
  - cardiac telemetry – beware prolonged QT interval (hypocalcaemia)
  - $NaHCO_3$ – alkalinizes urine to promote excretion of F^-
  - may also eliminate F^- by haemodialysis
  - hand injuries may require digital fasciotomy and intra-arterial infusion of calcium gluconate via the radial A
  - inhaled HF should be treated by respiratory support and nebulized calcium gluconate
- 2% TBSA involvement may be fatal

Alkyl mercuric compounds

Ethyl and methyl mercuric phosphates
Blisters containing liberated free mercury
Absorption and systemic poisoning
De-roof blisters and wash copiously

Hydrocarbons

Cell membrane injury by dissolving lipids

Erythema and blistering

Burns usually superficial

Beware systemic absorption – respiratory depression

Petrol

- three mechanisms of injury:
  - lipid solvent, endothelial cell membrane injury
  - leaded petrol leads to lead absorption (binds CNS lipids)
  - ignited petrol causes severe thermal injury

Phenol

- carbolic acid
- disinfectants
- binds irreversibly to albumin
- ingestion of 1 g may prove fatal
- necrosis and gangrene after prolonged skin contact
- dermatitis and depigmentation
- copious water irrigation followed by polyethylene glycol (antifreeze)
- phenol also an ingredient in tar which may be removed with toluene

Hot bitumen burns

Baruchin. *Burns* 1997

- mixture of petroleum-derived hydrocarbons, mineral tars and asphalt
- used at 100–200 °C, hence thermal and chemical injury
- cool the burn wound at the scene until the bitumen is cold and hard
- de-roof blisters with any attached bitumen
- dress bitumen adherent to other areas with liquid paraffin
- bitumen is slowly dissolved and absorbed by the overlying dressing

Highly reactive elements

- **phosphorous**
  - white phosphorous ignites on contact with air
  - military agent, also in fertilizers
  - burns at the skin surface until immersed in water
  - systemic toxicity (hepatorenal)
  - painful, necrotic yellow wounds
  - garlic odour
  - irrigation and removal of particles – UV light assists identification
  - then irrigation with copper sulphate to form cupric oxide (black film)
  - hypocalcaemia and hypophosphataemia
  - monitor ECG

Infusion agents. Severe extravasation injury

Burd. *BMJ* 1985

11% of children and 22% of adult patients receiving i.v. fluids experience extravasation injury

Radiological contrast media, hypertonic solutions and cytotoxic drugs may cause extensive soft tissue necrosis

Patients at extremes of age most at risk

Use 11 blade for irrigation ports

Hylase 1500 units in 10 ml normal saline followed by further irrigation

Scar management

Avoid the development of permanent joint changes by early scar release

Maintain a full passive range of movement and optimize active joint mobilization

Splint in a position of function throughout early treatment and later rehabilitation

Hypertrophic scars
- become apparent 6–8 weeks after grafting
- pressure therapy accelerates maturation of the scar by a process linked to a reduction in tissue perfusion and oxygenation
- effective pressure range is 15–40 mmHg
- pressure garments should be commenced within 2 weeks of grafting and maintained as long as the scar is immature or hypertrophic (>1 year) – head and neck compression devices in children impair mandibular growth
- digital pressure therapy may be achieved in the digits with coban tape
- develop at sites of delayed wound healing including deeper burns, infected wounds or those allowed to heal by secondary intention
- also high risk skin types and anatomical location
- abundance of disorganized type 1 collagen
- high TGF-β3:TGF-β1 and -2 ratio
- silicone gel sheet hydrates (?) and softens scars
- intralesional triamcinolone enhances collagenase activity and dampens fibroblastic activity
- axsain cream (capsaicin) is effective against scar itching – substance P inhibitor
- moisturizing pressure massage throughout
- excision with postoperative radiotherapy

Ambulation maintains joint movement, muscle mass and bone density

Resurfacing with free tissue transfer, expanded skin or Integra

Burn reconstruction

Rehabilitation is the process by which a person attains their maximal potential following injury

Pursue realistic goals

Reconstruction should be postponed until all wounds have matured unless there is a progressively deforming force, e.g. eyelid ectropion

Priorities:
- prevention of deformity
- restoration of active function
- restoration of cosmesis

Regional reconstruction:
- head and neck
  - aesthetic units
  - useful FTSG donor sites:
    - upper eyelid
    - nasolabial fold
    - pre-/postauricular area
    - scalp
    - supraclavicular fossa
- facial burns
  - conservative approach initially
  - debride in cosmetic units with a dermatome
  - thick unperforated sheet SSG from the scalp
  - suture grafts in cosmetic units
  - immediate pressure garment
  - inspect grafts twice daily and aspirate haematomas as required

Reconstructive surgery using Integra

Dantzer. *Br J Plastic Surg* 2001

Review of 31 patients who underwent Integra grafting for functional reconstruction of a scarred area or tumour site
- Age range 3–77 years
- A well-vascularized wound bed was obtained with 'perfect' haemostasis
- Meshing of Integra was avoided but where there was a risk of haematoma the Integra was hand perforated
- Integra was secured with stitches or staples and a tie-over pressure dressing applied at mobile sites
- Ultra-thin split skin grafts replaced the silicone layer after a mean of 22 days

Results
- Good functional reconstruction obtained
- Complications included:
  - Infection (five patients)
    - Total loss in one patient
    - Transparency of silicone allows for easily identification of infected ares
      - Must be excised and antibiotic therapy instituted
  - Haematoma (1)
  - Detachment of silicone (2)
  - Incomplete graft take (3)
- Areas up to $750\,cm^2$ can be treated in a single session
- Treated areas are supple and non-adherent to underlying structures
- Uniform skin colour and texture
- No hypertrophic scarring

Reconstruction of special areas

Facial reconstruction after burn injury
Evans. *BJPS* 1995

Reconstruction of full-thickness facial burn with marked hypertrophic scarring and contracture

FTSG release of eyelids early had failed to prevent ectropion

Free circumferential radial forearm flap to the right cheek

Pedicled groin flap inset into donor defect to cover tendons

Lateral arm flap raised but too bulky for nasal reconstruction

Free circumferential radial forearm flap to the left cheek

Tagliacozzi flap to the nasal dorsum but this failed to cover tip

Free dorsalis pedis flap to the nasal tip

Total face reconstruction with one free flap
Angrigiani. *PRS* 1997

Bilateral extended scapular–parascapular free flap used to reconstruct five full-thickness full-face burns

Nasal resurfacing achieved with a separate technique

Flap is not large enough to resurface the neck

Bilateral microvascular anastomoses of superficial circumflex scapular arteries to facial vessels

Acceptable donor area on the back is grafted

Scalp alopecia

McCauley classification

- type I – single alopecia segment
  - a – <25% – **single expander**
  - b – 25–50% – **single expander/over-inflation**
  - c – 50–75% – **multiple expanders**
  - d – >75% – **multiple expanders**
- type II – multiple areas of alopecia amenable to tissue expansion correction
- type III – multiple areas of alopecia not amenable to tissue expansion
- type IV – total alopecia

Serial excision (<15% of scalp)

Rotation flaps

Tissue expansion

Trunk and genitalia

Burned breast tends to be fuller and lacks natural ptosis necessitating mastopexy of the uninjured side and multiple scar releases

If implants required then site subpectorally

Skate flap nipple reconstruction

Perineal burns should be managed conservatively as for facial burns, except electrical injuries

Avoid long-term urethral catheterization – suprapubic catheters are preferred

Avoid excision of penile skin especially

Reconstruction of the burned breast with Integra

Palao. *Br J Plastic Surg* 2003

Burns to the nipple–areolar complex in adolescence may disturb breast growth

- Breast bud lies deep and so is relatively preserved
- Tight scar contracture on the anterior chest impairs development

14 breasts in 12 patients (12–27 years of age) were treated for childhood burn scars using Integra

- Careful preservation of the inframammary fold
- Integra placed upon mammary gland tissue, fascia or hypodermis
  - Overlapped at junctions to avoid scar hypertrophy
  - Dressed with gauze impregnated with povidone–iodine and nitrofurazone
    - Regular wound inspection
    - Dressings changed twice weekly
- Unmeshed autografts around day 28
- Antibiotic prophylaxis

Results

- 100% Integra take
- no infections
- good aesthetic reconstruction
- improved scar quality
- adnexal structures do not appear to regenerate in the Integra neo-dermis so some patients complain of dryness at reconstructed sites
  - managed by moisturising creams
- pruritis may be due to infiltartion of the neodermis by eosinophils

Hands

Early excision of FT and DD burns with preservation of dorsal veins where possible
Sheet autograft
High priority compared with other body sites burned
Vigorous physiotherapy and appropriate splinting, avoiding wrist hyperextension (develop compression neuropathies)
Palmar burns rarely need debridement
Dorsal scar contracture treated by full scar excision and lateral arm or radial forearm free flap – can include PL tendon graft
Release of burn syndactyly
Nail growth may be delayed for up to 6 months – after this time nail bed grafts may be required
Extensor tenolysis, joint fusions

Burns of the hand and upper limb

Smith. *Burns* 1998
Deep partial thickness and full-thickness burns should be debrided as soon as possible, ideally within 72 h
Early surgery has been shown to result in better function and especially less re-operation
Preserve fat and dorsal veins wherever possible
Sharp dissection may be easier than tangential excision for even deeper burns

Non-viable digits may be allowed to separate rather than debrided – mummified tips rarely a source of infection

Sheet SSG or unexpanded mesh

Proximal interphalangeal joint is the most commonly exposed joint

Cover exposed tendons and joints with free, pedicled or local flaps

May need to consider primary arthrodesis

Palmar burns treated conservatively, or thick SSG if absolutely necessary

Limb elevation and splints

Physiotherapy – active and passive movements – but avoid precipitating heterotopic bone formation by over-aggressive mobilization of shoulder and elbow

May require regional anaesthesia to encourage movement (BPB)

Psychiatric considerations

Established psychiatric disturbances may have led to the burn injury, e.g. suicide attempt

Altered perception due to substance abuse or withdrawal

Delirium may be a psychological reaction to injury or a manifestation of metabolic derangement, e.g. hypoglycaemia, hypoxia, sepsis, pain

Symptoms:
- psychosis
  - delusions
  - hallucinations
  - paranoia
  - rare in children
- post-traumatic stress syndrome
  - poor sleep
  - hypervigilance
  - flash-backs
  - nightmares
  - depression
  - panic attacks
  - guilt (e.g. sole survivor)
- longer-term problems
  - self-consciousness
  - poor self-esteem
  - phobias
  - anxiety
  - enuresis
- children and adolescents eventually appear to become well adjusted

Comfort Care
Platt. *Burns* 1998

Questionnaire-based survey of 'comfort care' policy in the UK

Priorities for determining suitability for resuscitation were:

- age and TBSA
- TBSA full-thickness burn (including special areas)
- smoke inhalation
- preburn morbidity

Suicidal intent was given low priority

Patients' wishes taken into account but often treatment had been initiated including sedation and intubation

Joint decision between consultant and relatives

7 Breast surgery (cosmetic breast surgery, reconstruction, reconstruction of abdomen and perineum)

Breast surgical anatomy
Breast augmentation: silicone breast implants
Breast reduction
Mastopexy
Breast reconstruction
Gynaecomastia
Chest wall reconstruction
Poland's syndrome
Pectus excavatum and pectus carinatum
Abdominal wall and perineal reconstruction
Posterior chest wall

Breast surgical anatomy

Blood supply
- internal thoracic – 60%
- lateral thoracic – 30%
- intercostal vessels – 10%

Venous drainage
- internal mammary veins
- axillary vein
- intercostal veins
- superficial veins draining upwards to communicate with neck veins and medially to communicate with internal mammary veins

Lymphatic drainage
- predominantly to the axilla
- 3–20% via internal mammary chain

Nerve supply to the nipple – T4 intercostal nerves, lateral cutaneous branch

Breast augmentation: silicone

Breast implants

Silicone implant controversy

1895 – first breast augmentation procedure carried out in Germany – transplantation of a giant lipoma from the back into the breasts

1945 – Japanese prostitutes inject liquid silicone into breasts to satisfy American servicemen clients

1962 – Frank Gerow first to implant Dow Corning's sialastic mammary prosthesis. Patient remains satisfied with original implants to this day

1982 – van Nunen links silicone breast implants with connective tissue disease in three patients

1990 – David Kessler appointed as commissioner of the FDA

1991 – Marianne Hopkins awarded US$7.34 million for mixed connective tissue disease. Double mastectomy for fibrocystic disease 1976. Both implants replaced within a few months and again 10 years later (1986) after having developed mixed connective tissue disease. Had undergone autoAb screen before original implants in 1975

1992 – Dow Corning documents released. Memo orders sales staff to wash away evidence of gel bleed.

- FDA ban on silicone implants. Onus on manufacturers to prove safety of implants but no evidence that implants cause connective tissue disease. Cosmetic advantages only, no risks tolerated
- Spain and France ban silicone breast implants
- Frank Vasey publishes *The Silicone Breast Implant Controversy* claiming a connection with mixed connective tissue disease

1994 – breast augmentation – third commonest aesthetic procedure in the USA. Implant removal the fifth commonest 30 000 lawsuits against Dow Corning. 440 000 women register for class action settlement, 250 000 claim to have established disease

Manufacturers agree to pay US$4.25 billion to women with breast implants as part of a class action settlement. US$1 billion reserved for lawyers' fees

- women entitled to compensation who had, or developed within 30 years, any of ten connective tissue diseases providing the symptoms began or worsened after the implants were placed
- 36 years – scleroderma → US$1.4 million
- >56 years – mild Sjögren's → US $140 000
- non-specific aches and pains, objectively verified → US$700 000
- husbands entitled to compensation for emotional suffering

Medical devices agency (DoH) concludes no reason for a ban

Class action lawsuits against manufacturers of penile implants

Mayo Clinic study – no link. Criticized for accepting funding from the American Society of Plastic and Reconstructive Educational Foundation – contributions from Dow Corning and other implant manufacturers

1995 – France lifts ban on silicone breast implants, then reinstates it

- Dow Corning files for bankruptcy protection
- Dow Chemical ordered to pay US$14.1 million to one patient by a jury in Nevada
- FDA recognizes body of evidence against a link to mixed connective tissue disease but maintains ban due to potential local complications

- class action lawsuits against manufacturers of Norplant contraceptive
- Nurses' health study – no link

1998 – Independent Review Group (DoH – Professor Roger Sturrock, University of Glasgow) publishes review and finds no link

1999 – Channel 4 *Equinox* programme:

- silicone implant + chemical carcinogen in rat → 11% cancer incidence
- no implant + chemical carcinogen → 64% cancer incidence – Cynthia Su, Chicago University
- expanded tissue expander + chemical carcinogen in rat → low cancer incidence
- unexpanded TE + chemical carcinogen → medium cancer incidence
- no TE + chemical carcinogen → high cancer incidence
  - Si Ramasastry, University of Illinois
  - ?mechanical effect → low blood flow

General considerations

Silicone in implants is polydimethyl siloxane, a polymer of silicon

100 000–150 000 women in the UK are estimated currently to have breast implants

~1–2 million women in the USA have implants (~1%)

Silicone also found in:

- heart valves
- joint prostheses
- baby bottle nipples
- IV cannulae

Types:

- textured vs. smooth

  textured shell decreases capsular contracture

  rippling of implants more common with a thicker shell
- cohesive gel vs. liquid gel

  range of cohesiveness

  implant shell may be overfilled to increase projection

  avoid cohesive gel in very thin patients (rippling)
- silicone vs. saline
- non-biodimensional (anatomical) vs. biodimensional

  anatomical implants contain a cohesive gel

  potential for rotation after placement

Placement – subglandular vs. submuscular:

Subglandular placement

- Suited to most cosmetic situations
- Natural breast shape
- Fills out redundant skin envelope in the ptotic breast

Subpectoral placement

- Indicated in very thin patients
- Fewer problems with capsular contracture
- Higher rate of implant displacement and asymmetry
- May be subjected to unwanted displacement or compression with contraction of the overlying pectoralis major muscle

- Double bubble deformity may develop at the inframammary fold in the ptotic breast (consider augmentation – mastopexy)

Incision:

- inframammary
- axillary
- peri-areolar
- endoscopic (inflatable saline implants)
  - axillary
  - transumbilical

Complications:

- **general**
  - infection ~2%
  - haematoma ~3%
  - scars
  - thromboembolic disorders (DVT/PE)
- **specific**
  - capsule formation
    - all implants have a surrounding capsule, capsular **contracture** is the problem
    - synovial metaplasia of capsular tissue in up to 40%
  - rupture
    - cumulative risk ~2% per year
    - MRI (stepladder sign) then USS are best radiological techniques for diagnosing rupture; Ahn. *PRS* 1994
    - lifespan of the implant cannot be guaranteed
  - gel bleed
    - bleed phenomenon due to escape of silicone oil from an implant with no evidence of a hole or tear in the outer shell
    - intracapsular and asymptomatic in the majority
    - may be related to lipid infiltration of the silicone elastomer
  - aesthetic complications
    - asymmetry
    - rippling
    - palpable edge
    - final result too big or too small
  - problems with pregnancy, lactation and breast feeding
    - all unaffected although oesophageal motility problems in children breast fed by mothers with silicone implants – unproven
    - patients may experience lactorrhoea post-augmentation
    - nipple sensation altered in ~20%
  - mixed connective tissue disorders (the silicone controversy)
    - Overall risk of connective tissue disorders is the same as the background population risk
  - implications for induction and detection of breast cancer

    No evidence to suggest induction of breast cancer

    Mammographic visualisation of breast cancer may be difficult but is possible with displacement techniques

    Breast cancer in patients with implants have the same survival as patients without implants and detection occurs at a similar stage

Breast augmentation: choosing the optimum incision, implant and pocket plane

Hidalgo. *Plastic Reconstruc Surg* 2000

Single author experience following augmentation mammaplasty in 220 patients in New York reviewed:

- commonest augmentation procedure included:
  - smooth saline-filled implant
    - deflation necessitated replacement in 4 patients within 3 years
    - overinflation of saline implants by 15% helps to reduce rippling
    - intra-operative sizers used to judge implant size
  - axillary incision
    - best suited to low volume saline implant augmentation in the submuscular plane
  - submuscular placement
    - decreases capsular contracture risk
    - subpectoral placement facilitated by inferomedial release of muscle
    - adjustable strap should be worn above the implants to prevent upward implant displacement
    - author's preferred plane in most patients
- secondary augmentation most commonly incorporated:
  - textured silicone gel implants
    - use in USA limited to secondary revisions and selected primary cases only (e.g. congenital deformity)
  - periareolar incision
    - considered the best choice of incision for lowering the level of the inframammary fold (but avoid double bubble deformity!)
    - also a good option in the tubular breast where concurrent circumareolar mastopexy is indicated
    - provides good access to the pocket for capsulectomy
    - avoid in the small or lightly pigmented areola
  - submuscular pocket
- nipple position asymmetry common pre-operatively and is often magnified by augmentation mammaplasty but the implants should still be placed in symmetrical pockets

Dual plane breast augmentation

Tebbets. *Plastic Reconstruct Surg* 2001

Patients with a pinch thickness of 2 cm or greater in the upper pole of the breast are suitable for retromammary implant placement

All patients with less than 2 cm in the upper pole required muscle coverage to avoid underfill rippling at this site

The dual plane pocket is created by:

- releasing the inferior insertion of pectoralis major at the inframammary fold (type 1)
  - the insertion of pectoralis major is divided with needle point cautery parallel to the inframammary fold and 1 cm above it
    - this allows the pectoralis muscle to retract 2–4 cm upwards
  - do not divide the muscle along the sternum except for white tendinous insertions
    - avoids visible retraction of muscle along the sternum and a palpable implant edge
  - used in patients where
    - the entire breast parenchyma is above the inframammary fold

- there are tight attachments of parenchyma to muscle
- a short nipple–inframammary fold distance of 4–6 cm under stretch
- plus division of muscle-breast parenchyma attachments to a point level with the inferior edge of the nipple–areolar complex (type 2)
  - used in patients where
    - most of the breast is above the inframammary fold
    - there are looser attachments of breast to muscle
    - and the nipple–inframammary fold distance is 5–6.5 cm under stretch
- or to the superior edge of the nipple–areolar complex (type 3)
  - used in patients
    - with glandular ptosis
    - very loose attachments (gland easily slides off pec major)
    - markedly stretch nipple–inframammary fold distance
    - constricted lower pole (tuberous breast deformity)

Induction of breast cancer

Polyurethane coating of some implants could break down under human body conditions to form a toluene derivative → sarcomas in rats – now withdrawn – polyurethane coating around silicone shell of saline implants initially thought to decrease capsular contracture
Induction of breast cancer – **no known risk over and above that of the general female population**

Berkel. *N Engl J Med* 1992

>11 000 women with implants (not polyurethane-coated)
Predicted number of patients with cancer (according to incidence in general population) and implant = 86
Observed number of women with cancer and an implant = 47
Hence lower than the risk associated with the general population
?Women with implants are a population already at low risk and implants do not substantially increase the risk

Deapen and Brodie. *PRS* 1993

Retrospective study of >3000 women with implants
Age, race and socio-economic factors within the follow-up period → expected number of breast cancers = 32
Observed breast cancers = 21

Detection of breast cancer

?Delayed diagnosis due to high false-negative mammography rate
Saline implants more radiolucent than silicone but both fairly radio-opaque → higher dose of radiation
Hence, difficulties visualizing the entire breast
Microcalcification obscured by implant
Microcalcification within the capsule

Silverstein. *Cancer* 1990

35 patients with implants who developed cancer

34/35 presented with **palpable** disease

41% false-negative mammography rate (normally ~5–10%)

Presence of an implant did not preclude radiotherapy or FNA/Trucut biopsy

Difficulty in imaging breast

- compression and displacement techniques visualize ~60% of breast if subglandular and ~90% if submuscular (Eklund)
- capsular contracture makes compression and displacement techniques difficult

Recommendations for patients at high risk of developing breast cancer (positive family history):

- warn that implants may delay diagnosis
- mammogram before implant placement if >30 years
- submuscular placement
- regular screening

Carson. *PRS* 1993

37 cases of breast cancer in augmented patients

35/37 presented with palpable disease

~50% false-negative mammography rate

Birdsell. *PRS* 1993

Study of >13 000 women in Alberta

Same 5-year survival and same incidence of lymph node disease in augmented and non-augmented women with breast cancer

Hence, no difference in pathological stage at diagnosis

Tumours in augmented patients were **smaller**

Augmented patients were ~12 years **younger** at diagnosis

Breast cancer and augmentation mammaplasty

Shons. *Plastic Reconstruc Surg* 2001

1 in 8 women in North America develop breast cancer at some point in their lives

Hence, of 203 000 women who underwent augmentation mammaplasty in 1997, 25 000 will develop the disease

- Although the presence of an implant may make the radiological diagnosis difficult due to either false-negatives or false-positives, those women in whom breast cancer does develop present at a similar stage, including nodal disease, and have equivalent survival compared with non-implanted women
- Patients with implants are more likely to require open biopsy for histological diagnosis than percutaneous needle techniques
- Small breast volume and distortion of tissue due to the presence of the implant capsule may make wide local excision of the tumour difficult. Patients with implants are more likely to undergo mastectomy rather than lumpectomy
- Adjuvant radiotherapy encourages the development of a firm capsule around an implant
- sentinel lymph node biopsy is unreliable in patients who have undergone axillary placement of their implant

Breast augmentation: cancer concerns and mammography

Jakubietz. *Plastic Reconstruc Surg* 2004

- Review of the literature concerning breast augmentation and breast cancer
- Patients with breast implants are not at a greater risk than the general population for developing breast cancer
- Early detection of occult cancer is possible in augmented patients
- Submuscular placement allows for greater mammographic visualization.
- Eklund views (displacement techniques) should be used when obtaining mammograms in augmented patients and should be interpreted by experienced radiologists
- Silicone and saline implants demonstrate the same radiodensity on mammograms
- The current recommendations for getting screening/pre-operative mammograms are no different for augmented patients

Surgical treatment of breast cancer in previously augmented patients

Karanas. *Plastic Reconstruc Surg* 2003

- As the augmented patient population ages, an increasing number of breast cancer cases among previously augmented women can be anticipated
  - is breast conservation therapy feasible in this patient population?
  - can these patients retain their implants?
- retrospective review of 58 patients between 1991 and 2001
  - 30 patients (52%) were treated with a modified radical mastectomy with implant removal
  - 28 patients (48%) underwent breast conservation therapy
    - lumpectomy, axillary lymph node dissection, and radiotherapy
    - 22 patients initially retained their implants
      - 11 patients ultimately required completion mastectomies with implant removal
      - implant complications (2)
      - local recurrences (5)
      - inability to obtain negative margins (4)
      - implant-related complications – contracture, erosion, pain, and rupture (9)
- breast conservation therapy with maintenance of the implant is not ideal for the majority of augmented patients – mastectomy with immediate reconstruction might be a more suitable choice

Capsular contracture

Baker classification of capsular contracture (1975):
- Class I – no contracture
- Class II – palpable contracture
- Class III – visible contracture
- Class IV – painful contracture

Pathogenesis of contracture – theories:
- subclinical *Staphylococcus epidermidis* infection (betadine wash-out shown to reduce colonization rates)
- fibroblastic foreign body type reaction

Reducing capsular contracture:
- use of textured implants; Malata. *BJPS* 1997; Hakelius. *PRS* 1997
- subpectoral placement

Treatment:

- capsulotomy/capsulectomy (capsulectomy reduces breast parenchymal volume)
- closed capsulotomy → implant rupture
- no guarantee that capsulectomy will prevent recurrent capsule formation

Calcification within the breast capsule may make interpretation of mammography difficult – may be mistaken for malignant disease

- chalky white exudate around implant

Capsular contracture: the Bradford study

Textured or smooth implants for breast augmentation? A prospective controlled trial

Coleman DJ, Foo IT, Sharpe DT. *BJPS* 1991

53 patients entered into a prospective study

Smooth or textured implants were placed in the submammary plane

Assessed at 12 months

Adverse capsular contracture (Baker grades 3 and 4) in 58% of breasts augmented with smooth surface implants

8% of breasts in the textured surface implant group

Textured or smooth implants for breast augmentation? Three year follow-up of a prospective randomized controlled trial

Malata CM, Feldberg L, Coleman DJ *et al. BJPS* 1997

Study reviewed, after 3 years, 49/53 patients who underwent subglandular breast augmentation mammoplasty in a randomized double-blind study with textured or smooth silicone gel-filled implants in 1989

Adverse capsular contracture was 59% for smooth implants and 11% for textured ones

Eight patients (31%) with smooth prostheses underwent breast implant exchange for severe capsular contracture between the 1- and 3-year assessments

Revisional surgery rate of only 7.4% (2/27 patients) for the textured group

Effect of textured implants in reducing capsular contracture in augmentation mammoplasty found at 1 year is maintained at 3 years, and suggest that it may be long-lasting

The effect of Biocell texturing and povidone-iodine irrigation on capsular contracture around saline-inflatable breast implants

Burkhardt and Eades. *Plastic Reconstruc Surg* 1995

Prospective, controlled, blinded 4-year trial

60 patients, two independent variables:

- texturization
- betadine antibacterial irrigation

Incidence of fibrous capsular contracture around saline-inflatable implants following retromammary augmentation

Textured devices irrigated with betadine → 4% contracture

Smooth devices irrigated with saline solution → 50% contracture

Betadine wash-out and textured implants both independently reduce contracture

Mondor's disease

Superficial thrombophlebitis
Treat with warm compresses and NSAID

Implant rupture

Rupture of silicone breast implants: causes sequelae and diagnosis [review]

Brown. *Lancet* 1997

Intra- or extracapsular rupture – intracapsular rupture → no change in shape or size of the breast

Strength of the silicone elastomer shell decreases with age

Causes of rupture:

- iatrogenic – mammography, closed capsulotomy
- trauma
- idiopathic

Extracapsular spread of silicone reported in up to about one-quarter of patients → silicone granulomas

- skin and nipple ducts
- lymph nodes
- distant sites

USS screening for implant rupture in patients without symptoms is unnecessary but ruptured implants should be removed

Robinson. *Ann Plast Surg* 1995

Explanted series ~300 patients (592 implants) → 63% rupture or bleed rate irrespective of whether patients complained of symptoms or not – explanted due to silicone controversy

Included all implants of between 1 and 25 years

Only 50% of women could expect to have their prosthesis intact by 12 years

Recommended that implants should be electively replaced at 8 years

Silicone granulomas

Austad. *Plastic Reconstruc Surg* 2002

A silicone granuloma is a foreign body type reaction to the presence of silicone

- aggregates of macrophages and polymorphs
- may show necrosis
- persists until the foreign body is degraded as much as possible
- palpable mass in the breast tissue

Rare occurrence, not always associated with implant rupture

- Incidence of silicone granulomas not known but thought to be between 0.1 and 0.5%
- may be associated with low grade *Staphylococcus epidermidis* infection
- excised granulomas should be submitted for culture

Microscopic subclinical silicone granulomas may also occur

- fragments of silicone found in the capsules of 46 of 54 textured implants in one study

Anatomical distribution usually limited to the breast

- may also occur outside the breast on the chest wall or upper limb

- silicone lymphadenopathy reported may years after the placement of an implant or MCP joint prosthesis
  - almost exclusively in the axilla

No evidence to suggest that silicone granulomas bear any relationship to any form of systemic disease

Most silicone granulomas are excised simply to exclude a malignant breast lump

Mixed connective tissue disease

Definition

Human **adjuvant disease** is an atypical array of rheumatoid-like symptoms (associated with abnormalities of the immune response, auto-antibody formation, and chronic inflammation) mediated by silicone acting as an immunological adjuvant

Landmark papers

Post-mammoplasty connective tissue disease. Van Nunen. *Arthritis Rheum* 1982

- first report of connective tissue disorder in three patients within 2.5 years of receiving silicone breast implants: SLE, RA and a mixed connective tissue disorder
- previous reports had linked connective tissue disorder with injections of liquid paraffin into the breast
- none of the patients reported wished to have their implant removed

Gabriel. *N Engl J Med* 1994

- Mayo Clinic study – 'Olmsted County'
- 5/749 women with implants developed connective tissue disease
- 10/1498 controls developed connective tissue disorders

Sanchez-Guerrero. *N Engl J Med* 1995

- nurses' health study – questionnaire of nurses in the USA
- 90 000 women evaluated of whom ~1% had implants
- no increased incidence of connective tissue disorders in women with implants

Nyren. *BMJ* 1998

- comparison of >7000 breast augment patients with >3000 breast reduction patients
- recorded first hospitalization rates for connective tissue diseases
- no difference found
- paper reviewed in *BMJ* Editorial same issue

Miller. *PRS* 1998

- CRP, RF, anti-nuclear Ab and anti-streptinolysin O titres measured pre-operatively in 218 patients and post-operatively over 13 years
- no increase in levels in women with either saline or gel-filled implants

Background risk

High incidence of rheumatoid-like symptoms in the general population

- fibromyalgia ~5%
- RA ~2%

- SLE ~143/100 000
- scleroderma ~113/100 000

By chance alone, of women in the USA with breast implants:
- 30–50 000 → fibromyalgia
- 10–20 000 → RA

Studies examining patients suffering from SLE, RA and scleroderma have all found that, in these patients, the number with implants is no higher than the estimated percentage of women in the population with implants, i.e. ~1% in the USA

Long term health status of Danish women with silicone breast implants
Breiting. *Plastic Reconstruc Surg* 2004

Retrospective study comparing three cohorts of women:
- breast augmentation ($n = 190$)
  - majority silicone implants in submammary pocket
  - unilateral implants for asymmetry in 26 women
  - 19 patients had undergone explantation following an average of 15 years
  - 13 women had undergone exchange of implants
- breast reduction ($n = 186$)
- population controls ($n = 149$)

Data indicated no difference between any cohort in:
- smoking
- alcohol consumption
- education
- marital status
- use of contraceptive, analgesic, antiallergic or cardiac drugs
- positive autoimmune antibody tests
  - seropositivity for antinuclear Ab, rheumatoid factor and IgM Ab recorded in 5–10% of women in each group
- incidence of breast cancer

Implant cohort compared with breast reduction and population controls:
- patients with implants had slightly more pregnancies and younger at first delivery
- lower body mass index
- breast pain reported more commonly (3 ×)
  - 18% of patients reported severe pain associated with Baker IV capsular contracture
- higher self-reported use of hormone replacement therapy and antidepressant and anxiolytic drugs
  - increased risk of suicide amongst augmentation mammaplasty patients reported elsewhere (Koot. *BMJ* 2003)
- fatigue and Raynaud-like symtoms were similar in implant and reduction cohorts
  - reported more frequently than in the population control group

Contamination of breast milk with silicon
Semple. *PRS* 1998

Theoretical risk of silicone breakdown products (e.g. silicon) entering breast milk in patients with implants in a submammary pocket

Reports of abnormal oesophageal motility in children breast-fed by women with implants

This study measures elemental silicon in breast milk of patients with and without implants

Silicon levels were the same in each group

Silicon was $10 \times$ higher in cows' milk and even higher in infant formulas

Grain, rice and beer also have high levels of silicon

Silicone levels in breast and capsular tissue

Weinzweig. *PRS* 1998

Silicone levels in breast tissue were the same in patients with implants as those without

Capsule silicone levels were significantly higher than breast tissue levels

Capsule silicone levels were higher in patients with gel-filled implants than in those with saline implants

There was no relationship between the level of capsular silicone and the incidence of connective tissue disease

Management of the breast after explantation

Rohrich. *PRS* 1998

Options following explantation:

- explantation and capsulectomy alone
  - presence of microcalification or silicone granulomas makes detection of breast cancers more difficult if the capsule is left behind
  - may be possible to remove entire capsule while maintaining the implant inside
  - dissection of a subpectoral capsule is achieved by anterior then posterior capsulectomy
- re-implantation
  - if intending to replace the implant with a *saline* implant then subpectoral placement is preferred to avoid rippling
  - (capsul**ectomy** or -**otomy**?)
- mastopexy – related to the degree of ptosis

Tuberous breast deformity

Tuberous breast deformity
Heimburg. *BJPS* 1996

'Tuberous'/'tubular'/'constricted' all describe the same deformity

But distinguish from a hypoplastic breast – more easily treated by augmentation $\pm$ TE

Unilateral or bilateral – asymmetry common

Fewer ducts and less breast tissue in the inferior quadrants

Classification:

- type 1 – hypoplasia of the inferior medial quadrant
- type 2 – hypoplasia of both inferior quadrants
- type 3 – hypoplasia of both lower quadrants + subareolar skin shortage
- type 4 – severely constricted breast base

Surgical options:

- type 1 – augmentation with a submammary implant
- type 2

- augment plus internal flap – 'unfurling' of breast tissue on the chest wall, turned downwards to augment the lower half of the breast
- may be performed through an inferior circumareolar incision
- types 3 and 4
  - augment plus internal flap plus skin importation:
    - **skin importation avoids 'double bubble' deformity**
    - Z-plasty across the inframammary fold
    - thoraco-epigastric flap
    - tissue expansion
  - circumareolar mastopexy and tissue expansion
- breast reduction may be considered in an adequately sized breast

Self-assessment: Discuss how you would manage a patient with unilateral tubular breast deformity

History
- age, partnership status, children/breast feeding history
- do you prefer the larger or the smaller breast size (contralateral reduction or mastopexy versus ipsilateral augmentation) – and do you want to avoid scars on the normal breast?
- family history of tubular breast
- breast cancer history – lumps, nipple discharge, previous breast surgery, mammogram, family history
- smoker, drugs, etc.

Examination
- reclined for breast cancer examination – hand behind head, palpate each quadrant for lumps, feel the axilla
- sit up for aesthetic examination – symmetry, ptosis (Regnault classification), degree of tubular breast deformity (Heimberg classification)
- determine the level of the inframammary fold on the affected side
- feel for a Poland's and look at the hand

Management options
- augmentation of the tubular breast
  - classes 1–3 → tissue expansion then augmentation via inframammary or infra-areolar incision trying to avoid a double bubble
  - class 4 → as above but may need to import skin to break up the constricted base at the abnormal inframammary fold – thoraco-epigastric flap
- contralateral reduction
- contralateral mastopexy ± augmentation

Aesthetic reconstruction of the tuberous breast deformity

Mandrekas. *Plast Reconstr Surg* 2003
- tuberous breast deformity was first described in 1976 by Rees and Aston
- characterized by:
  - a constricting ring at the base of the breast
  - deficient horizontal and vertical development of the breast
  - herniation of the breast parenchyma toward the nipple–areolar complex
  - areola enlargement
- Embryologically

- breast tissue comes from the mammary ridge, which develops from the ectoderm during the fifth week
- most parts of this ridge disappear, except for a small portion in the thoracic region that persists and penetrates the underlying mesenchyme (10 to 14 weeks)
- no further development occurs until puberty
- as a result of the ectodermal origin of the breast and its invagination into the underlying mesenchyme, the breast tissue is contained within a fascial envelope, the superficial fascia, consisting of two layers:
- the superficial layer of the superficial fascia (outer layer covering the breast parenchyma)
- the deep layer of the superficial fascia (the posterior boundary of the breast parenchyma and lies on the deep fascia of the pectoralis major and serratus anterior muscles)
  - penetrated by fibrous attachments – suspensory ligaments of Cooper – which join the two layers of the superficial fascia and extend to the dermis of the overlying skin and the deep pectoral fascia
- critically, the superficial layer of the superficial fascia is absent in the area underneath the areola
- there is also a constricting fibrous ring at the level of the periphery of the nipple–areola complex that inhibits the normal development of the breast
- approach to surgery from embryological principles:
  - periareolar incision
  - re-arrangement of the inferior parenchyma by division of the constricting ring
  - and creation of two breast pillars.
  - in cases of volume deficiency, a silicone breast implant is placed in a subglandular pocket
  - dough-nut mastopexy to address the size of the nipple-areola complex
  - used in 11 patients (21 breasts) with good results

Self assessment: How would you counsel the patient regarding a silicone implant?

Rationale for submammary placement and textured silicone implant:
- more natural feel to a silicone implant
- submammary placement takes up skin envelope
- avoids ugly contractions of overlying pectoralis
- in thin patients may consider submuscular placement – also may increase success of mammography and encourage less capsule formation

Early complications
- infection
- haematoma
- extrusion

Late complications
- scar-related
- rupture – Robinson: 50% rupture rate at 12 years – older implants
- gel bleed – remains intracapsular and usually asymptomatic
- capsule formation – all form capsules (subclinical *Staphylococcus* infection? → reduced with betadine wash-out; fibroblast response – Bradford studies smooth vs. textured) – Baker classification
- asymmetry of shape and volume

- migration of implant – too high
- lactation and nipple sensation may be affected
- issues regarding induction of breast cancer → less than predicted incidence in patients with implants; Berkel. *NEJM*; Deapen and Brodie. *PRS*, both early 1990s; also new research from the USA – compression → decreased BF and ?fewer cancers in animals; also polyurethane coating (?less capsule but → toluene derivative and sarcomas in rat) no longer used
- issues regarding the detection of breast cancer (Silverstein, cancer – 40% false-negative mammography rate, patient should have a mammogram first and if there is a family history of breast cancer choose submuscular placement); but displacement and compression techniques (Eklund) → 60% visualization of breast (submammary placement) and 90% visualization (submuscular placement)
- issues regarding the silicone controversy – two large studies – Mayo Clinic (700 patients, Gabriel. *NEJM* 1994) and nurses health study (90 000 nurses, Sanchez-Guerrero. *NEJM* 1995) both showed no increased incidence; initial reports (van Nunen, Australia 1982) largely anecdotal, incidence of connective tissue diseases in the population is high (fibromyalgia 5%, RA 2%, scleroderma, SLE 0.10 and 0.14%) so risk with implant no greater than background risk; everyone exposed to high levels of elemental silicon in diet and medical devices, higher levels in infant formula milk than in milk of mothers with implants

Breast reduction

Cup size:
- measured by:
  - inframammary circumference = Chest–nipple circumference = AA
  - chest–nipple circumference = inframammary circumference + 2 cm = A
  - + 2 cm = B cup
  - + 2 cm = C cup, etc.
- 32–34-inch chest → one cup size = 100 g
- >36-inch chest → one cup size = 180–200 g

Gigantomastia: >2.5 kg reduction per breast

Macromastia: <2.5 kg reduction per breast

Virginal breast hypertrophy: seen only in pubertal and prepubertal females

Indications in the patient with large breasts:
- mastalgia
- secondary back, shoulder and neck pain
- psychological
- submammary maceration and infection

Techniques

Liposuction – alone or in combination

No pedicle
- **Thorek 1922**
- breast amputation and free nipple graft

Central mound/glanduloplasty; Balch. *PRS* 1981

Dermoglandular pedicle

- horizontal pedicle
  - Strombeck. *BJPS* 1960
  - horizontal bipedicle, inverted T scar
  - Skoog. *Acta Chir Scand* 1963
  - horizontal unipedicle, inverted T scar (Wise pattern)
- lateral pedicle
  - Duformentel. *Ann Chir Plast* 1965
  - lateral pedicle and lateral scar
- vertical pedicle
  - McKissock. *PRS* 1972
  - bipedicle, inverted T scar
  - Weiner. *PRS* 1973
  - superior pedicle
  - Lejour. *Ann Chir Plast Esthet* 1990
  - superior vertical pedicle, vertical scar only
  - Robbins. *PRS* 1977
  - inferior pedicle, inverted T scar
  - Regnault. *PRS* 1980
  - glanduloplasty technique
  - inferolateral resection, B-shaped scar

Lassus technique

Plast Reconstr Surg 1996

Initial markings indicate position to which the nipple must move (A) and a second point 2–4 cm above the inframammary fold (B) defining the inferior limit of skin resection

Vertical lines marked to connect these points after medial and lateral displacement of the breast

Keyhole pattern incorporated to mark inset of nipple–areolar complex

Superior dermal pedicle – must be thin and include adequate tissue above the nipple to avoid venous congestion

Nipple raised on pedicle then central breast parenchymal excision undertaken

No skin underming

Nipple inset temporarily and margins of rescection closed

Framing sutures then sited to generate desired breast shape

Margins inked and framing sutures removed

Secondary resection undertaken along inked margins

Vertical scar closed and pleated to ensure that scar does not descend below inframammary fold

Lejour technique

Ann Chir Plast Esthet 1990

Modification of the Lassus technique

Incorporates a vertical pedicle

Circumareolar and superior vertical scar

Relies upon substantial postoperative skin contraction and inferior breast remodelling

Some numbness to the nipple itself post-operation due to the superior pedicle (nerves enter inferolaterally)

Vertical vs. Wise pattern breast reduction: patient satisfaction, revision rates, and complications

Cruz-Korchin. *Plast Reconstr Surg* 2003

A prospective, randomized study to compare the outcome of inferior pedicle/Wise pattern reduction with medial pedicle/vertical pattern

- reduction in moderate resections averaging 500 g per breast ($n = 207$)
- vertical scar revision rate 11%
- complications similar in both groups
- overall patient satisfaction not significantly different
- vertical mammaplasty ranked significantly higher by patients in regard to scars and overall aesthetic results
- vertical scar breast reduction for moderate macromastia provides better cosmetic results but is associated with a significantly higher revision rate

The vertical mammaplasty: a reappraisal of the technique and its complications

Berthe. *Plast Reconstr Surg* 2003

- Criticisms of the vertical mammaplasty as described by Lejour are
  - delayed healing on the vertical scar
  - risk of seromas
  - haematoma
  - glandular necrosis
  - increased need for secondary corrections
- 170 consecutive vertical mammaplasty procedures (330 breasts) reviewed
  - minor complications observed in 30% (minor skin edge necrosis)
  - major complications in 15% (glandular necrosis and severe infection)
  - surgical revision for scar or volume correction necessary in 28%
- original technique then modified by
  - decreasing the skin undermining
  - avoiding liposuction in the breast
  - primary skin excision performed in the submammary fold at the end of the operation if the skin could not be puckered adequately
- review of modified technique in 138 consecutive patients (227 breasts)
  - minor complications observed in 15%
  - major complications in 5%
  - no significant change in secondary scar and volume corrections (22%)

Benefits and pitfalls of vertical mammaplasty

Beer. *BJPS* 2003

Survey of US plastic surgeons has shown that only 12% undertake vertical mammaplasty but is more popular in Europe

Complications following Lejour mammaplasty similar to T scar breast reduction according to most studies

Review of Lassus reduction technique in 170 patients

- median resection weight 380 g (range 60–1262 g)
- mean operation time 3 h 10 mins

Early complications in 21% including:

- haematoma 4%

- infection 4%
- wound dehiscence 12%
  - infra-areolar area prone to dehiscence
- nipple necrosis 0.7%

Late complications in 26%:

- inadequate reduction 3%
- shape problems 5%
- minor asymmetry (1/4 patients)
- problems with the vertical scar
  - hypertrophy
  - broad
  - dog ears
  - too long – breast/nipple too high 15% and scar appears below the new inframammary fold

Benefits

- long-lasting and enhanced projection
- reduced scarring

Complications

general
infection
haematoma
dehiscence (T-junction)
scarring (including hypertrophic)
DVT/PE
Specific
mild asymmetry
nipple loss – partial/complete
nipple sensation – increased/decreased
lactation and breast feeding compromised (but ~70% can still lacatate) following inferior
    pedicle technique
fat necrosis
revisional surgery (dog ears)
scar hypertrophy

Pathological findings in breast reduction surgery
Titley. *BJPS* 1996

~25% of all breast reductions show abnormal pathology, although most of these are due to
fibro-adenosis

42% of plastic surgeons (BAPS) had experience of at least one patient with unexpected breast
cancer at some time

Incidence of breast cancer in women <28 years of age is ~8 in 100 000

If sending specimen for histopathology must indicate area from which separate blocks of
tissue have been removed – 60% of breast cancer occurs in the upper outer quadrant

Evidence to suggest that BBR reduces Ca risk

- ?removes microscopic disease
- ?reduces potential foci – ductal and lobular tissue

In patients <30 years of age there is no need to send tissue for histology unless there is a strong family history or the tissue appears macroscopically abnormal

Breast cancer in reduction mammoplasty
Jansen. *PRS* 1998

Analysis of 5000 breast reductions by Snyderman in 1959 → 19 cancers (0.38%)

This survey of plastic surgeons in New Orleans revealed four cancers after 2500 reductions (0.16%)

Sending specimens for pathology **is** appropriate

> Self-assessment: Describe how you would classify approaches to breast reduction, and manage and counsel your patient

Operation performed for macromastia or gigantomastia

Aim to achieve smaller breasts with shape and volume symmetry

Classified according to the type of pedicle and the type of skin markings

Pedicle types:
- dermoglandular
  - vertical bipedicle – McKissock
  - superior – Weiner
  - inferior – Robbins
  - lateral – Duformentel
- glanduloplasty – central mound – Balch
- free nipple grafts – Thorek
- liposuction

Skin incisions:
- inverted T
- B-shaped (Regnault)
- vertical scar – Lassus/Lejour

History – full breast cancer history (lumps, nipple discharge, previous surgery, mammogram history, family history), intentions to breast feed, current size and ideal size, symptoms related to large breasts including psychological, marital history, scar history

Examination:
- cancer examination – lumps, nodes, scars, etc.
- aesthetic examination – size, shape, symmetry, degree of ptosis (Regnault), sternal notch–nipple distance, nipple–inframammary fold distance, general body habitus

Investigations:
- pre-operative mammogram depending on history
- bloods – Gp&S, Hb

Explain nature of operation, drains, post-operative pain relief, expected duration of stay, dressings and sports bra for 6 weeks

Risks and complications:
- early
  - infection

- haematoma
- T-junction dehiscence
- DVT and PE
- late
  - scar distribution and hypertrophy
  - skin necrosis
  - nipple-related complications:
    - sensation increased or decreased
    - partial or total loss
  - shape and volume asymmetry
  - fat necrosis
  - breast feeding difficulties
  - revisional surgery to dog ears

Breast reduction surgery and breast cancer risk

Tarone. *Plast Reconstr Surg* 2004

- Lifetime risk of a developing breast cancer is estimated to be one in eight females (American Cancer Society)
  - Median age at diagnosis is approximately 60 years old
- 0.1% of women are carriers of BRCA1 or BRCA2 (BRCA1/2)
  - Of women who developed breast cancer before age 42, 25% have a definable hereditary component
  - 50% of BRCA1 carriers treated by lumpectomy and radiotherapy recurred or developed a second cancer in the same breast
- 100 000 breast reductions were undertaken in the USA in 2002
- Women with increased body mass index tend to have more fatty tissue and elevated peripheral oestrogen
  - associated with increased breast cancer risk in post-menopausal (though *not pre-menopausal*) women
  - most US breast reduction patients younger than in the UK
- Five studies were reviewed:
  - three cohort studies from Scandinavia
  - one cohort study from Ontario, Canada
  - one small case-control study from the United States (10 cases, 13 controls)
- Each study concluded that the risk of breast cancer was less in the breast reduction patients than in the controls (relative risk, 0.2 to 0.7)
  - Scandinavian studies found
    - almost no reduction in risk in women under 40 (at the time of breast reduction)
    - substantial reductions in women aged over 40
- Prophylactic mastectomy shown to decrease cancer risk by 90–100%
- Tamoxifen has been shown to decrease the risk of breast cancer among BRCA1/2 mutation carriers by 50–62 %
- Bilateral oophorectomy before menopause by 25–53%.
- Women screened annually by mammography have a low risk of breast cancer-related mortality, and screening remains a reasonable option for high-risk women

Occult breast carcinoma in reduction mammaplasty specimens: 14-year experience

Colwell. *Plast Reconstr Surg* 2004

Reduction mammaplasty is commonly performed for

- bilateral macromastia
- congenital asymmetry
- contralateral symmetry following cancer surgery/reconstruction

History:

- Maliniac first described the association of breast cancer and reduction mammaplasty, incriminating his free nipple graft as the source of ductal stasis and subsequent carcinoma
- Tang *et al.* (*PRS* 1999) documented invasive carcinoma in 0.06 per cent of 27 500 breast reductions from the Ontario registry
- Other studies have reported occult breast cancer in 0.06 per cent to 0.4 per cent of breast reduction specimens

Incidence of breast cancer in breast reductions performed in one institution over a 14-year period

- 800 reduction mammaplasties performed between 1988 and 2001
- Six cancers were detected (0.8%)
  - three were invasive (0.4%)
  - three were ductal carcinoma *in situ* (0.4%)
- trend toward higher detection rates in the reconstruction group (1.2%) compared with the macromastia (0.7%) or congenital asymmetry (0%) groups
- pre-operative mammography invariably negative

Mastopexy

Regnault classification of ptosis:

- first degree – nipple descends to the level of the inframammary fold
- second degree – nipple falls below fold but remains above lowest contour of breast
- third degree – nipple reaches the lowest contour of the breast
- pseudoptosis – loose, lax breast but nipple remains above inframammary fold

Breast reduction-type markings: Regnault, Lejour, inferior pedicle, also cirumareolar (Benelli)

De-epithelialization within markings

Glanduloplasty

Breast parenchyma sutured to chest wall

Resiting of the nipple–areolar complex as for reduction surgery

Augmentation:

- restores superior breast volume in the ptotic breast
- an alternative to mastopexy – fills out skin redundancy only in the low volume breast
- combined with mastopexy:
  - skin excision required for more severe ptosis in the low volume breast
  - implant fills out the remaining volume
  - excise inferior breast tissue rather than in-fold and place implant in a subglandular pocket or submuscularly

Breast reconstruction

Breast cancer

Epidemiology

- 30 000 new cases of breast cancer diagnosed annually in the UK
- Half are in the <65-year age group
- Half of these require mastectomy
- Hence 7500 breast reconstructions per year + prophylactic reconstructions

Breast cancer genes

- *BRCA1* and *BRCA2* genes for breast cancer account for 2–3% of breast cancer cases
- tumour suppressor genes that have become mutated
- More than four cases of breast cancer when <60 years of age within one family → likely to be genetic
- two-to-three cases only → likely to be due to chance only
- Carriers are likely to develop breast cancer before 50 years of age and have a lifetime risk of ~85%
- Other as yet unidentified genes may also contribute to risk
- Carriers may elect to undergo subcutaneous mastectomy and reconstruction

Screening

- Identifies six cancers for every 1000 women screened
- Pre-menopausal breast is dense and difficult to screen by mammography – hence screening not currently offered to those <50 years of age, although some studies have indicated that this may be worthwhile
- MRI is a sensitive investigation in the premenopausal breast and is currently performed within a MRC trial in carriers of the *BRCA* gene
- USS good for differentiating solid vs. cystic lesions and guided biopsy
- High-resolution USS can pick up some cancers and can monitor tumour response to chemo-/radio-Rx
- MRI imaging of implants → linguine sign where the implant has pulled away from the capsule leaving multiple parallel lines (stepladder sign)
- MRI operated with silicone or water suppressed sequences
- Snowstorm appearance of ruptured implant on USS

Pathology

- 75% invasive ductal – DCIS → microcalcification on mammogram
- 5% invasive lobular
  - LCIS → no mammographic changes
  - a marker of invasive disease rather than a precursor
  - tendency to bilaterality (40%) and multifocality (60%)
- Special types generally have a good prognosis
  - medullary (numerous lymphocytes) <5%
  - mucinous (bulky mucin-forming tumours) <5%
  - tubular (well-differentiated adenocarcinoma)
  - phyllodes (mixed connective tissue and epithelial tumour, fern-like cellular pattern)

Staging

- **TMN classification** – main landmarks (~5-year survival%)

- stage 1 – tumour <2 cm confined to the breast (T1) (85%)
- stage 2 – mobile axillary nodes (N1) (65%)
- stage 3a – fixed axillary nodes (N2) (40%)
- stage 3b – chest wall or skin involvement (T4) 25%
- stage 3b – internal mammary nodes (N3)
- stage 4 – distant metastases (M1) (10%)
- Tis – Ca *in situ* or Paget's disease of the nipple with no associated tumour
- T1 – <2 cm
- T2 – 2–5 cm
- T3 – >5 cm
- T4 – extension to chest wall or skin
- N0 – no regional lymph node metastasis
- N1 – ipsilateral axillary lymph nodes
- N2 – fixed ipsilateral nodes
- N3 – internal mammary lymph node(s)
- M0 – no distant metastasis
- M1 – distant metastasis (includes metastasis to supraclavicular lymph nodes)

Tumour excision

- lumpectomy + radiotherapy + node sampling or clearance
- skin-sparing mastectomy for extensive DCIS
- modified radical mastectomy (includes in-continuity axillary clearance, leaves pectoralis major) may be incorporated into a breast reduction type marking with contralateral surgery for symmetry
- quadrantectomy may be treated by circumareolar-orientated mobilization of the breast mound and direct closure of the overlying skin
- concept of 'mirror' surgery to achieve symmetry
- thoraco-epigastric flaps (based on the superior superficial epigastric A and V) may be used for skin following lower quadrant resection
- axillary tail transposition flap used for the upper outer quadrant, also inverted T breast reduction

Neo-adjuvant therapy

- neo-adjuvant chemo-Rx downstages tumour size and treats systemic disease
- downstaging tumour size may increase the changes of breast-conserving surgery
- neo-adjuvant radio-Rx may also be used except where local tissues are required for flap closure
- overall response rate to neo-adjuvant chemo-Rx ~80% with complete response in ~30%, but no evidence of a survival advantage
- but there is a significant morbidity rate associated with chemo-Rx
- radio-Rx usually used postoperatively

Angiosarcoma of the breast

Georgiannos. *BJPS* 2003

Sarcomas account for <1% of all breast cancers

Four cases of angiosarcoma of the breast reported

- Two patients were young (20 and 35 years of age)
- Two patients were older (45 and 64 years) – both of these had received radiotherapy for breast cancer

All patients ultimately treated by mastectomy after incisional or excisional biopsy each case

All patients alive and disease free (3–7 years post-mastectomy)

Prognosis is generally related to histological grade and excision margins

- high grade median disease free survival 15 months

Skin-sparing mastectomy. Kroll. *Surg Gynecol Obstet* 1991, Carlson. *Ann Surg* 1997, Slavin. *PRS* 1997, Hidalgo. *PRS* 1998

Removes breast, nipple/areolar complex and biopsy scar

Superior aesthetic result

- preserves native breast skin (except skin overlying a superficial Ca)
- preserves inframammary fold
- less need to alter the contralateral breast

Improves psychological response to mastectomy

All forms of mastectomy leave behind **some** breast tissue

Local recurrence rate is proportional to **stage** of disease and tumour biology rather than type of surgery

- SSM used safely in the treatment of invasive Ca without compromising local control
- Average time to local recurrence ~2–4 years
    - 30% of recurrences occur within the first year
    - 50% have occurred within the first 2 years
- Most recurrence occurs in skin
- Local recurrence is a marker for disseminated disease: all patients with local recurrence eventually die of disseminated disease

Incidence of skin flap necrosis same as for non-SSM

Indications:

- prophylactic
- DCIS
- stage 1 and 2 invasive breast Ca
- phyllodes tumour
- where immediate reconstruction is planned
    - latissimus dorsi + implant
    - free or pedicled TRAM

Classification:

- type 1 – nipple/areolar complex only (prophylactic)
- type 2 – nipple/areolar complex + separate scar excision
- type 3 – nipple/areolar complex + in-continuity scar excision
- type 4 – nipple/areolar complex within a breast reduction (large breast, unsuitable for TRAM, contralateral reduction planned)

May need a separate incision for axillary sampling/clearance and/or microsurgery

Nipple reconstruction after 3 months removes obvious 'patch'

Breast reconstruction

Immediate versus delayed – delay reconstruction where there is an inflammatory carcinoma

Breast reconstruction is a process, often involving a number of procedures, rather than a one-off operation

Contralateral breast plays a major role in the selection of the reconstruction technique:

- post-lumpectomy deformity (Clough)
  - If there is a late change in the breast, always check for recurrence – examination and MRI scan
  - asymmetry only → contralateral breast reduction
  - deformity requiring partial breast reconstruction → implant or autogenous
  - deformity relating to surgery and/or radio-Rx requiring mastectomy and total reconstruction

Maximizing the size of a breast reconstruction using latissimus without an implant:

- fleur-de-lis skin paddle – but poor scar
- take all the fat along with the muscle
- orientate the skin paddle perpendicular to the pedicle axis

TRAM reconstruction

- Bilateral pedicled TRAM reconstruction for bilateral mastectomy – quicker and less complicated than bilateral free TRAMs
- Can use in the presence of a midline scar
- For a unilateral breast reconstruction, the procedure of choice is a free flap
- Incidence of fat necrosis 7–16%
- Gynaecological Pfannenstiel incisions do not usually compromise the flap (recti are spread apart at operation/caesarean section) but a general surgical Pfannenstiel approach usually cuts the muscle
- Mesh does not interfere with pregnancy
- Beware in the obese and smokers
- Immediate reconstruction is usually safer, quicker and more aesthetic
- If performing delayed reconstruction consider using the internal mammary arteries

DIEP flap

- First described by Allen 1994
- Always throw away zone 4 or will get fat necrosis
- Sacrificing the recti adversely affects the functioning of the internal obliques – need resistance against which to contract → decrease in rotational strength
- Recti responsible for initiating the first 35–40° of abdominal flexion only, also responsible for raising intra-abdominal pressure
- 10–20% of patients do not return to their job/hobbies after a TRAM
- Must preserve segmental nerves if raising a DIEP flap to keep the recti innervated – otherwise no point in preserving the muscle
- Duplex Doppler pre-operatively to define perforators and create a 'road map'
- Vessels at tendinous intersections are usually larger
- Flap may be made sensate

Superficial inferior epigastric flap

- Described by Arnez; vessels are very small
- If delaying a pedicled TRAM must also cut these vessels

Lateral transverse thigh flap

- Uses TFL muscle on lateral circumflex femoral vessels
- But leaves a significant contour defect

S-GAP flap

- First described by Allen 1995
- Avoids raising the superior gluteal flap on a large vein which is difficult to size match for breast reconstruction

Rubens flap

- Based on the DCIA
- Must repair abdominal wall muscles back to the iliac crest
- Long consistent pedicle

Small breast

- Becker prosthesis, expandable anatomically shaped implants (below) or TE then implant
  - Following skin-sparing, mastectomy must be placed in a subpectoral pocket
  - Over-inflate to achieve ptosis when replaced by implant
  - Capsulotomy at time of implant placement if a troublesome capsule has developed
  - Avoid making pocket too high
  - Chest wall radiotherapy is given to ~20–30% of patients after mastectomy – the presence of a breast implant increases the chance of capsular contracture
- Latissimus dorsi + implant (+ contralateral implant if very small breast)

Moderate breast

Becker prosthesis or TE then implant

Latissimus dorsi + implant

Pedicled TRAM (Hartrampf)

Free DIEP flap

Where only zones 1 and 3 are required – supply to contralateral side is unreliable on the non-dominant superior pedicle

Ipsilateral pedicle → acute angle → compromises venous flow

Contralateral pedicle generally preferred, but either possible

Large breast

Bipedicled TRAM

- but significant donor defect
- overcomes problem of the midline scar

Free TRAM

- Anastomosing end–end to the circumflex scapular vessels saves latissimus dorsi as a lifeboat
- Anastomosing end–end to the thoracodorsal artery proximal to the serratus branch also preserves latissimus dorsi (retrograde flow from intercostal supply to serratus)
- Utilizes zones 1–4

If unsuitable, contralateral breast reduction and other technique

- pedicled TRAM (or DIEP flap)
- latissimus dorsi + implant

Reconstruction of both breasts

Bilateral pedicled or free TRAM/DIEP flaps, lat dorsi, implants

Twenty free S-GAP flap sensate breast reconstructions

Blondeel. *BJPS* 1999

Skin/fat flap vascularized by a single perforator from the superior gluteal artery

Identify position of perforator before surgery by Doppler

Anastomoses to internal mammary vessels in third intercostal space

Second choice to DIEP flap

- Indicated in patients in whom a DIEP flap is impossible
  - scarring
  - insufficient abdominal tissue

Advantages:

- large calibre, long vascular pedicle – no need to perform the difficult dissection of the (short) superior gluteal pedicle
- hidden scar
- no functional morbidity at donor site
- leaving muscle behind avoids exposure of sciatic nerve
- made sensate by coaption of sensory nerves entering the flap from above (dorsal branches of lumbar segmental nerves) to the fourth intercostal nerve

One hundred free DIEP flap breast reconstructions. Blondeel. *BJPS* 1999

Maintains abdominal flexion and rotation strength compared with TRAM

No need to dissect right down to the external iliac artery – the pedicle is long enough to be divided at the lateral border of the rectus abdominis muscle (but uses the internal mammary vessels)

- An **ipsilateral** flap is required if anastomosing to the internal mammary vessels
- A **contralateral** flap is required if anastomosing to the thoracodorsal vessels

Majority of flaps were isolated on one or two perforators

Vascular anatomy:

- Lateral branch of the DIEA connected these perforators in 50%
- Medial and lateral branches equally dominant in 15%
- One common vessel in ∼30%
- Zone 4 may need to be discarded if the flap is nourished predominantly by lateral perforators

Innervated by branches of 10th and 11th intercostal nerves

Raise the pedicle side first, preserving the other side as a lifeboat

When raising bilateral flaps, dissect out the distal perforators first – if these are damaged, the flap can still be raised as a pedicled TRAM

Expandable anatomical implants

Mahdi *et al.* (McGeorge). *BJPS* 1998

McGhan anatomically shaped implants inserted subpectorally

Muscle splitting approach through the mastectomy wound for immediate reconstruction

Inframammary approach for delayed reconstruction

Dissect at least 1 cm inferior to the inframammary fold to avoid the implant riding high

Anatomical shell makes up 50% of final volume

Remaining volume in lower pole achieved by expansion via a port in axilla

- Port is designed to stay in permanently
- Commence expansion 2 weeks post-operatively

16/20 patients underwent surgery to match up the normal breast at the time of expander insertion (based upon the anticipated size and shape of the reconstructed breast)

Internal mammary vessels for free flap breast reconstruction. Two papers. Ninkovic and Arnez. *BJPS* 1995

Axilla may be scarred due to surgery or radiotherapy and thoracodorsal vessels may have been disrupted

Shorter pedicle required for internal mammary anastomosis

Internal mammary vessels are very fragile but good size match for deep inferior epigastric vessels

Lie 1.5 cm lateral to the lateral border of the sternum

Third or fourth costal cartilage is removed subperichondrially to facilitate recipient vessel dissection in the third–fourth space

>80% of TRAM flaps were ipsilateral

Advantages

- Allows for improved positioning of the flap on the chest wall
- Spares latissimus dorsi as a lifeboat
- Zone IV lies lateral rather than medial
- Avoids further dissection of the axilla which may worsen lymphoedema

Disadvantages

- Respiratory movement during anastomosis
- Compromises blood supply to sternum if the other internal mammary vessels have been used in cardiac surgery
- Risks iatrogenic pneumothorax

Endoscopic delay of the pedicled TRAM flap

Codner. *Plast Reconstr Surg* 1995

Performed in 'high risk' patients undergoing pedicled TRAM breast reconstruction – obesity, smokers, radiation, abdominal scars

Performed either open or endoscopically

TRAM flaps in patients with abdominal scars

Takeishi. *Plast Reconstr Surg* 1997

Free TRAM flaps were preferred and performed wherever possible

Patients with low transverse scars (Pfannenstiel) were explored and if the DIEA was not intact then an ipsilateral pedicled TRAM flap or free contralateral TRAM flap was raised

In all patients with lower paramedian scars the vessels had been divided

In patients with lower midline scars the flap was designed higher up on the abdomen so that 5–7 cm of unscarred skin formed a bridge above the umbilicus – leaves a high, mid-abdominal, transverse scar

Subcostal incisions meant that the ipsilateral flap had to be free because of fear of prior division of the superior pedicle

Appendicectomy scars do not compromise the TRAM flap

Carcinoma of the male breast

Benedetto. *Plast Reconstr Surg* 1998

1% of all breast cancers

~1% is bilateral

Aggressive tumour

Delayed diagnosis but symptoms and signs as for female cancer

Mean age at diagnosis ~60 years

Pathological types and incidences same as for female breast cancer except invasive lobular – only seen in association with Klinefelter's

Neoplastic cells are hormone dependent: aetiology relates to hyperoestrogenic states

Higher incidence of positive internal mammary nodes compared with female disease

Reconstruction depends on stage at diagnosis, e.g. stage 4 lesions may need chest wall reconstruction

Almost impossible to close margins after radical or modified radical mastectomy – need local thoraco-epigastric FC flap or distant latissimus dorsi

Local recurrence or death after excision of phyllodes tumours of the breast

De Roos. *BJS* 1999

Uncommon tumour

20% recurrence rate

90% 5-year survival

Low-to-high-grade malignancies

Low recurrence after radical surgery

Higher recurrence where resection margins were involved

Size and grade of tumour were prognostic for metastatic death

The transverse myocutaneous gracilis free flap in autologous breast reconstruction

Wechselberger. *Plast Reconstr Surg* 2004

The myocutaneous gracilis free flap:

- transverse orientation of the skin paddle
- proximal third of the medial thigh
- in selected patients provides a moderate amount of tissue for autologous breast reconstruction
- the donor-site morbidity is similar to that of a classic medial thigh lift

Ten patients underwent autologous breast reconstruction with 12 transverse myocutaneous gracilis free flaps

- no free-flap failure
- no functional donor-site morbidity

Valuable alternative for immediate autologous breast reconstruction after skin-sparing mastectomy in patients with

- small and medium-sized breasts
- inadequate soft-tissue bulk at the lower abdomen and gluteal region
- desire for no visible scar at the latissimus or any other donor site

Breast reconstruction by the free transverse gracilis flap

Arnež. *BJPS* 2004.

Type II myocutaneous free flap

Pedicle:

- ascending branch of the medial circumflex femoral artery (from the profunda femoris artery)
- only 5–6 cm long (internal mammary vessels preferred site of anastomosis)
- 1.6 mm diameter
- enters the proximal third of the muscle 10 cm below the inguinal ligament

Skin paddle:

- orientated transversely over the upper part of the muscle
- maximum width 10–12 cm

Indication:

- small – moderate-sized breast

- large hips/thighs
- skin sparing mastectomy reconstruction
- patients keen to avoid abdominal, back or gluteal scars

A 10-year retrospective review of 758 DIEP flaps for breast reconstruction
Gill. *Plast Reconstr Surg* 2004

Review of 758 deep inferior epigastric perforator flaps for breast reconstruction, with respect to risk factors and associated complications

- Risk factors that demonstrated significant association with any breast or abdominal complication:
  - smoking
  - post-reconstruction radiotherapy
  - hypertension

Results

- 12.9% developed fat necrosis
  - 19 cases (2.5%) of partial flap loss
  - 4 cases (0.5%) of total flap loss
  - 45 flaps (5.9%) returned to the operating theatre
    - 29 flaps (3.8%) because of venous congestion
    - venous congestion was unrelated to the number of venous anastomoses
- Post-operative abdominal hernia or bulge occurred in only five reconstructions (0.7%)
- Complication rates were comparable to those in retrospective reviews of pedicle and free TRAM flaps

Aesthetic subunits of the breast
Spear. *Plast Reconstr Surg* 2003

- Surgery for breast cancer has traditionally addressed the breast as if it were a geometric circle with associated quadrants
- Cosmetic reconstruction should not follow geometric patterns but should emphasize perceived contour and normal clothing lines
- A subunit principle in breast reconstruction planning may significantly improve the appearance of the result
  - Aesthetic subunits illustrate the placement of scars along natural lines that maximise the advantages of camouflage afforded by clothing
- Review of 10 years of autogenous reconstruction in 264 patients
  - Favorable subunits of the breast in terms of post-operative appearance and camouflage of scars included the:
    - nipple
    - areola
    - expanded areola subunits
  - For larger skin defects, most favourable subunits were:
    - infero-lateral area
    - lower half of breast
    - total breast subunits
- Augmentation mammaplasty techniques have always instinctively emphasized hiding scars in natural lines
  - inframammary fold

- edge of the areola
- the axilla
- Aesthetic subunits of the breast are outlined by tissue, colour, or texture changes
  - breast skin to areola
  - areola to nipple
  - breast skin to chest skin at the inframammary fold
  - anterior axillary line
  - breast to sternal skin
- The best aesthetic units are expanded concentric circles around the nipple
  - The eye is accustomed to viewing a circular areola, and a large concentric circular subunit is also acceptable
  - The areolar margin is the ideal transition for this subunit in a subcutaneous mastectomy on the breast
- Less aesthetic units include:
  - the upper inner quadrant
  - the medial half
  - the inferomedial quadrant
- The aesthetic lines for scar placement in breast reconstruction should incorporate the inframammary fold, the areola, or the anterior axillary line as much as possible

Internal mammary perforating vessels in microsurgical breast reconstruction
Haywood. *BJPS* 2003
Rationale is to use perforators from the internal mammary vessels as recipient vessels for microsurgical breast reconstruction
- Obviates need for the removal of costal cartilage to access the main vessels
- Perforators from the second and third intercostal spaces used
  - diameter 1.5 mm – good match for DIEP perforators
- Some perforators amenable to dissection superficial to pectoralis major
- Other perforators demanded dissection through pectoralis major
- DIEP, SGAP and SIEP flaps used for reconstruction
- Suitable recipient vessels found in 21 of 44 cases
- No flap loss but four patients required re-exploration of anastomoses
- Disadvantages of internal mammary anastomosis
  - Technically difficult (deep)
  - Removal of a segment of cartilage leads to visible contour deformity
  - Potential for pneumothorax
  - Removes possibility of later use as a bypass graft

Nipple reconstruction

nipple sharing
skate flap
- central full-thickness flap with subcutaneous fat
- two lateral de-epithelialized skin flaps
Areolar complex
- FTSG from groin but natural pigmentation often fades with time
- tattooing

Analysis of nipple/areolar involvement with mastectomy: can the nipple be preserved?

Simmons. *Ann Surg Oncol* 2002

Histological evaluation of the nipple/areolar complex from 217 mastectomy patients between 1990 and 1998

- 10.6% of patients overall had involvement of the nipple
  - central tumour location – 27.3% had nipple involvement
  - non-central location – 6.4% had nipple involvement
- Two patients (<1%) had involvement of the areola
  - Both patients had tumours >5 cm, located centrally below the areola and had > two involved axillary nodes

Areolar skin does not contain ductal cells or breast parenchymal tissue

- Areolar sparing SSM may be considered in selected patients but not preservation of the nipple

Histological analysis of the mastectomy scar at the time of breast reconstruction

Soldin. *BJPS* 2004

Review of mastectomy scar histology in 63 patients who underwent delayed breast reconstruction

- 45 patients showed no sign of recurrence at the time of reconstruction
  - Three patients had bilateral reconstruction = 48 mastectomy scars
  - No evidence of malignancy in any of the mastectomy scars
- Five patients had local tumour recurrence
  - further tumour clearance in three patients
  - breast reconstruction in two patients

Up to 90% of local recurrence following mastectomy occurs within 3 years

Local recurrence is detectable clinically hence routine histological evaluation of the mastectomy scar at the time of reconstruction is unnescessary, especially after 3 years

> **Self-assessment:** A patient is referred from your general surgical colleague with a biopsy proven invasive ductal carcinoma of the left breast, with a view to surgery and immediate reconstruction. What would be the optimal management of the tumour itself and the reconstruction?

History

- age, occupation, marital status
- duration of the lump, rate of growth, time since biopsy
- family history of breast disease
- last mammogram
- any other aches/pains, e.g. backache (metastases)
- general health, current medications
- previous operations – laparotomy, abdominoplasty, etc.
- current bra size
- **what does the patient want?**
- **what does she *not* want?**

Examination

- oncological examination – site, size, chest wall fixation, skin involvement, nodes

- thorough examination of the contralateral breast
- aesthetic examination – contralateral breast volume, shape, ptosis
- abdominal scars, rectus divarication, skin laxity
- skin laxity overlying latissimus, back scars
- determine TMN stage

Investigations

- CXR (staging)
- investigations directed at sites suspicious of metastatic spread, e.g. liver USS, CT head, etc.
- routine bloods, etc.

Treatment

- Options depend upon both the:
  - oncological management and
  - contralateral breast
- Reconstruction can either be:
  - designed to match the contralateral breast, or
  - contralateral breast can be modified to match the reconstruction

Tumour

- All patients get tamoxifen generally
- Widespread DCIS or prophylactic mastectomy → SSM, leave nodes, no radiotherapy
- Small lump, invasive with limited DCIS → lumpectomy, node clearance, adjuvant radiotherapy – can be designed with breast reduction markings
- Small lump, widespread DCIS → SSM, node clearance, adjuvant radiotherapy
- Big lump → neo-adjuvant CMF chemotherapy, mastectomy, node clearance, adjuvant radiotherapy

Reconstruction

- largely dictated by the size of the contralateral breast
  - autologous tissue
    - free TRAM
    - pedicled TRAM
    - pedicled latissimus dorsi – can also be used to fill out lumpectomy deformity
    - DIEP/S-GAP/Rubens
  - implant reconstruction
    - TE then implant
    - Becker or expandable implant
    - implant only
  - combination – pedicled latissimus dorsi + implant
- nipple reconstruction
  - nipple – sharing or skate flap
  - areolar – tattoo or FTSG

Inverted nipple correction

Purse-string suture for nipple projection

Peled. *Plast Reconstr Surg* 1999

Simple technique for the correction of inverted nipple

- Performed under local anaesthesia

- (Nipple everted with a skin hook and) traction suture placed at nipple apex
- fibrous bands released using an 18-gauge needle introduced at the 6 o'clock position and swept medially and laterally in a horizontal plane
- through the same hole, a 4–0 clear monofilament nylon suture is placed and used to create a subcuticular purse string around the nipple, exiting every 5 mm through the skin and reintroduced through the same hole
- purse string tension adjusted, tied and buried at starting point

Gynaecomastia

Abnormal breast development in the male
Aetiology

Physiological

Neonatal, pubertal and senile gynaecomastia
- ?androgen–oestrogen imbalance
- affects up to 75% of pubertal males – 75% resolve within 2 years
Hypogonadism
- pituitary disorders (decreased GRH)
- androgen insensitivity syndrome (5-α-reductase deficiency)
- Klinefelter's – XXY – (20–60 × increased risk of breast cancer)
Systemic disease
- liver disease (e.g. cirrhosis) and hyperthyroidism → increased serum hormone binding globulin (decreases free androgens)
- renal disease → increased LH and oestrogens
- general debility → interferes with pituitary–hypothalamic axis, e.g. burns

Pathological

Hormone-producing tumours
- seminomas, teratomas, choriocarcinomas of testis → hCG
- Leydig, Sertoli and granulosa theca cell of testis → oestrogen
- lung, liver, kidney tumours → GRH
Male breast cancer

Pharmacological

Drugs
- spironolactone, cimetidine, digoxin, metoclopramide, tricyclics, methyldopa, marijuana, steroids (adrenal suppression)
- drugs used vs. prostate cancer:
  - LHRH analogues → increased testosterone then decreased due to negative feedback: Zoladex
  - anti-androgens: cyproterone acetate
  - oestrogens: stilboestrol

Classification

Grade I – subareolar 'button'

Grade II
- a – moderate enlargement, no skin excess
- b – moderate enlargement with extra skin

Grade III – marked enlargement with extra skin

Surgical treatment

Grade I – circumareolar incision, excise 'button'

Grade II
- a – liposuction alone or in combination with excision of a disc of breast tissue via a circumareolar incision
- b – excision of skin using donut mastopexy technique, excision of breast disc and liposuction to feather edges

Grade III – breast reduction
- inferior pedicle markings
- horizontal skin ellipse with nipple–areolar vertical bipedicle leaving transverse scar

Complications

Early
- haematoma
- infection

Late
- dishing
- inadequate correction of gland volume or skin excess
- nipple stuck to chest wall
- scarring

> **Self-assessment:** A 20-year-old male is referred with gynaecomastia. What is gynaecomastia, what causes it and how would you manage this patient?

Gynaecomastia is abnormal breast development in the male

Causes can be physiological, pharmacological or pathological:
- physiological
  - neonatal, pubertal, senile
    - imbalance between oestrogens and androgens
    - usually resolve
  - hypogonadism
    - pituitary hypogonadism
    - androgen insensitivity (5-α-reductase deficiency)
    - Klinefelter's XXY
- pharmacological
  - spironolactone
  - cimetidine
  - digoxin

- steroids
- prostate cancer drugs
  - LHRH analogues – Zoladex
  - anti-androgens – cyproterone acetate
  - oestrogens – stilboestrol
- marijuana
- pathological
  - tumours
    - testis – Sertoli, Leydig, teratomas
    - liver
    - kidney
    - lung
    - male breast cancer masquerading as gynaecomastia
  - disease states
    - cirrhosis
    - renal failure
    - thyrotoxicosis (increased serum hormone binding globulin)
    - burns

History
- age of onset
- rate of growth
- psychological effects
- pain
- nipple discharge
- general state of health
- drug history (any of the above + aspirin, warfarin, etc.)
- scar history
- smoker

Examination
- cancer examination
- aesthetic examination and grade/degree of gynaecomastia
  - I – subareolar button
  - II – general breast enlargement, little (b) or no (a) skin excess
  - III – general breast enlargement with skin excess
- size of nipple–areolar complex
- examination of thyroid, abdomen (liver, kidneys) and genitalia/testes

Investigations
- hormone screen
- CXR
- investigations directed towards aetiological factors

Treatment
- treat the aetiological factor
- surgery under general anaesthesia
- markings
- LA infiltration
  - I – subareolar disc excision ± liposuction (UAL ideal)
  - II – (a) breast disc excision + liposuction or (b) donut mastopexy technique

- III – breast reduction (inverted T or vertical bipedicle with a horizontal scar) and liposuction
- post-operative drain

Systematic approach to surgical treatment of gynaecomastia

Fruhstorfer. *BJPS* 2003

Gynaecomastia is benign enlargement of the male breast

Occurs in up to 38% of young males

Medical therapy:
- Used during the active proliferative phase of breast development
- danazol
- tamoxifen
- clomiphene
- testolactone

Surgical treatment:
- failed medical management
- longstanding gynaecomastia
- techniques:
  - liposuction
    - alone or in combination with other techniques
  - UAL
  - Open excision via a semi-circular circumareolar incision between 3 o'clock and 9 o'clock
    - Bevelled excision at the margins of the breast disc
  - Skin reduction
    - Lejour markings

Classification and management of gynecomastia: defining the role of ultrasound-assisted liposuction

Rohrich. *Plast Reconstr Surg* 2003

Gynaecomastia has an incidence of 32 to 65% of male population

Medical management has had limited success

Surgical therapy, primarily through excisional techniques, has been the accepted standard but subjects patients to large, visible scars

Ultrasound-assisted liposuction (UAL) has recently emerged as a safe and effective method for the treatment of gynecomastia
- Particularly efficient in the removal of the dense, fibrous male breast tissue while offering advantages in minimal external scarring

Review of 61 patients with gynaecomastia from 1987 to 2000
- UAL effective in treating most grades of gynaecomastia
- Excisional techniques are reserved for severe gynaecomastia with significant skin excess after attempted ultrasound-assisted liposuction
- UAL better than conventional liposuction in addressing dense, fibrous lipodystrophy

Three histological patterns with varying degrees of stromal and ductal proliferation:
- florid pattern: increased numbers of budding ducts in a highly cellular fibroblastic stroma
- intermediate type: overlapping of the fibrous and florid histological patterns
- fibrous type: extensive stromal fibrosis with minimal ductal proliferation

Male breast cancer:
- 1% of all breast cancer occurs in men

- Patients with Klinefelter syndrome have up to a 60 × greater risk of developing breast cancer (incidence 1:400 to 1:1000)
- No increased risk for breast cancer in patients with gynaecomastia compared with the normal male population
- Liposuction and excisional techniques of gynaecomastia surgery do not impair detection of male breast cancer

Principle

- Ultrasonic energy transmitted by means of excited piezoelectric crystals placed on terminal ends of suction cannulae to emulsify fat while preserving adjacent nervous, vascular, and connective tissue elements
  - Emulsification is effected through cavitation of fat cells in tumescent fields

Technique

- subcutaneous infiltration of a wetting solution
- UAL
- evacuation and final contouring by conventional suction-assisted lipectomy
- endpoints for UAL (time and loss of resistance) differ from those for standard suction-assisted lipectomy (pinch and contour)

Advantages

- Selective emulsification of fat leaving higher density structures, such as fibroconnective tissue, relatively undamaged (more efficient fat removal)
- At higher energy settings, UAL is effective in removal of the denser, fibrotic parenchymal tissue that suction-assisted lipectomy is inefficient in removing
- UAL performed in the appropriate subdermal plane affects the dermis, allowing for skin retraction in the post-operative healing period
- reduced physical demand

New classification system based on the amount and character of breast hypertrophy and the degree of ptosis

- Grade I: minimal hypertrophy (<250 g of breast tissue)
- Grade II: moderate hypertrophy (250 and 500 g of breast tissue)
  - IA and IIA for primarily fatty breast tissue
  - IB and IIB for primarily fibrous breast tissue
- Grade III: moderate – severe hypertrophy (>500 g of breast tissue) and grade 1 ptosis
- Grade IV: severe hypertrophy (>500 g of breast tissue) and grade 2 or 3 ptosis

Treatment

- Suction-assisted lipectomy can be used in grade IA and grade IIA
- UAL is effective in all grades of gynaecomastia
- if removal of redundant skin and/or resistant lipodystrophy is still required after ultrasound-assisted liposuction, excision is delayed for 6 to 9 months to allow for maximal skin retraction and healing

Chest wall reconstruction

Reconstruction may be required following:

- clearance of a breast cancer (including phyllodes) or other chest wall malignancies – palliative surgery may be acceptable

- sternotomy wound dehiscence
- radiation-induced ulceration
  - Radiation → scarring → stiffer tissues → less tendency to paradox post-resection
  - Difficult to distinguish between radiation ulcers and tumour on biopsy – whole of the area needs to be excised anyway
  - Post-radiation defects need to be reconstructed with flaps which bring their own blood supply – pedicled or free muscle flaps ideally
  - Hence the 'reconstructive ladder' does not apply
  - Allow at least 6–12 weeks following cessation of all radiotherapy before considering reconstruction
- congenital spinal defects or spinal surgery
- trauma
- Poland's syndrome
- intrathoracic transposition
  - bronchopleural fistula
  - post-pneumonectomy empyema
    - occurs due to incomplete obliteration of the hemithorax following pneumonectomy
    - Clagett's procedure useful: allow cavity to granulate then fill with antibiotic solution

Tumour excision:
- tie off internal mammary vein first
  - thin-walled vessel
  - avoids intra-operative haemorrhage

Flaps for chest wall reconstruction:
- pectoralis major advancement flaps
- pectoralis major turnover flaps based on parasternal perforators
- pedicled latissimus dorsi
- pedicled TRAM
- breast sharing
- omentum (based on right gastro-epiploic artery)
- serratus anterior for intrathoracic transposition

Paradoxical chest movement:
- skeletal reconstruction if two or more ribs removed (elderly)
- skeletal reconstruction if three or more ribs removed (athletes)
- Marlex mesh/methyl methacrylate sandwich
- cement layer ~0.5 cm thick

Chest wall reconstruction in 500 patients
Arnold. *PRS* 1996

Indications: tumour, infection, radiation, trauma

Latissimus dorsi myocutaneous flap originally described by Tansini in 1906 for closure of a chest wall defect

Muscle flaps include pectoralis major, latissimus dorsi, serratus, external oblique, rectus and trapezius in that order of frequency

Omentum used in 50 patients as a salvage flap

Skeletal defects reconstructed with mesh or autologous rib

Central back defect can be closed using bilateral latissimus dorsi advancement flaps

Make sure that resection of irradiated tissues is adequate

'Cyclops flap' (breast sharing) for chest wall reconstruction
Hughes. *PRS* 1997

Axial pattern flap based upon the lateral thoracic artery

Breast tissue advances across the midline to leave the nipple in a central position

Useful in situations where:

- scarring in the axilla precludes a pedicled latissimus dorsi or microvascular anastomosis
- and the chest wall defect precludes use of the internal mammary arteries (may also be lost due to previous cardiac surgery), e.g. full-thickness excision of chest wall
- or the patient may be unfit for a major procedure

In the discussion – poor aesthetic result but worth keeping in mind

Intrathoracic flaps for the management of empyema
Perkins. *BJPS* 1995

Evacuate, obliterate and sterilize the pleural cavity

Evacuation performed by chest drain or open drainage

Packing/dressing to achieve a granulating cavity may be required for ~2 weeks

Finally closure of bronchopleural fistula and obliteration of dead space with
a muscle flap

- pedicled latissimus dorsi precluded by lateral thoracotomy incision on that side
- free muscle flaps to the thoracodorsal vessels then indicated:
  - contralateral latissimus dorsi
  - de-epithelialized TRAM

External oblique myocutaneous flap
Bogossian. *PRS* 1996

Large myocutaneous rotation flap from the whole of the ipsilateral upper quadrant of the abdomen

Extend ~3 cm beyond the midline

Raised superficial to the rectus sheath then, more laterally, deep to the external oblique muscle

Laterally based on perforators from intercostal vessels at the posterior axillary line

Reliable flap, quick to raise without turning, donor site closes directly, no abdominal hernia (rectus intact)

Flap is sensate

Sternotomy dehiscence

Early

- often minor due to superficial wound infection
- lay cavity open and dress
- may need to remove wire

Late

- often major including dehiscence of the sternum
- need to know whether the LIMA was used

Reconstructive options:

- vertical rectus (if LIMA was used → use **right**-sided flap)
- omentum (but can be very thin)
- pectoralis major advancement or turnover
- bilateral bipedicled pectoralis major/rectus flaps
- latissimus dorsi free flap

Secondary sternal repair using bilateral PMA flaps and sternal suture Perkins. *BJPS* 1996

Technique involves use of no. 1 PDS interosseus sutures and bilateral pectoralis major **advancement** (PMA) flaps

- Sternum sutured first (unicotical) – if, after debridement, the sternum could not be closed directly then VRAM or pectoralis major turnover flaps or omentum was used
- Raise the muscle only as far laterally as the site of the internal mammary artery (if present) perforators – 6 cm from the midline
  - These maintain blood supply to this part of the muscle – too far away from the thoraco-acromial pedicle
  - Where the internal mammary A has already been harvested, the muscle is considered to have been delayed
  - Where the internal mammary A is present, this keeps the turnover flap as a lifeboat
  - Pectoralis major turnover flaps do require an intact internal mammary A – based on the intercostal perforators
  - VRAM may be vascularized by the cardiophrenic A (anastomoses with intercostal arteries) in the absence of the internal mammary but unreliable
- Mobilized muscles approximate to the midline

Breast reduction and PMA flaps for sternal dehiscence de Fontaine. *BJPS* 1996

Bilateral PMA flaps combined with breast reduction and free nipple graft

Reduces breast weight and thus tension on wound closure

Preserving the internal mammary perforators maintains perfusion to the mobilized muscle and also to the medial breast dermoglandular flap of the reduction

Sternal wound reconstruction

Schulman. *Plast Reconstr Surg* 2004

Poland's syndrome

First described in a post-mortem examination by Poland 1841

1:25 000 live births

Male:female ratio=3:1

Involves the right side in 75% of cases

Aetiology – theories

- intra-uterine vascular insult or hypoxia during the stage of limb bud development (weeks 6 and 7)
- genetic – familial tendency reported, although mostly sporadic

Chest wall defects

- deficiency of pectoralis major (total aplasia or loss of sternocostal head)
- variable deficiency of pectoralis minor, serratus, latissimus dorsi, deltoid, supra- and infraspinatus
- breast hypoplasia or aplasia with a smaller nipple–areolar complex or absent nipples
- deficiency of subcutaneous tissue
- contraction of the anterior axillary fold
- abnormalities of the anterior portion of the second–fourth ribs
- thoracic scoliosis
- pectus excavatum
- Sprengel's deformity

Limb abnormalities

- shortening of digits and syndactyly (simple, complete) – brachysyndactyly – middle phalanges most affected
- hypoplasia of the hand and forearm
- foot anomalies

Cardiovascular abnormalities

- dextrocardia
- hypoplastic or absent vessels (subclavian, thoraco-acromial, thoracodorsal)
- consider angiography before breast reconstruction with a latissimus dorsi flap

Other associated abnormalities

- renal hypoplasia
- congenital spherocytosis
- increased incidence of leukaemia

Patients present for chest wall management at adolescence or early adult life

Men complain of deficient anterior axillary fold

- Latissimus dorsi muscle transposition corrects axillary fold
- Tendon re-inserted into bicipital groove
- Beware hypoplastic muscle or absent thoracodorsal vessel – may consider angiography first

Women complain of breast maldevelopment – correction of the breast hypoplasia – conventional silicone breast augmentation

Chest wall management in the male patient with Poland's syndrome Marks. *BJPS* 1991

Compared customized silicone implant reconstruction with both latissimus dorsi and silicone implant **plus** latissimus dorsi

Patients lack the sternal head of pectoralis major

Axillary approach to latissimus dorsi

Muscle raised and transferred via a subcutaneous tunnel to the chest wall

Tendon of latissimus dorsi was sutured beneath the clavicular head of pectoralis major

Superior long-term results when a silicone implant was used in combination with muscle transposition

Over-correction initially but optimum result after atrophy of the muscle (despite maintaining the thoracodorsal nerve)

Pectus excavatum and pectus carinatum

Pectus excavatum

= funnel chest

Present in early childhood

Male:female ratio = 3:1

Association with Marfan's syndrome

Most patients are asymptomatic but some may have cardiopulmonary compromise

Correction of pectus excavatum

- midline sternal incision or bilateral inframammary incisions
- partial costal cartilage resection/overlapping, sternal elevation, and retrosternal strut (titanium, dexon)
- silicone implant for less severe deformity – 3D reconstructive CT used to guide custom-made implant design

Pectus carinatum

= barrel or pigeon chest

Correction of pectus carinatum – Lester's method: partial costal cartilage resection/overlapping and wedge osteotomy of the sternum to achieve sternal depression

Surgery of chest wall deformities
de Matos. *Eur J Cardiothoracic Surg* 1997

Patients <15 years of age

Most asymptomatic

- secondary back problems in later life due to poor posture and spinal scoliosis
- psychological morbidity
- some patients have dyspnoea and abnormal respiratory function tests
- a minority of patients have associated congenital cardiovascular anomalies (ASD, VSD, pulmonary stenosis, etc.)

70% had pectus excavatum, 30% pectus carinatum

Subperichondrial resection of abnormal costal cartilages – turned over

and replaced

Anterior transverse sternal osteotomies

Steel rod (Steinmann pin) internal stabilization – removed after 6–12 months

Sternal turnover procedures have been described incorporating costal cartilages

but → problems of avascular necrosis (large bone graft)

Position of the sternum is the result of abnormal growth of the costal cartilages

Abdominal wall and perineal reconstruction

Indications

fungating colonic tumours

traumatic abdominal wall defects

necrotizing fasciitis

laparotomy wound dehiscence

fungating carcinomas of anus or rectum

carcinomas of uterus or cervix

vulval carcinoma

post-radiation ulcers

burn scar contractures

fistulae – vesicovaginal

Choice of flaps for the perineum

Muscle flaps bring the best blood supply but FC flaps are sensate

Rectus femoris myocutaneous flap can be applied to most situations of perineal reconstruction but leave a poor donor site scar

Pedicled flap for the groin and ischium – TFL

Gracilis muscle or myocutaneous flap

Posterior thigh FC flap

Rectus abdominis muscle, TRAM (high skin paddle but include umbilical perforators) or VRAM flaps based on the DIEA

- useful for reconstructing large perineal defects
- transferred through the pelvis or subcutaneously
- disinsertion from the pubis allows greater mobility

Free flaps – latissimus dorsi, TRAM – anastomosed to inferior gluteal vessels

Need a mesh to support the abdominal wall

- can allow to granulate and will accept a SSG
- poor long-term graft stability
- first used during the Vietnam war

Full-thickness abdominal wall reconstruction using an innervated lat dorsi flap (Ninkovic. *PRS* 1998) or autologous fascial grafts (Disa. *PRS* 1998)

Congenital
- exomphalos
- can use expanded myocutaneous flaps

Acquired
- trauma
- tumour
- infective processes, e.g. necrotizing fasciitis
- large hernias

Determine what is missing: skin, muscle, fascia

Reconstructive options in acquired defects

- either as definitive closure or as a first stage:
  - debridement and immediate SSG
  - allow to granulate/vacuum closure and SSG
- pedicled flap from the abdomen (± tissue expansion)
- distant flap from the thigh region
  - TFL, rectus femoris, sartorius, gracilis
  - limited by size and arc of rotation
  - only suitable for lower defects
- free latissimus dorsi myocutaneous flap
  - innervated by coaption of the thoracodorsal nerve to intercostal nerves supplying rectus abdominis – provides muscle contraction to the abdominal wall and can avoid a mesh
  - vascular anastomosis to the superior epigastric artery and VCs

Marlex mesh to prevent hernia

If contraindicated by the presence of potentially contaminated tissue use autologous fascia lata grafts instead of mesh but leave behind the tendon of the iliotibial tract to maintain lateral knee stability

Abdominal wall expansion in congenital defects
Byrd. *PRS* 1989

TE used to reconstruct the lower abdominal wall defect of two children with cloacal exstrophy

TE placed in the space between transversus abdominis and internal oblique from within the lateral part of the rectus sheath – the aponeurosis of internal oblique splits to encircle the rectus sheath

Expanded over ~10 weeks, GA each time

One patient suffered from colonic dysmotility and constipation during the course of the expansion

An algorithm for abdominal wall reconstruction

Rohrich. *Plast Reconstr Surg* 2000

Aim of reconstruction is the restoration of functional integrity of the abdominal wall

Consider pre-operative pulmonary function tests and assess the effect on respiration of closing the abdominal wall (e.g. large incisional herias)

Wait until local tissue inflammation (due to bowl fistulae, trauma, surgery or infection) has subsided before attempting reconstruction

- Vacuum assisted closure will assist in reducing the defect while stabilising the wound

Assess size of defect

- Small defects often closed directly by undermining and local advancement, small random pattern fasciocutaneous flaps or skin grafts
- Larger defects may be reduced by VAC then managed as above
- Defects >15 cm may require axial pattern flaps, tissue expansion or reconstruction using distant pedicled or free flaps

Fascial reconstruction

- fascial defects reconstructed using

- free or vascularized fascia lata (TFL flap)
- prosthetic materials (e.g. nylon mesh)
- collagen substitues (e.g. Permacol^{TM} – acellular porcine collagen)

Wound closure in large defects:

- midline: component separation or lateral relasing incisions to advance faciocutaenous flaps medially
- lateral defects:
  - Upper third
    - superiorly based rectus abdominis from the other side
    - external oblique
    - extended latissimus dorsi flap
    - extended TFL
  - Middle third
    - rectus abdominis (including extended deep inferior epigastric flap)
    - external oblique
    - TFL, rectus femoris
  - Lower third
    - inferiorly based rectus abdominis (including extended deep inferior epigastric flap)
    - internal oblique
    - TFL, rectus femoris, vastus lateralis, gracilis, groin flap

Free tissue transfer

- Recipient vessels include
  - deep inferior epigastric vessels
  - deep circumflex iliac vessels
  - internal mammary vessels
- Donor muscles include latissimus dorsi and TFL (innervated muscle transfer described by Ninkovic as above)
- May be applied to upper, middle and lower third defects

Posterior chest wall

Spina bifida

Spinal surgery wound dehiscence

Upper third – trapezius myocutaneous flap based on transverse cervical A

Middle third – latissimus dorsi based on thoracodorsal pedicle

Lower third:

- latissimus dorsi turnover flap
- gluteus maximus or S-GAP flap
- bipedicled FC flaps

Also

- tissue expansion
- vacuum closure and SSG

Management of massive thoracolumbar wounds following scoliosis surgery

Mitra. *Plast Reconstr Surg* 2004

Series of 33 patients (11–65 years) with large thoracolumbar wounds following scoliosis surgery

- exposure of metalwork
- dead bone/osteomyelitis
- bone graft
- large dead space

Principles of management:

- expedient return to theatre for early signs of infection
  - pain, tenderness, erythema, pyrexia
  - wound irrigation and primary closure
  - specimens for culture
- advanced infection and wound breakdown
  - thorough excisional debridement of non-viable bone and soft tissue
  - myocutaneous extended latissimus dorsi flap raised for soft tissue cover
    - the fasciocutaneous extension of the flap, beyond the inferior muscle edge, is de-epithelialized and turned in to the defect to help obliterate dead space
  - skin graft to secondary defect
  - closed suction drainage
  - lower wounds closed using the whole of the gluteus maximus muscle islanded on the superior gluteal vessels and rotated in to the defect
    - insertions on the iliac bone, sacrum and gluteal fascia are divided
    - also released laterally from iliotibial tract and the femur
    - all patients reconstructed with this flap were non-ambulatory
  - lower wounds may also require inferiorly based fasciocutaneous skin flaps to supplement closure
- metalwork was retained in all patients

8 Head and neck oncology and reconstruction, facial reanimation, maxillofacial trauma, craniofacial surgery

Reconstruction of the cheek

The cheek is divided into three zones:

- *zone 1*: suborbital zone from the lower eyelid down to the gingival sulcus and from the nasolabial fold to the anterior sideburn
- *zone 2*: pre-auricular zone from the tragus to the anterior sideburn and from the junction of the helical rim with the cheek down to the mandible
- *zone 3*: buccomandibular – area inferior to the suborbital zone and anterior to the pre-auricular zone

Suborbital zone

Examples of reconstructive options:
- direct closure with a vertically orientated scar
- FTSG
- local flaps including Limberg, V–Y, McGregor flap, cervicofacial flap
- see also lower eyelid reconstruction, p. 367

Pre-auricular zone

Examples of reconstructive options:
- direct closure (facelift-type undermining)
- local flaps: Limberg flap, hatchet flap, anteriorly based cervicopectoral flaps, deltopectoral flaps
- distant flaps: pectoralis major and latissimus dorsi myocutaneous flaps
- free flaps: radial forearm, scapular flap

Buccomandibular zone (cheek proper)

Examples of reconstructive options:
- skin only: direct closure, FTSG, local flaps and distant flaps as above
- lining: tunnelled nasolabial flap, tongue flap, flaps which epithelialize including buccal fat flaps, galeal flaps (with periosteum) and masseter cross-over flaps
- skin and lining: double skin paddle pectoralis major, deltopectoral flap, free flaps including radial forearm ($\pm$ bone, tendon), scapular flap
- flaps in combination for reconstructing lining and skin separately

Cervicofacial flap

Used for reconstruction of zones 1 or 3

Inferiorly based as a rotation flap moving post-auricular skin anteriorly on to the cheek

Posteriorly based as a rotation flap moving neck skin upwards on to the cheek

Include platysma in the flap

Plane of dissection is deep to SMAS

Anchor to zygomatic or infra-orbital periosteum to prevent ectropion

Reconstruction of the eyelids and correction of ptosis

Anatomy

Skin and orbicularis (anterior lamella)

Tarsal plate and conjunctiva (posterior lamella)

Orbicularis oculi
- orbital fibres effect screwing up of the eyes
- palpebral fibres responsible for blinking

Tarsal plates (upper and lower) are condensations of the orbital septum – hence, dense fibrous tissue **not cartilage**

- suspensory ligament of Lockwood completes the ligamentous attachments to the globe
- numerous glands of Moll
- height of the upper lid tarsal plate is ~8–12 mm

Lateral and medial condensations form the lateral and medial canthal **ligaments**

Levator palpebrae superioris

- Attaches to the upper tarsal plate via the levator aponeurosis (~15 mm in length) to form the anterior lamella
- Levator muscle 45 mm in length
- Acts to open the eye by elevating the upper lid
- Supplied by the superior division of the oculomotor nerve
- Crossed by the superior transverse ligament (of Whitnall) in its upper part – acts as a check to levator retraction

Müller's muscle lies deep to levator

- Supplied by sympathetic fibres travelling in the oculomotor nerve
- Effects fine adjustment on lid height
- Paralysis (cut, Horner's syndrome) causes 2–3 mm of ptosis
- Maintains tone of raised eyelids
- Involved in the sympathetically mediated startle response (eye opens wide)
- May help to transmit the action of levator to the tarsal plate

Lacrimal gland

- secretomotor fibres from superior salivary nucleus
- relay in pterygopalatine ganglion
- travel in zygomatic branch of VII

Accessory lacrimal glands

- meibomian glands – lubricate lid margins
- glands of Zeis
- glands of Moll

Lacrimal apparatus

- Opens at the punctum in the inner canthus
- Upper and lower lacrimal canaliculi lead from the punctum to the lacrimal sac, travelling beneath the upper and lower limbs of the medial canthal ligament
- Lacrimal sac drains into the nasolacrimal duct
- Lacrimal sac is pulled open during contraction of the palpebral fibres of orbicularis (blinking) and closes by elastic recoil
- Valves prevent reflux of fluid (along the canaliculi), which exits via the nasolacrimal duct to drain into the inferior meatus of the lateral wall of the nose

Dry eyes

Smokers

Age

Postmenopausal

Antihistamine treatment

Sicca syndrome

Eyelid tumours

Mainly BCCs

Tumours of accessory lacrimal glands likely to be variants of BCCs

Only 10% of lid tumours occur on the upper lid

Lower lid BCCs mainly at medial and lateral canthi

Recurrent BCCs should be excised with frozen section control of margins

SCC accounts for ~2%

LM ~1%

Consider biopsy before definitive excision and reconstruction to confirm histology

Excision under frozen section control

Lacrimal gland tumours

50% are pleomorphic adenomas

- high risk of local recurrence following tumour spillage
- **Do not biopsy**
- slow growing
- painless growth
- no inflammatory signs
- treat by total gland excision

25% are adenoid cystic carcinomas

- spreads diffusely along tissue planes
- locally aggressive
- almost always recurs locally
- Swiss cheese appearance histologically
- basaloid changes associated with very poor prognosis (20% survival at 5 years, otherwise 70% at 5 years)
- requires total gland excision and orbital exenteration

25% miscellaneous including adenocarcinomas, malignant change in a pleomorphic adenoma or muco-epidermoid tumours. Requires total gland excision and orbital exenteration

Reconstruction of the lower lid

Defects between one-quarter and one-third of the eyelids can be closed directly after wedge excision. May require lateral canthotomy if tight – provides ~5 mm advancement

Local flaps:

- bipedicled Tripier flap (includes muscle)
- Fricke flap
- glabellar flap
- upper eyelid transposition flaps (unipedicled Tripier)
- nasolabial flap
- cheek flap, e.g. McGregor (transposition with Z-plasty) or Mustardé (cheek rotation)

Hughes flap – anterior lamellar advancement from upper lid button-holed through the lid beneath the lashes to reconstruct the lower lid

- **But** inadvisable to take full-thickness tissue from the upper lid to reconstruct the lower lid – it cannot afford it!

- Cutler–Beard flap is similar but from the lower to the upper lid

Tenzel flap – rotation flap based high above the outer canthus – alternative to McGregor flap

Local tissue provides best colour and texture match

FTSG from postauricular sulcus or upper lid

>50% defects may require small two-layer composite chondromucosal graft from the nasal septum

- Lower lid defects very rarely require cartilage support in reconstruction – thick cheek or forehead skin will usually suffice
- Conjunctiva can usually be advanced into a lower lid defect such that mucosal grafts are rarely required

Laissez faire – small defects heal by secondary intention

Islanded flap for reconstruction of the lower lid

Nakajima. *BJPS* 1996

Pedicle based on the lateral canthus and a small portion of orbicularis

Skin island described on the lateral cheek and rotated 180° into the lower lid

Lined with palatal mucosal graft (but leave periosteum intact)

Donor site dressed with a tie-over collagen sponge for 10 days

Hard palate mucosa is thicker and more durable than oral mucosa

Enables reconstruction of the entire skin of the upper or lower lid as an aesthetic unit

Similar flap described by Heywood and Quaba. *BJPS* 1991

Upper lid reconstruction

Graft muscle defects – re-innervation almost always successful

Local flaps similar to lower lid reconstruction

Required for defects >25%

Greater need for chondromucosal septal grafts or grafts of conchal cartilage

Abbé-type flap from the lower lid (Heuston lid switch)

- most suited to defects >50% of the upper lid
- donor defect reconstructed with one of the above techniques
- technically complex
- but may be the **best option** for the large upper lid defect
- two-stage technique

V–Y myotarsocutaneous advancement flap for upper lid reconstruction

Okada. *PRS* 1997

Suited to defects of 25–50% where the lateral canthus remains intact

Advances full-thickness lid tissue except orbicularis which forms the pedicle

Single-stage reconstruction

Avoids the need for chondromucosal grafts

Moves tissue from laterally medially, the stem of the Y in the lateral canthus

Surgical reconstruction in cryptophthalmos

Weng. *BJPS* 1998

Feature of Fraser syndrome

Absence of the upper eyelid

Microphthalmos

Skin membrane – passes from the forehead to the cheek, partially or completely over the affected eye adhering to the globe

May accompany cleft anomalies

Presentation during childhood → may be blind in the affected eye

AR inheritance + organ system abnormalities = Fraser syndrome

Eyelid reconstruction involves a composite chondromucosal graft and flap cover

Intraorbital tissue expansion in congenital anophthalmia

Dunaway. *BJPS* 1996

Developing globe is a stimulus to the growth of the bony orbit

Anophthalmia → absent stimulus

Spherical expander positioned within the muscle cone

Port tube passed through a hole in the lateral orbital wall via the infratemporal fossa to the scalp

Tarsorrhaphy then performed

Intra-orbital tissue expansion restores growth stimulus

- in combination with releasing osteotomies in children >2 years (expansion over a short period). Osteotomies reduce the resistance to expansion and help prevent expander extrusion
- alone, over a prolonged period, in neonates – removed at ∼7 years

Facilitates insertion of a size-matched prosthesis

Still need to reconstruct lids

Report of ten cases of anophthalmos and microphthalmos

Management of orbitofacial dermoids in children

Bartlett. *PRS* 1993

Most are subcutaneous, a minority have deeper extension

84 patients retrospectively reviewed

Three anatomical locations:

- frontotemporal – outer eyebrow area – 65%
  - slow growing
  - soft
  - non-fixed
  - asymptomatic
  - subperiosteal excision, splitting orbicularis oculi
  - need no work-up
- orbital – 25%
  - females twice as common as males
  - may adhere to frontozygomatic or medial sutures
  - easily dissected free
  - no transosseous extensions – rarely need work-up
- nasoglabellar – 10%
  - mass ± punctum (fine hair growth or sebaceous debris from punctum)
  - may have splitting of the nasal bones
  - midline glabellar lesions had no deep extension ($n = 2$)

- dorsal nasal lesions → occult naso-ethmoid and cranial base abnormalities on CT
- these need radiological work-up and may need bicoronal approach

Classification of dermoid cysts:

- acquired (implantation type)
- congenital (teratoma type)
- congenital (inclusion type)

 Orbitofacial dermoids are of the congenital inclusion type – embryonic lines of fusion

Conjunctival defects

Advancement

Grafts from the other side

Hard palate mucosa

Nasal mucosa

Eyebrow defects

Hair-bearing FTSG

Pedicled flap based on superficial temporal vessels

Pinch grafts

Ptosis

Normal lid level is covering 1–2 mm of the upper limbus of the cornea

Ptosis is an abnormal droopiness of the upper lid

Beard's classification of ptosis

Congenital:

- absence of levator
- blepharophimosis syndrome
- lid lag commonly accompanies a congenital ptosis
- leave alone until ~5 years unless:
  - severe ptosis obstructing visual field leading to amblyopia
  - corneal exposure risking ulceration

Acquired:

- neurogenic
  - oculomotor N lesion (levator palpebrae superioris)
  - Horner's syndrome (correct with 10% phenylephrine hydrochloride)
  - demyelination
  - traumatic ophthalmoplegia or ophthalmoplegic migraine
- myogenic
  - senile ptosis – stretching of the levator aponeurosis and muscle with age
  - myaesthenia gravis (Tensilon test)
  - muscular dystrophy
  - steroid ptosis
- traumatic
  - injury to levator mechanism
  - also post-cataract surgery – damage to superior rectus muscle – used for insertion of a stay stitch to immobilize the eye → scarring

- mechanical
  - lid tumour
  - dermatochalasis (excess redundant skin)
- pseudoptosis
  - appearance of ptosis rather than true ptosis, e.g. with enophthalmos

Assessment:

- look for a lid crease – site of aponeurosis insertion, lost in disinsertion syndrome
- measure ptosis in mm (compare with other eye distance between mid-pupillary point to lid margin, normally ~5 mm):
  - mild: 1–2 mm
  - moderate: 3 mm
  - severe >4 mm
- observe levator function – measure from down gaze to up gaze with frontalis immobilized (should be 15–18 mm)
- look for Bell's phenomenon – eyes rotate upwards when closed. Some patients do not have a Bell's phenomenon – in these patients be much less aggressive with ptosis correction: over-correcting → corneal exposure during sleep
- look for lagophthalmos (incomplete closure of the lids). Avoid over-correcting as above

Treatment:

- good levator function (>10 mm)
  - mild ptosis <2 mm → **Fasanella–Servat** procedure. Invert the tarsal plate, clamp with artery forceps and excise a 2-mm caudal segment (includes aponeurosis attachment) then oversew
  - mild-to-moderate ptosis >2 mm → **aponeurosis surgery**, e.g. resection or plication of the aponeurosis
- poor levator function (<10 mm) or ptosis >3 mm
  - moderate ptosis, poor levator function 4–10 mm → **levator shortening** (resection or plication) **or advancement**
  - severe ptosis, very poor levator function <4 mm → **suspension surgery** frontalis sling (fascia lata sling connecting frontalis to tarsal plate)
- Note that local anaesthetic with adrenaline causes partial lid retraction
  - blocks somatic innervation of levator
  - activates sympathetic innervation of Müller's muscle
  - hence final position of lid needs to be 1–2 mm of over-correction

Complications:

- under-correction
- over-correction and corneal exposure

Surgical treatment of lagophthalmos in facial palsy

Inigo. *BJPS* 1996

Complications of lagophthalmos

- dryness
- corneal keratitis
- conjunctivitis

Treatment approaches

- cross facial nerve grafts to re-innervate orbicularis (but where paralysis is long-standing this alone is ineffective)
- artificial tears

- protective lenses
- lateral tarsorrhaphy
- canthoplasty/canthopexy
- gold weight
- temporalis turnover flap (but may cause involuntary closure during chewing)

This paper describes levator lengthening using autologous conchal cartilage

Cartilage graft sutured between tarsal plate and levator aponeurosis

Width of graft required to reduce the palpebral fissure by 1 mm is ~4 mm

Levator lengthening for the retracted upper lid

Piggott. *BJPS* 1995

Occurs with Graves' disease or occasionally following upper lid blepharoplasty

Two main approaches:

- Müller's muscle division via a conjunctival incision
- division of levator aponeurosis and Müller's muscle via a skin incision

This technique lengthens the levator aponeurosis

'Castellated' flaps designed in the aponeurosis and sutured end–end

Length of each flap = desired correction +1 mm

This technique not suited to skin loss problems, e.g. burn scar contracture

Blepharophimosis

Congenital malformation occurring either in isolation or in combination with other developmental abnormalities

May have AD inheritance

Reduced vertical and transverse dimensions of the palpebral aperture due to a combination of upper lid ptosis with epicanthic folds and telecanthus

May also have mild hypertelorism

Usually require brow suspension to correct ptosis

Jumping man flap (originally described by Mustardé) used to correct epicanthic folds or Roveda correction

May need craniofacial surgery for hypertelorism

Self-assessment: Outline the management of a patient with a droopy eyelid

---

Take a history

Age, occupation

Patient's concerns – function vs. aesthetic

Medical history in an attempt to ascertain cause of ptosis as per Beard's classification:

- Has it been there since birth?
- **Congenital** – blepharophimosis syndrome, congenital absence of levator
- **Acquired**:
  - **neurogenic**: any history of problems with the eye or neck (stellate ganglion); any history of multiple sclerosis?
  - **myogenic**: any history of myaesthenia gravis (worse at any particular time of day – later on suggestive of myaesthenia), muscular dystrophy or steroid medication?
  - **mechanical**: any lumps/swellings on the lid?

- **trauma**: any history of an injury to the eye or cataract surgery or blepharoplasty? Any history of atopic episodes (suggestive of blepharoptosis)
- if none of the above and in an elderly patient likely to be **senile** ptosis or **pseudoptosis** due to other conditions, e.g. myxoedema
- smoker/diabetic/general health/drugs – aspirin/warfarin
- any history of dry eyes

Examination
Look
- brow ptosis (level in relation to the supra-orbital rim)
- dermatochalasis
- lid crease
- measure the level of ptosis (mild 1–2; moderate 3–4; severe >4 mm)

Move
- levator function (should be ∼15 mm) – brow immobilized
- lagophthalmos
- Bell's phenomenon
- extra-ocular movements

Test
- acuity
- pupils
- Schirmer's test

Surgical options

Levator function	Degree of ptosis	Procedure
Good (>10 mm)	Mild (1–2 mm)	Fasanella–Servat
Good (>10 mm)	Moderate (3–4 mm)	Aponeurosis surgery
Poor (4–10 mm)	Moderate (3–4 mm)	Levator surgery
Very poor (< 4 mm)	Severe (>4 mm)	Suspension surgery

Ectropion

Classification and treatment:
- **involutional** → lid shortening by wedge excision ± lower lid blepharoplasty (Kuhnt–Symanowski)
- **mechanical** (e.g. lid tumour) → excision of the lesion provoking the ectropion
- **cicatricial** → release scar (Z-plasty, FTSG or flap)
- **paralytic** (VII) → can treat as for involutional, also canthoplasty and sling suspension, also Kuhnt–Symanowski

Inferior retinacular lateral canthoplasty
Jelks. *PRS* 1997

Lateral canthoplasty: techniques and indications
Glat. *PRS* 1997

Anatomy

- Upper and lower tarsal plates are attached via the lateral canthal tendon (or 'retinaculum') to Whitnall's tubercle inside the lateral orbital rim
- Lateral canthal tendon is continuous with the levator aponeurosis in the upper lid and the suspensory ligament of Lockwood in the lower lid

Main indications for canthoplasty:

- correction of horizontal lid laxity or ectropion from paralysis or atony
- prevention of cosmetic blepharoplasty lower lid retraction

Main techniques:

- **tarsal strip procedure**
  - horizontal lid shortening
  - used for horizontal lid laxity, paralytic and atonic ectropion
  - tarsal strip/dermis strip raised and anchored to the superolateral orbital rim
  - ± pentagonal wedge excision
- **inferior retinacular lateral canthoplasty**
  - suspension of the inferior limb of the lateral canthal tendon to the periosteum of the superolateral orbital rim at a level equal to the upper edge of the pupil
  - upper eyelid approach (via a simultaneous upper lid blepharoplasty)
  - cosmetic canthoplasty – mild lid retraction in the lateral segment
    - used in conjunction with blepharoplasty to avoid post-operative lower lid retraction – or frank ectropion
    - used to correct lid retraction/ectropion following blepharoplasty without canthoplasty

Entropion

In children – leave alone, will resolve

In adults – Kuhnt–Symanowski blepharoplasty – same aetiology as involutional ectropion

Thyroid eye disease

Management is predominantly medical

Autoimmune reaction to extra-ocular muscles and fat

May need emergency orbital wall decompression

Olivari procedure: lateral canthoplasty and excision of retrobulbar fat using a blepharoplasty approach

Reconstruction of the lips

Anatomy

Muscles

- orbicularis oris
  - extrinsic fibres intermingle with buccinator, decussate at the modiolus
  - intrinsic fibres – incisive and mental slips
  - acts to form a whistling expression

- elevators
  - levator labii superioris alaeque nasi
  - levator labii superioris
  - levator anguli oris
  - zygomaticus minor
  - zygomaticus major
- depressors
  - depressor anguli oris
  - depressor labii inferioris
  - mentalis

Nerves
- motor
  - upper lip – buccal branch of VII
  - lower lip – marginal mandibular branch of VII
  - orbicularis supplied by both
- sensory
  - upper lip – infra-orbital N (maxillary branch of V)
  - lower lip – mental N, termination of inferior alveolar N (mandibular branch of V)

Blood supply
- labial branches of facial A

Pathology

Upper lip lesions tend to be BCCs
Lower lip lesions tend to be SCC (only 5% of SCCs occur on the upper lip)
Commissural and mucosal SCCs have a higher propensity for metastasis
Tumour size and thickness also correlate with metastatic potential
Excision margins should be 5–10 mm for SCC
May need to combine surgery with radiotherapy

Staging of lower lip SCC

As for intra-oral SCC if involving mucosa
T_1 tumour <2 cm
T_2 tumour >2–4 cm
T_3 tumour >4 cm
T_4 tumour invades adjacent structures (bone, tongue, skin of neck)

Upper lip reconstruction

Loss of up to one-quarter of the upper lip may be closed directly
Anaesthesia by bilateral infra-orbital nerve blocks (7 mm below the inferior orbital margin in line with the medial limbus)
Advancement flaps may be combined with crescentic perialar excisions
Abbé flap
- midline upper lip defects closed directly lose the normal philtral appearance – may be better to use an Abbé flap, especially in women

- also useful for lateral defects up to 50% of the upper lip

Karapandzic flap

- 'neurovascular fan flap'
- transfers skin, muscle and mucosa
- oral circumference advancement technique
- needs an intact commissure
- introduces no new tissue – hence, leads to microstomia but will stretch up
- incision in skin and superficial facial muscles
- preserve neurovascular supply to orbicularis when dividing radial elevators or depressors
- achieves correct muscle orientation
- preserving nerves allows only limited advancement so usually needs to be bilateral
- limited mucosal incision

Lower lip reconstruction

Ideally should remain sensate and with a good sulcus created by innervated muscle to prevent drooling

Loss of up to one-third of the lower lip may be closed directly

Anaesthesia by bilateral mental nerve blocks (infiltrated into the mucosa of the lower buccal sulcus in line with the lower canines, nerve may also be visible at this site with the lower lip on the stretch)

In situ SCC may be treated by lip shave and mucosal advancement (may need incisional release to convert into a bipedicled flap) or CO_2 laser

Defects one- to two-thirds of the lower lip:

- Abbé–Estlander flap (defects of the commissure/lower lateral lip)
- Karapandzic flap
- Gilles fan flap
    - half way between a Karapandzic flap and a McGregor flap
    - **advances** rather than rotates into defect
    - commissure moves medially
    - no new tissue
    - myocutaneous flap
    - muscle is denervated
    - lower lip still shortened but less so than with Karapandzic flap
    - cut vermilion ends sutured together
- McGregor flap
    - myocutaneous flap
    - three equally sized squares
    - **rotates** around the commissure
    - commissure remains in the same place
    - introduces **new tissue** into the lip to avoid microstomia
    - lip becomes devoid of vermilion and functioning muscle but theoretical risk of drooling rarely observed
    - vermilion may be reconstructed by mucosal advancement or tongue flap
- Johanson's step technique
    - allows for approximation of margins following central excision by creating step cuts along the nasomental folds

- defects up to 50%
- larger defects lead to microstomia

Defects > two-thirds of the lower lip:
- bilateral McGregor or other flaps
- Webster–Bernard flaps
  - vermilion reconstructed by mucosal advancement
  - similar to Freeman's cheiloplasty – excisional triangles based more laterally on the cheek
  - avoid simultaneous neck dissection
- Steeple flap
  - islanded composite cheek flap based on the facial artery
  - but flap is denervated, hence sensory and motor loss
  - avoid simultaneous neck dissection
- free tissue transfer

Lip replantation
Walton. *PRS* 1998

Retrospective review of 13 separate reports of lip replantation

All due to bite injuries (11 dog, two human)

Main dog culprits were German Shepherd ($n = 3$) and Labrador (3)

Upper:lower ratio $= 2{:}1$

Anastomoses of labial vessels <1 mm diameter

Vein not feasible in one-half of patients

Operating time 2.5–12 h

Venous congestion in all patients
- leeches used post-operatively in 11/13
- 10/13 systemically heparinized
- 11 patients required blood transfusion

Use of leeches associated with visible chevron scars

All replants survived

12/13 required subsequent scar revision(s)

Better aesthetic and functional result than other methods of reconstruction

Reconstruction of the oral commissure (electrical burns)
Donelan. *PRS* 1995

Commissure reconstruction is difficult because it is a highly specialized area
- thin mobile lip segment
- moves dynamically and symmetrically

Local flaps bring in too much bulk

In burns a conservative approach is adopted initially with secondary reconstruction (including scar contracture release) at a later stage

Author describes the use of an anteriorly based ventral myomucosal tongue flap to reconstruct the **lower lip portion** of the commissure
- provides good volume of tissue
- pedicle divided at 2 weeks
- but awkward tongue position and significant swelling post-operatively

- soft or liquid diet several days post-operation

Upper lip portion of the commissure reconstructed with a Gilles–Millard flap

- superiorly based flap raised from the scarred commissure and rotated upwards to lengthen the upper lip
- scar release performed through the flap incisions

Nasal reconstruction

Aims

- good cosmesis
- patent airway
- reconstruction of skin, support and lining

Reconstruction of cosmetic units where there is >50% skin defect in any one unit

Mainly BCC, SCC less common (ratio = 10:1)

BCC margins should be ~3 mm minimum for nodular BCCs on the nose, up to ~10 mm for histologically confirmed morphoeic lesions

Bone and cartilage act as barriers to penetration

Bone is less commonly invaded than cartilage because there is a loose plane between it and the overlying skin

Reconstruction of the skin

Healing by secondary intention or direct suture

SSG

- Prone to contracture but acts as a window to monitor recurrence
- Consider resurfacing the whole nose as a single cosmetic unit

FTSG (pre-/postauricular)

Composite grafts

- skin and cartilage
  - McLaughlin 1954
  - helical rim, root of helix
  - limited to <1.5 cm in size
  - maximize area of dermal contact to optimize take
  - notches usually develop either side of these grafts
- skin and fat

Local flaps

- banner flap (local transposition flap)
- Rieger rotation flap (rotates dorsum tissue inferiorly based on a lateral pedicle); similar to a hatchet flap or glabellar flap
- median glabellar advancement flap
- bilobed flap
- nasolabial flap – one- or two-stage
- V–Y flaps from the cheek
- Islanded nasolabial flap

Pedicled flaps from the forehead ('Indian technique') for total nasal skin reconstruction

- May be used to drape over small full-thickness defects and simultaneously reconstruct large skin defects (the raw deep surface of the flap re-epithelializes from surrounding lining mucosa)
- May need to consider delaying the flap
- Can thin the flap distally because vessels become more superficial as they near the hairline
- Usually requires 7.5 × 7.5 cm of scalp to provide for total nasal skin reconstruction (accounts for 35–45% of the forehead)
- Pre-operative (or intra-operative) subgaleal tissue expansion may be useful
  - increased vascularity
  - thinner flap
  - provides more lining with less bulk
  - facilitates direct closure of the donor defect
  - but may undergo secondary shrinkage
- flap thinning is safe ~1 month post-operation (intradermal steroid injections causing fat atrophy may also be used)
- forehead flap
  - based on supratrochlear vessels
  - useful where lining and support are not needed
  - may be taken high into the scalp in male pattern baldness
  - subperiosteal dissection from a point 2 cm above the supra-orbital rim to the medial canthus to preserve supratrochlear vessels
- seagull forehead flap (Millard)
  - modified forehead flap
  - lateral extensions for covering alae
- scalping rhinoplasty (Converse, 1942)
  - based laterally on superficial temporal vessels
  - makes use of 60–70% of the whole forehead, arching into anterior scalp
  - can prefabricate with cartilage grafts inset into the forehead
  - pedicle divided after 2–3 weeks

Distant flaps from the arm ('Italian technique') for total nasal skin reconstruction

- medial arm skin flap, proximally based
- original description distally based (Tagliacozzi, 1597)
- pedicle divided after 3 weeks
- historical interest only

Free flaps

- radial forearm flap
- may include bone
- microsurgical replantation of an amputated nasal skin has been described

Reconstruction of the lining

In-turning of pedicled forehead flaps

Skin grafts to the inner raw surface of pedicled forehead flaps

In-turning of external nasal skin (similar to a trap-door flap)

Nasolabial flaps

Septal hinge flap – anteriorly based, leave enough septum to provide support

Reconstruction of the skeleton

Ideally provided at the same time as skin/lining reconstruction
Midline support

- 'L'-shaped costochondral strut from the nasal radix and angulated to contact the anterior nasal spine but produces a wide columella
- cantilever bone graft screwed to the nasal radix with a small subjacent bone wedge to provide projection; avoids wide columella (Jackson, 1983). Ideally, use calvarial graft – less prone to resorption and may be harvested via the skin flap incisions
- Hinged septal flap – similar to the 'L'-shaped strut but made from septum

Lateral support – free cartilage grafts

Reconstruction by prosthesis

Branemark osseo-integrated prosthesis
Prosthesis suspended on spectacles
Debilitated or elderly patients

'Distal' dorsalis pedis flap for nasal tip reconstruction
Bayramicli. *BJPS* 1996

Used in a patient with tip loss requiring free cartilage grafts and unwilling to undergo staged procedures or have a forehead scar
Flap based on dorsalis pedis artery and tributaries to the long saphenous vein
Skin raised from the dorsum of the second toe and the first and second web spaces
Anastomosis into the superior labial A and facial V
Donor defect split skin grafted
Flap may be used with cortex from the second metatarsal to provide support where necessary
Very long pedicle
Thin flap with good aesthetic result
Useful in the burned patient where unscarred tissue must be imported
May get hair growth which can be treated by electrolysis

Nasal reconstruction in arhinia
Meyer. *PRS* 1997

Arhinia is extremely rare and may be associated with CNS abnormalities
Total arhinia includes loss of the entire olfactory system
Failure of invagination of nasal placodes hence no nasal cavities (choanal atresia)
Approached in three stages:

- construction of skin (forehead flap), septum (costochondral graft) and lining of the septum (in-turned de-epithelialized flaps) and raw surfaces of the forehead flap (nasolabial flaps)
- drilling out of the maxilla to provide a communication into the oropharynx and allow nasal breathing while eating; lined by buccal mucosal flaps and reconstruction of alae with composite conchal grafts
- widening of nasal airways using a burr, lined with FTSG using fibrin glue and stenting with silicone spacers

Reconstruction of the ear

Pathology

70% of tumours due to actinic damage

Mainly SCC with a higher metastatic potential than other facial SCC and a predilection for spread to internal jugular and parotid nodes

BCCs uncommon outside the conchal fossa, but may also be found on the posterior surface and lobe

Tumours readily spread locally

More common in men – women's ears protected by hair

Other tumours include melanoma and adnexal tumours (adenocarcinoma, adenoid cystic) but are rare and require amputation of the pinna and possibly neck dissection

Clinical classification of auricular defects (Tanzer)

I. Anotia

II. Complete hypoplasia (microtia)

    A. with atresia of the external auditory canal

    B. without atresia of the external auditory canal

III. Hypoplasia of the middle third of the auricle

IV. Hypoplasia of the superior third of the auricle

    A. constricted (cup or lop) ear

    B. cryptotia

    C. hypoplasia of the entire superior third of the auricle

V. Prominent ears

Reconstruction in microtia

Ears are 85% fully grown by 4 years of age

By 6 years of age an adult-sized ear can be reconstructed

Auricular reconstruction for mirotia

Walton and Beahm. *Plast Reconstr Surg* 2002

Tanzer technique

- Stage one: transverse re-orientation of lobular remnant
- Stage two: costal chondral framework carved from sixth–eighth costal cartilages and buried beneath mastoid skin
- Stage three: elevation of construct to create retroauricular sulcus with full thickness skin graft in to sulcus
- Stage four: reconstruction of tragus by composite graft from normal ear

Brent technique

- Tanzer technique modified in sequence
- *Stage one*: formation of a high profile cartilaginous framework as above and placement in to a mastoid pocket (use of suction drains emphasises underlying cartilage shape)
- *Stage two*: transposition of the lobule (occasionally combined with stage three)
- *Stage three*: elevation of the construct as above with placement of a banked piece of cartilage behind the ear to increase projection

- *Stage four*: tragus reconstruction and excavation of conchal bowl

Nagata technique

- *Stage one*: formation and placement of a cartilginous framework with transposition of the lobule to include tragal reconstruction
- *Stage two*: after 6 months, elevation of the construct with placement of a further crescent of costal cartilage in the post-auricular sulcus to increase projection. Temporoparietal fascial flap and SSG from occipital scalp used to resurface sulcus
- Only two stages but greater risk to skin vascularity from increased dissection and more cartilage required from the chest leading to secondary donor site deformity, minimized by leaving perichondrium intact at the donor site

Complications of ear reconstruction for microtia

- Hair growth on the new ear resulting from placement in hair bearing skin where there is a low hairline (laser depilation)
- Inelastic skin compromising aesthetic result
- Infection and haematoma
- Complications arising out of use of a temporoparietal fascial flap
  - alopecia and visible scar
  - scalp numbness
- Donor site complications
  - pneumothorax
  - chest wall scar and deformity
  - pain
- Skin necrosis and extrusion of the cartilage framework
- Resorption of the cartilaginous framework

Reconstruction following acquired loss (tumour)

Conchal/antehelical defects reconstructed by:
- FTSG
- trap-door flap
- islanded retro-auricular flap

Upper third defects reconstructed by:
- helical advancement (Antia and Buch)
- banner flap – from posterior sulcus based at the root of the helical rim
- pocket technique – two stage – suture cut edge into an adjacent skin incision along with a chondral cartilage or rib graft then release with a FTSG at 6 weeks

Middle third defects reconstructed with:
- composite grafts of contralateral helical rim
- ipsilateral conchal cartilage graft covered both posteriorly and anteriorly by a transposition flap from retro-auricular skin
- direct closure using either wedge excision or helical advancement (Antia and Buch)
- large rim defects reconstructed with tubed bipedicled flaps created in postauricular skin, transferred at two later stages

Lower third defects (lobe reconstruction):
- two-stage approach: inset free edge into adjacent skin then release with an adjacent local flap
- one-stage approach (below)

Reconstruction of the amputated ear

Banking of cartilage beneath retro-auricular skin – but flattens out

Banking of cartilage subcutaneously as a prefabricated flap, e.g. forearm

Dermabrasion of anterior skin and draping with a retro-auricular flap

Temporo-parietal fascial flap coverage of denuded cartilage

Fenestration of cartilage and resiting as a composite graft – prone to fail

Microvascular replantation – but technically difficult

Management of the burned ear

Early debridement reduces the risk of infection and chondritis

Topical antibiotics, cleansing and avoidance of pillow friction

Non-viable areas may separate spontaneously

Aggressive debridement of areas of chondritis and FTSG or fascial flaps

Reconstruction with a prosthesis

Branemark prosthesis

Correction of the cauliflower ear
Vogelin. *BJPS* 1998

Cartilage splits into two leaves with haematoma between them

Untreated haematoma fails to resorb but becomes calcified

Bat ear type of approach, resecting calcified haematoma and posterior leaf of cartilage

Anterior leaf resculpted by anterior scoring to recreate antihelix

Prevention by early drainage

Tissue expansion for ear reconstruction
Chana. *BJPS* 1997

TE used to generate additional skin in difficult or salvage situations

Where large amounts of unscarred skin are available, then TE is not used

If excessive scarring prevents even TE, then a temporoparietal flap may be required but does lead to a loss of definition of the cartilage framework

Retro-auricular rectangular expander placed via a remote incision in the temporal hairline

Slow expansion commenced after 2 weeks and upon completion left for 2 weeks before removal

Removal accompanied by capsulectomy (simplified by hydrodissection)

Cartilage framework inserted through expander incision and suction drains used to facilitate draping of skin over framework

Complications in 30% including extrusion, infection, haematoma

Hair depilation using the ruby laser

Correction of Stahl's ear
Ono. *BJPS* 1996

'Third crus' projecting from the antehelix with flattening of the helical rim

Anterior wedge excision of skin and cartilage

Closure with helical advancement and a small cartilage graft (from conchal fossa) inset behind approximated cartilage edges

Other approaches include splinting from the neonatal period (similar to bat ears)

One-stage lobe reconstruction
Alconchel. *BJPS* 1996

Anterior skin of antihelix/helix reflected inferiorly to form upper part of posterior surface of lobe

Islanded skin flap raised from posterior sulcus based upon medial subcutaneous pedicle

Upper apex of flap inset into free edge of antihelical flap and lower apex turned inferiorly and up to cover anterior surface

Avoids two-stage approach

Donor defect closes directly (could be closed with a FTSG if necessary)

Ear reduction
Gault. *BJPS* 1995

Aims: achieve symmetry or reduce congenitally large ears

Excision of crescent-shaped skin and cartilage from the scaphal hollow and advancement of the helical rim

Excess helical rim is then excised at the root of the antihelix

Total ear replantation
Kind. *PRS* 1997

Vein grafts from branches of the superficial temporal vessels

Direct anastomosis to the superficial temporal vessels achieved by dissecting these out distally then reflecting them back into the operative field (but sacrificing the superficial temporal vessels precludes later use of a temporoparietal flap)

Direct anastomosis to the postauricular vessels

Venous drainage often inadequate because of small calibre vessels and low flow

Leeches often used post-operatively, especially in artery-only ears

Heparinization also used to augment replant survival

May need multiple transfusions

Ear replantation without microsurgery
Pribaz. *PRS* 1997

Technique of de-epithelialization by dermabrasion and placement in a retro-auricular pocket

Remove from pocket after 2 weeks and allow spontaneous re-epithelialization

Other techniques include

- excision of posterior skin and cartilage fenestration (Baudet)
- banking the cartilage framework in a forearm pocket for later transfer as a composite free flap; Sciavon. *PRS* 1995. But flap bulk obscures definition therefore consider transfer as a fascial/cartilage flap and SSG

Neck anatomy

Fascial layers

Deep cervical fascia split into four layers:

- investing fascia
  - deep fascia beneath subcutaneous fat
  - surrounding the parotid gland investing fascia splits into superficial and deep layers as the parotid fascia
  - thickened to form the stylomandibular ligament
- prevertebral fascia
  - forms a layer over which the pharynx and oesophagus can freely slide
  - covers the muscles that form the floor of the posterior triangle
  - hence also covers the brachial plexus trunks and subclavian artery but **not** the subclavian vein
  - pierced by the four nerves of the cervical plexus
- pretracheal fascia
  - separates the trachea from the overlying strap muscles to allow free gliding of the trachea
  - blends laterally with the carotid sheath
  - encloses the thyroid gland
  - pierced by the thyroid vessels
- carotid sheath
  - envelopes the carotid arteries (common and internal), the internal jugular vein (thin) and vagus nerve
  - adherent to the deep surface of sternocleidomastoid

Triangles of the neck

Posterior triangle

Borders
Posterior border of SCM, middle third of clavicle, anterior border of trapezius
Subdivided by the posterior belly of omohyoid into an upper occipital triangle and a lower supraclavicular triangle

Roof
Investing fascia

Floor
Prevertebral fascia (deep to this lie splenius capitis, levator scapulae, scalenus posterior, scalenus medius and scalenus anterior; also the three trunks of the brachial plexus)

Contents
Lymph nodes
- Occipital nodes
- Supraclavicular nodes
- Lowermost deep cervical nodes

- Thoracic duct enters the junction of the internal jugular and subclavian veins behind the internal jugular vein on the left side

Nerves

- Accessory nerve (upper third SCM – lower third trapezius) lies within the roof of the triangle (investing fascia)
- Cutaneous branches of cervical plexus
  - lesser occipital C2
  - greater auricular C2,3
  - transverse cervical C2,3
  - supraclavicular C3,4
- Muscular branches of the cervical plexus
  - C1 travelling with XII forming the superior root of the ansa
  - C2,3 forming the inferior root of the ansa
  - C2,3 to SCM
  - C3,4 to trapezius
  - C3,4,5 as the phrenic nerve to the diaphragm
  - Lies on scalenus anterior beneath the prevertebral fascia
  - May be joined by the accessory phrenic N, a branch from the N to subclavius from the brachial plexus

Vessels

- Transverse cervical and suprascapular vessels from the thyrocervical trunk (off the subclavian A, terminates as the inferior thyroid A)
- Subclavian A low down in the triangle
- External jugular vein

Anterior triangle

Borders

Anterior border of SCM, lower border of the mandible, midline

May be subdivided into four further triangles by the digastric and omohyoid muscles:

- carotid (jugulodigastric)
- digastric (submandibular)
- submental
- muscular

Suprahyoid region within the paired anterior triangles is of surgical relevance

Roof

Platysma and deep cervical fascia

Contents

Hyoid bone and thyroid cartilage
Thyroid gland
Parathyroid glands
Submandibular and sublingual salivary glands

Trachea and oesophagus

Muscles (see below)

Suprahyoid muscles

Digastric and stylohyoid

Mylohyoids – deep to the above

Geniohyoids – between mylohyoids

Hyoglossus muscles – extrinsic muscles of the tongue (see tongue)

Infrahyoid strap muscles

Sternohyoid and omohyoid

Thyrohyoid and sternothyroid – lie deep to the above

Nerves

X within the carotid sheath and superior laryngeal branch

Lingual branch of V3:

- mandibular nerve has two branches from the main trunk
  - meningeal N
  - N to medial pterygoid
- four branches from its anterior division
  - three motor Ns (temporalis, masseter, lateral pterygoid)
  - one sensory N – the buccal N – supplies a 'thumb print' area below the zygoma
- three sensory branches from its posterior division
  - auriculotemporal
  - inferior alveolar
  - lingual

XI (apex of the triangle)

XII

Ansa cervicalis

Arteries

Common carotid A

- no branches proximal to its bifurcation
- bifurcates at C4 (upper border of thyroid cartilage)

Internal carotid A – no branches in the neck

External carotid A

- three anterior branches:
  - superior thyroid A
  - lingual A
  - facial A
- two posterior branches
  - occipital A
  - posterior auricular A
- one deep branch – ascending pharyngeal A
- two terminal branches:
  - maxillary A
  - superficial temporal A

Veins

Internal jugular vein

- lies lateral to the internal carotid A
- tributaries:
  - inferior petrosal sinus
  - pharyngeal plexus

Facial, lingual, superior and middle thyroid veins

Lymph nodes

Deep cervical nodes (closely adherent to internal jugular vein throughout its course)

Submandibular nodes

Submental nodes

Branchial cyst

Classic presentation is a soft, cystic mass anterior to SCM in the anterior triangle

Straw-coloured fluid with cholesterol crystals

Usually well encapsulated but can extend to the lateral pharyngeal wall

Suprahyoid region

Incorporates the area described by the digastric (submandibular) and submental triangles combined:

- above the hyoid bone and posterior belly of digastric
- mylohyoids, and laterally the hyoglossus muscles, forming the floor
- platysma and investing fascia forming the roof

Anterior jugular veins drain into the external jugular veins in the posterior triangle

Submental and submandibular lymph nodes

Submandibular and sublingual salivary glands

Submandibular duct

Lingual nerve spiralling around (crossing twice) the submandibular duct

Hypoglossal nerve crossing twice the kink in the lingual A. Supplies all the muscles of the tongue, extrinsic and intrinsic, except palatoglossus (pharyngeal plexus)

Muscles

Digastric

Mastoid process – intermediate tendon (lesser horn of hyoid) – mandible

Anterior belly supplied by nerve to mylohyoid (V3)

Posterior belly supplied by VII

Depresses mandible

Stylohyoid

Styloid process – greater horn of hyoid

Supplied by VII

Retracts/elevates hyoid when swallowing

Mylohyoid

Mylohyoid line of mandible – anterior surface of hyoid

Supplied by nerve to mylohyoid (V3)

Forms a stable gutter-shaped floor to the mouth

Geniohyoid

Genial tubercle of mandible – body of hyoid

Supplied by C1 fibres in XII

Protracts/elevates hyoid when swallowing

Sternohyoid

Inferior border of hyoid – manubrium

Divaricate around the thyroid cartilage

Supplied by ansa cervicalis (C1–3)

Depresses the larynx

Omohyoid

Inferior border of hyoid – (between SCM and carotid sheath) – clavicle – transverse scapular ligament

Supplied by ansa cervicalis (C1–3)

Depresses the larynx

Thyrohyoid

Greater horn of hyoid – oblique line of thyroid cartilage

Supplied by C1 fibres in XII

Depresses the larynx

Choice of recipient artery in the head and neck

Superficial temporal

Occipital

Facial

Lingual

Superior thyroid

Choice of recipient vein in the head and neck

External jugular

Formed by the posterior auricular vein joining the posterior division of the retromandibular vein.

Retromandibular vein formed by the superficial temporal vein and the maxillary vein

Drains into the subclavian vein

Facial

Anterior facial vein joins the anterior division of the retromandibular vein to form the common facial vein

Common facial vein divides into two – one division drains into the internal jugular vein while the other receives the anterior jugular vein before draining into the external jugular vein

Management of neck nodes

TMN Staging of intraoral cancers

Tis – carcinoma *in situ*

T1 – <2 cm

T2 – 2–4 cm

T3 – >4 cm

T4 – extension to bone, muscle (including extrinsic muscle of tongue), skin, neck, etc.

N0 – no evidence of regional lymph node involvement

N1 – mobile ipsilateral node <3 cm

N2

- N2a – mobile ipsilateral node 3–6 cm
- N2b – multiple ipsilateral nodes
- N2c – mobile contralateral or bilateral nodes

N3

- any node >6 cm
- fixed nodes

M0 – no evidence of distant metastases

M1 – distant metastases

Node levels

Level I – submandibular triangle

Level II – jugulodigastric (upper deep cervical)

Level III – mid deep cervical

Level IV – lower deep cervical

Level V – posterior triangle

Enlarged supraclavicular node:

- primary site usually below the clavicle
- breast, bronchus, stomach, pancreas

Enlarged level nodes III–V:

- primary site usually in the mid-neck
- thyroid, larynx, pharynx

Enlarged jugulodigastric node – oral cavity, face and scalp

Multiple enlarged nodes

- Consider a lymphoma
- Check other node basins and liver/spleen

Classification of neck dissection

Radical

Crile 1906

Indications:

- recurrent tumours
- level II node encasing accessory node ± extracapsular spread
- post-irradiation field

'Modified radical' or 'functional'

Type 1: accessory nerve only preserved (Bocca, 1975)

Type 2: preserve XI and the internal jugular vein

Type 3: preserve XI, internal jugular vein and SCM (Skolnik, 1967)

Type of functional dissection performed depends upon clearance of the tumour and is often determined on-table

Functional neck dissection is indicated wherever possible, except for the above indications for radical dissection

Extended radical

Paratracheal dissection

Parotidectomy

Selective

Hanley 1980

Often performed to gain 'access'

Suprahyoid dissection

Removes level I submental and submandibular nodes from the suprahyoid region

Supra-omohyoid dissection

Anterior tongue and floor of mouth tumours

Performed **en passant** while gaining access to the tumour. Removes nodes in levels I–III along with occipital nodes in the posterior triangle

3.5% failure rate (Jayton Shah)

- do not have to worry about the thoracic duct
- spares SCM, XI and internal jugular vein

Not suitable for parotid and tonsillar tumours as these all drain preferentially to level IV and V (and tip of tongue to level IV)

Posterolateral neck dissection

Removes occipital nodes along with posterrior triangle (V) and jugulodigastric chain (II–IV)

Modified radical neck dissection (type 2) – operative steps

Secure the airway by tracheostomy if bilateral neck dissection is being performed

- vertical or horizontal incision
- second tracheal ring
- Bjork flap
- cuffed Shiley tube size 8

Position the patient with the neck extended and the head turned away from the operative side

'Y' incision (Conley) with a curved vertical limb to avoid contracture (McFee incision if the neck has already been irradiated)

- Raise the skin flaps deep to platysma and preserving the marginal mandibular and cervical branches of VII in the upper flap
- Identify and preserve the external jugular vein for a venous anastomosis if required
- Define the posterior border of the posterior triangle (trapezius)

- Identify the spinal accessory nerve and dissect this along its course through the posterior triangle and through the sternocleidomastoid (SCM) muscle
- Clear the apex of the posterior triangle, delivering this tissue benath the accessory nerve to remain in-continuity with the rest of the posterior triangle
- Divide SCM from its sternal and clavicular attachments to expose the internal jugular vein
- Advance the dissection of the posterior triangle on a broad front, dividing branches of the cervical plexus while identifying the phrenic nerve
- The dissection procedes over the IJV (identifying the vagus nerve in the carotid sheath)
- Divide the inferior belly of digastric and develop a plane beneath it by finger dissection in to the anterior triangle
- Advance the dissection now superiorly to the submandibular area, dividing the superior belly of omohyoid
- Taking care to avoid injury to marginal mandibular nerve branches, the submandibular gland is freed, ligating tWharton's duct and the facial artery twice in the process
  - The hypoglossal nerve is identified deep to the posterior belly of digastric
- Level II dissection can then be completed by division of SCM superiorly

Surgical education: neck dissection

Chummun. *BJPS* 2004

Cervical node metastases in patients with head and neck cancer reduces survival by 50%

Risk factors for metastases

- Site – anteriorly located tumnours within the aerodigestive tract less likely to metastasize compared with posteriorly located tumours
  - Highest risk of nodal metastases associated with tongue tumours
- T-stage
- Thickness (highest risk >8 mm thick, lowest <2 mm)
- Histology
  - Perineural invasion
  - Perivascular invasion

Radiotherapy reduces the risk of postoperative neck failure by >50%

Operative photographs and a description of the author's preferred technique

Complications of neck dissection

Intra-operative

- nerve injury (IX, X, XI, XII, lingual, phrenic)
- injury to the sympathetic chain leading to Horner's syndrome
- inadvertent vessel injury – especially internal jugular vein
  - air embolus

Early postoperative

- airway problems
- infection
- seroma
- haematoma
- carotid artery blow-out (salivary fistula, previous radiation therapy)
- skin flap necrosis (posterior flap)

- dehiscence and vessel exposure
- lymphatic fistula (1–2% of neck dissections):
  - repair damaged lymphatics if recognised intraoperatively
  - TPN dries up the drainage within 24 h
  - low fat diet
  - control protein levels and electrolytes

Late
- long-term complication is trigger point sensitivity at the site of division of branches of the cervical plexus
- scar contracture
- problems related to division of XI – shoulder pain and weakness
- glossopharyngeal nerve injury → difficulty swallowing

Radiotherapy

Positive neck dissections

Single large involved node

Extracapsular spread

Complications of radiotherapy to the head and neck:
- eyes → cataracts and dry eyes
- hearing → sensorineural loss
- salivary glands → xerostomia
- pituitary gland malfunction
- growth disturbances of the craniofacial skeleton in children
- fibrosis of facial soft tissues
- injury to dental roots
- TMJ ankylosis

Alternative to external beam radiotherapy is brachytherapy facilitated by the insertion of selectron rods at the time of surgery

If radiotherapy planned → OPT to look at health of teeth: if there are caries/root fillings then remove these before giving radiotherapy as subsequent dental infections will rapidly involve the mandible

Should a recurrence occur after a full course of radiotherapy then further radiotherapy is not possible

Reconstruction of the head and neck

Ariyan. *Surg Oncol Clin N Am* 1997

Five-year survival for hypopharyngeal SCC is <25% regardless of mode of treatment:
- gastric pull-up is palliative but allows rapid return to oral feeding
- jejunal free flaps are technically more difficult with more complications

Protection of the brain during and after intracranial surgery:
- pre-operative antibiotics
- pre-operative dexamethasone 4 mg 6 hourly
- post-induction drainage of 100–120 ml CSF → relaxation of the brain → less retraction needed during the operation

- controlled hyperventilation → decreased P_aCO_2 → cerebral vasoconstriction → decreased brain volume
- IV infusion of mannitol → decreased ICP

Pattern of lymph node metastases in intra-oral squamous cell carcinoma

Sharpe. *BJPS* 1981

Radical neck dissection specimens from 98 patients with intra-oral SCC were examined

Definition of 'functional' neck dissection in this paper was where the accessory nerve and SCM was preserved

No lymph node metastases were found in

- posterior triangle
- submental triangle
- salivary glands
- sternomastoid muscle

Node groupings

- Level I = submandibular triangle
- Level II = upper internal jugular (jugulodigastric)
- Level III = mid-internal jugular
- Level IV = lower internal jugular
- Level V = posterior triangle
- Levels III and IV were grouped together in this paper

Patterns of lymph node involvement:

- hard palate and maxilla → level I
- lower lip → levels I and II
- floor of mouth and alveolus → levels I and II
- tongue → levels I and II

No lower internal jugular nodes (levels III and IV) were involved in the absence of disease higher up

The more anterior the lesion the more likely that level I nodes would be involved first

The more posterior the lesion the more likely that level II nodes would be involved first

Functional neck dissection, preserving the accessory nerve in the posterior triangle, is oncologically safe

MRI diagnosis of cervical lymphadenopathy

Wilson. *BJPS* 1994

MRI capable of identifying all enlarged nodes >4–5 mm diameter (100% sensitive)

But cannot differentiate between benign and malignant lymphadenopathy (53% specific for malignant lymphadenopathy)

Clinical examination unreliable in many patients:

- 30% false-positive
- 40% false-negative
- misses nodes up to 2 cm in diameter, especially if deep to SCM

Clinically negative neck → MRI scan: if negative then dissection unnecessary

Clinically positive neck → FNA → LND if histologically confirmed

CT superior for assessing bony involvement

T1-weighted images:

- relaxation time for protons to align to the magnetic field

- tumours generally appear **darker** than normal surrounding tissues
- fat has high signal – bright
  - subcutaneous tissues
  - medullary cavity
- fluid has low signal – dark
- contrast – gadolinium
  - increases T_1 relaxation time
  - nodes become brighter (more iso-intense with fat)
  - hence not useful in this context

T_2-weighted images:

- relaxation time for protons to 'dephase'
- tumours generally appear **brighter** than normal surrounding tissues
- fat has low signal while fluid has high signal – opposite to T_1

Management of the occult primary

Clinically palpable node – T0N1

History

Full history of age, occupation, smoking, drinking, dental health, drugs, allergies, PMSH, systems review

Examination

Thorough head and neck examination including intra-oral examination

Differentiate a secondary node from a lymphoma (examine other node basins) or primary Ca in a branchial cyst

Investigations

FNA

CXR and OPT

Panendoscopy

- sites to look at:
  - nasendoscopy
  - pharyngostomy
  - oseophagoscopy
  - bronchoscopy
- sites to biopsy:
  - nasopharynx
  - tonsil
  - piriform fossa
  - base of tongue
  - floor of mouth
  - lymph node biopsy in the neck if FNA was equivocal

MRI scan

- use the information from the above investigations to direct the MRI scan
- T_2-weighted image shows peri-tumour oedema and so may slightly overestimate size
- sinister features for lymph nodes include:

- node >1.5 cm
- loss of capsule definition
- multiple nodes
- central necrosis

Surgical treatment

If N1 consider modified radical neck dissection **or primary radiotherapy**

If >N1 proceed to modified radical neck dissection

General principles

Frozen section histology is unreliable in previously irradiated tissues

~20% of tumours overall will recur despite clear margins

60% of tumours recur if margins are involved

Radiated tissues lose natural planes making dissection difficult

Field change in oral mucosa may lead to a high second (or more) primary rate

Hypopharyngeal tumours also have a high second primary rate

Mandible

Main blood supply is from periosteum (especially with advanced age) – inferior alveolar A supplies the teeth and alveolar part of the mandible only

Periosteal supply is from buccal and submandibular branches of the facial A

Following dental extraction

- cortical bone never regenerates so that cancellous bone is in contact with overlying mucosa
- alveolar resorption results in loss of alveolar height and approximation of gingival mucosa to the floor of the mouth at the myelohyoid line

Most intra-oral tumours *do not* involve bone

Access to excision of intra-oral tumours may require

- splitting the mandible
- Slaughter's pull through technique (stripping floor of mouth structures off the mandible by subperiosteal dissection and delivering them through a submandibular incision)

Mandibular osteotomy

Lip split in the midline with an incision curving around the chin:

- most aesthetic
- preserves sensation
- preserves motor control

Site of osteotomy:

- symphyseal
- paramedian
  - anterior to the mental foramen
  - allows genioglossus and geniohyoid muscles to remain attached to the mandible and maintains tongue stability

- good exposure
- lateral
  - posterior to the mental foramen
  - divides inferior alveolar N and A

Technique of osteotomy:

- vertical osteotomy. Usual site between the second incisor and the canine
- step osteotomy
  - risks exposing the dental roots
  - good osteosynthesis with two plates
- sagittal split. Inevitable exposure of the dental roots

Fixation:

- plate/screw
- intra-osseus wires

SCC invading the mandible

>90% of intra-oral tumours are SCC

Direct infiltration

- dentate mandible – via the periodontal membrane at the occlusal surface
- edentulous mandible – via the alveolar surface at tooth gaps
- post-irradiation mandible may be invaded at several sites
- spread within the mandible either through the medulla or permeative spread along the mandibular canal

Periosteum is resistant to tumour invasion but fails to protect to edentulous occlusal surface

Invasion of the dentate mandible is heralded by loosening of teeth

Radiographic changes suggesting invasion include new bone formation (except on the occlusal surface)

Involved bone loses haemopoietic marrow

Changes secondary to radiotherapy difficult to distinguish from tumour

Image by OPT, CT or MRI

Trismus (pterygoid involvement) and pain radiating to the ear or temple (auriculotemporal nerve) or lower lip (mental nerve) are poor prognostic signs

Principles of mandibular excision

Limit excision to what is required for adequate margins – controlled by frozen section

Difficult to determine degree of invasion of the mandible by tumour

Choice between rim resection and segmental resection

Vertical height of the mandible helps to determine which option to choose – shorter vertical height increases need for segmental resection

Rim resection only feasible in the non-irradiated mandible for early tumour spread or because stripping of overlying mucosa off the mandible is difficult or impossible as it is so densely adherent

Rim resection performed because the mandible itself is involved should be conducted below the mandibular canal such that the entire canal from mandibular foramen to mental foramen is resected, obviating tumour permeation along the inferior alveolar nerve

Alternatively, T3 or T4 tumours may require segmental resection

When the mandible has been irradiated, segmental resection is also advocated:
- difficulty in determining clinically the degree of involvement
- poor bone healing at an osteotomy site

Segment may be small, hemimandibulectomy or subtotal/total mandibulectomy

Temporomandibular joint should be preserved if possible during hemimandibulectomy

Pre-operative EUA may be necessary to stage the disease

Radical excision, immediate reconstruction and post-operative radiotherapy

Consider the fitness of the patient – if a curative operation is impossible on the grounds of unfitness then a non-operative approach alone may be preferred

Virtually all mandibular resection is accompanied by synchronous neck dissection whether or not there is palpable disease

Mandibular reconstruction

Aims
- enable normal chewing and swallowing
- maintain oral competence
- denture rehabilitation
- aesthetics

Jewer classification of mandibular defects (modified by Soutar):
- **central segment** – mental foramen to mental foramen, subdivided by the midline into left and right; requires a curvature
- **lateral segment** – mental foramen to the lingula preserving the posterior ascending ramus and the condyle; may be reconstructed with a straight piece of bone
- **ascending ramus**

Non-vascularized bone grafts

Bone segment iliac crest or rib grafts
- re-activation of the osteogenic potential of periosteal progenitor cells
- ingrowth of vessels
- removal of dead bone cells and repopulation of the existing Haversian canal network

Particulate bone and cancellous marrow (PBCM)

- harvested from the ilium
- provides marrow mesenchymal cells and endosteal osteoblasts
- PBCM still undergoes the same resorption–replacement cycle but resorption is less

Graft survival may be enhanced using pre- and post-operative hyperbaric oxygen
- in irradiated tissues this promotes vascularization from 30 to 80% of normal tissue levels
- should be considered whenever operating within an irradiated field, especially when bone grafting

If radiotherapy is contemplated mandibular reconstruction may need to be delayed unless there is a symphyseal defect – pull of the pterygoids can cause sleep apnoea

Must have adequate soft tissue cover

Complicated by
- resorption
  - calvarial bone retained longer than other bone grafts – intramembranous vs. endochondral ossification

- poor take due to hostile recipient bed (including previous radiotherapy – hypovascular, hypocellular, hypoxic tissues)
- preclusion of post-operative radiotherapy which may compromise 'cure'

Osteomyocutaneous flaps

Lateral trapezius/spine of scapula
- skin paddle can be orientated horizontally or vertically (along the paraspinous processes)
- based on transverse cervical vessels – preserve during ipsilateral neck dissection
- incorporates bone from the spine of the scapula and a skin paddle over the acromioclavicular joint
- preserve the suprascapular nerve – supplies supraspinatus, which initiates shoulder abduction

Pectoralis major/fifth rib or edge of sternum
- myocutaneous flap described by Ariyan 1979
- based on pectoral branch of thoraco-acromial A (50% of pectoralis major blood supply)
- also supplied by lateral thoracic A (40%) and superior thoracic A (10%)
- contraindicated by pectus excavatum
- plan incisions to allow for a deltopectoral flap
- inclusion of pleura for intra-oral lining (post-operative chest drain)

SCM/medial segment of clavicle
- based on occipital vessels
- also supplied lower segmentally by the superior thyroid A and the thyrocervical trunk
- skin paddle overlying clavicle used for intra-oral lining
- ~8 cm of medial clavicle may be raised
- contraindicated by cervical nodal disease which requires radical neck dissection, although the flap may be used where there is a single level I node treated by suprahyoid dissection
- indicated for benign defects in the mandible, dysplasia or primary mandibular tumours
- arc of rotation determined by point of entry of the XIth nerve
- viability of skin paddle ~35% but increased if the middle vessel is preserved
- may raise a bilateral flap incorporating the intervening manubrium

Vascularized bone

Radial forearm flap
- originally described by Soutar 1983 for mandibular reconstruction
- good for lateral and central segmental defects
- periosteal supply via perforators in the lateral intermuscular septum and vessels which pass through FPL
- bone segment lies between the insertion of pronator teres proximally and brachioradialis distally (~12 cm)
- remove only < third of the cross-sectional area to avoid subsequent fracture
- thin pliable skin for mucosal and skin reconstruction
- low volume of bone, unsuited to osseo-integrated implants

DCIA
- naturally curved – requires no osteotomy
- ideal bone flap but precarious skin paddle
- suited to hemimandible reconstruction
- can also raise a portion of the internal oblique muscle based on the ascending branch of the DCIA

● accommodates osseo-integrated implants

Free fibula

● longest length of bone available
● requires multiple osteotomies for subtotal mandibular reconstruction
● skin paddle useful for floor of mouth reconstruction. May be excised later on and replaced with expanded submental skin to reconstruct the beard
● short pedicle
● elderly patients may rely upon the peroneal artery for supply to the foot
● accepts osseo-integrated implants

Scapula flap

● thin, straight 12×3 cm bone segment from the lateral border of the scapula
● reliable skin paddle
● good for central (symphyseal) defects
● thin bone cannot accommodate osseo-integrated implants

Alloplastic materials

Bone substitutes such as hydroxyapatite are rigid, cannot support a prosthesis and do not remodel

Metal plates may be used as a temporary support only

Allogeneic bone including whole or hemimandible, split rib or iliac crest may be useful as a crib for PBCM autograft. Mandible allografts must be hollowed out to allow packing with autograft and holes burred through the cortex to enable suturing to host soft tissues and the ingrowth of vessels

Reconstruction of the posterior mandible using a rectus abdominis free flap

Kroll. *BJPS* 1998

Suitable in patients with poor tumour prognosis or poor general health

Also suitable where there has been TMJ excision – very difficult to reconstruct

Otherwise vascularized bone flaps are ideal

Posterior defects cause less morbidity than anterior defects

Good aesthetics and functional outcome reported

Secondary lengthening of the reconstructed mandible by distraction osteogenesis

Yonehara. *BJPS* 1998

Mandibular distraction osteogenesis originally described by McCarthy. *PRS* 1992

Two cases of distraction osteogenesis following free fibular mandibular reconstruction are reported

Lengthening of the mandibular arch produced by midline osteotomy with gradual widening of the gap

Oral cavity

Examination: gauze, glove, tongue depressor, light

Metachronous tumours ~10% therefore look for these

● **synchronous** tumours – detected within 6 months – up to 15%

- **metachronous** tumours – detected at >6 months. Sites affected in both include oropharynx, lung, oesophagus

Leukoplakia vs. erythroplakia vs. *Candida*

Leukoplakia

- dysplastic/keratotic mucosa
- ulceration indicative of invasive SCC
- dysplasia responds to CO_2 laser
- observe if only keratotic
- must biopsy

Leukoplakia more likely to develop into an SCC if there is speckled erythroplasia

Erythroplakia has a higher malignant potential than leukoplakia ($\sim$50%)

- considered as an *in situ* SCC
- affects the 'sump' areas of the oral cavity
- *Candida* (lichen sclerosis) usually scrapes off, is less keratotic and can be differentiated on biopsy

T_1 and low-volume T_2 tumours can be reasonably treated by brachytherapy alone as long as their distance from the mandible will avoid radionecrosis

- similar control rates
- superior function

Excision margins

- **do not compromise excision to preserve function**
- well-defined tumours should be excised with margins of at least 1 cm using a Colorado needle
- ill-defined tumours or those arising in previously irradiated tissues should be excised with margins >2 cm
- consider perineural spread along lingual or inferior alveolar nerves into the pterygopalatine fossa – divide nerves as close to the skull base as possible

>90% of intra-oral tumours are SCC

Salivary gland tumours of sublingual and minor mucosal glands are likely to be high-grade malignant including adenoid cystic and muco-epidermoid tumours

Also acral lentiginous melanoma of oral mucosa (but usually superficial) and sarcomata

Intra-oral adenoid cystic tumours

- excite little inflammatory response
- invade mandible without radiological change
- aggressive perineural spread
- skip lesions

Reconstructive options

- split skin grafts are suited to resurfacing hard palate defects
- nasolabial flaps
  - reliable, predictable, useful
  - reconstructs defects 6 × 3 cm
  - may be used bilaterally
  - two-stage technique (de-epithelializing a portion of the flap to make it a one-stage procedure compromises flap viability)
  - floor of mouth, ventral surface of tongue
  - difficult in the dentate subject
- pectoralis major myocutaneous flap
  - useful for high volume defects

- donor site pain may promote chest infection via basal atelectasis
- latissimus dorsi myocutaneous flap
  - large volume
  - reliable, safe, quick and simple
  - need to turn patient
- free flaps
  - variability of design
  - not acceptable to Jehovah's Witnesses
  - radial forearm flap most useful including fascial flap (+ SSG) for very low volume defects, e.g. hard palate fistulae

Other considerations
- airway management
  - tracheostomy
  - avoid neck tapes
- single large dose of steroid to reduce post-operative oedema
- flap regime:
  - warm, comfortable, well-filled
  - flap observations
  - consideration of δ-T
  - early return to theatre if concerned
  - if one flap fails, re-reconstruct with another flap: the indication for this type of reconstruction will not have changed
- irradiated carotid exposed to saliva risks blow-out
- post-operative NGT feeding
- infection prophylaxis
- psychological support
- speech therapy
- pain management

Squamous cell carcinoma of the floor of mouth: 20-Year review Hicks. *Head and Neck* 1997

T1 tumours have a ~20% risk of occult nodal disease – ELND often performed for reasons of access but also warranted for occult disease
Involved margins → ~40% recurrence locally (surgery alone)
Clear margins → ~10% local recurrence (surgery alone)
Postoperative radiotherapy advocated especially where:
- margins are involved
- multiple positive lymph nodes
- extracapsular spread
- perineural invasion

Role of radical surgery and postoperative radiotherapy in the management of intra-oral carcinoma Robertson *et al.* BJPS 1985

Comparison of two treatment modalities for floor of mouth and tongue tumours
1. radical surgery (including radical LND) + radical radiotherapy

2. non-radical surgery ($\pm$ LND) + radical radiotherapy

Radiotherapy carried out 4–8 weeks after surgery

Results in all patients (T_2 and greater, N0–3, M0):

1. Tongue	2. Tongue	1. Floor of mouth	2. Floor of mouth
44% 5-year survival	5% 5-year survival	41% 3-year survival	10% 3-year survival

Oral lesions rarely metastasize below the clavicle

- T1N0M0 lesions may be effectively treated using either surgery or radiotherapy alone
- T1N0M0 SCC tongue $\rightarrow$ 80% 5-year survival with only radiotherapy or surgery
- T3N0M0 SCC tongue $\rightarrow$ 30% 5-year survival with only radiotherapy or surgery

Surgery first:

- debulks 99% of tumour mass
- free tissue transfer facilitates postoperative radiotherapy
- allows accurate staging

Radiotherapy first:

- only debulks the tumour by $\sim$25%
- delays surgery
- eliminates the possibility for further radiotherapy if surgical margins are narrow or involved
- induces fibrosis
- telangiectasia develops late (>2 years)

Nasolabial flaps in oral reconstruction

Varghese. *Br J Plast Surg* 2001

Inferiorly based flap supplied by the facial artery, superiorly based flap by the infraorbital artery

Use of nasolabial flaps described in 224 paients for reconstruction of a variety of intraoral defects (including tongue, floor of mouth lip and oral commissure) following tumour resection

Division of flap pedicle undertaken at week 3–4

Inferiorly based flaps were more reliable except where the facial artery was ligated during simultaneous neck lymphadenectomy

Retromolar trigone

Area between the upper and lower third molar teeth, medial to the ascending mandibular ramus and the medial pterygoid muscle

Inside of the medial pterygoid is the pterygomandibular raphe which blends posteriorly with the superior pharyngeal constrictor muscle

Lingual nerve lies anterior to the medial pterygoid

Site of development of SCC

Lymphatic drainage to the jugulodigastric and submandibular nodes

Tumour extension more commonly occurs to the floor of the mouth/tongue and to the faucial area more common than spread to the palate or buccal (cheek) mucosa

Almost invariably present with bony involvement (ascending ramus) → infiltration of mandibular canal and inferior alveolar nerve

Also involved are medial pterygoid, masseter and tendon of temporalis → trismus

Faucial tumours

Considerations of pathology, excision and reconstruction given to tumours of the retromolar trigone are similarly given to tumours of the fauces (tonsillar fossa and pillars)

Faucial tumours are both SCC and malignant lymphoid tumours (tonsil)

SCC are keratinizing or non-keratinizing. Non-keratinizing tumours are lymphoepithelioma and TCC

Faucial tumours spread laterally through the pterygomandibular raphe/constrictors to invade the medial pterygoid but rarely the mandible; also medially to the floor of mouth/tongue and anteriorly to the retromolar trigone

T_2 tumours or less have a 40% cure rate with radiotherapy alone

Surgical approach
- 'Y'-shaped neck dissection incisions
- mandibular 'swing'

Resection of the tumour and involved bone
- rim resection
- rim, anterior ascending ramus, coronoid process. Includes mandibular canal and inferior alveolar N
- entire ascending ramus including condyle (articulates in TMJ)

Reconstruction
- soft tissue
  - radial forearm free flap
  - pectoralis major myocutaneous flap
- bone
  - strip of radius in the radial forearm flap
  - may be unnecessary even where the ramus has been completely removed

Tongue and oropharynx

Tongue

Total glossectomy mainly reserved for:
- T_3/T_4 tumours
- post-radiotherapy recurrence
- where >50% of the tongue is involved, high risk of perineural and perivascular spread. Lingual A and N and hypoglossal N often involved contralateral to the tumour precluding hemiglossectomy

EUA is often necessary to establish the degree of spread within the mouth

MRI imaging, including the neck nodes, also helpful

T_1 tumours usually demand excision possibly with direct closure or SSG and no neck dissection

T_2 tumours usually demand ipsilateral neck dissection and reconstruction with a small volume free flap, e.g. radial forearm flap

T_2 tumours of the tip of the tongue usually demand bilateral neck dissection (35% incidence of occult nodal disease in the N0 neck)

Involvement of extrinsic muscles of the tongue $= T_4$ tumour

High incidence of involved neck nodes often requiring bilateral neck dissection. Stage I or II SCC $\rightarrow$ 42% occult metastases in neck nodes

Tongue may be approached via

- submandibular 'visor' incision and a pull-through technique sparing the mandible
- lip split and 'Y' incision (for synchronous neck dissection) combined with a paramedian mandibular osteotomy

If tumour fixes the tongue to the hyoid then this must also be removed. Suspend later to facilitate swallowing

Consider frozen section control of margins

Total glossectomy reconstruction

- laryngeal suspension – hyoid to mandible
- reconstruction of the mucosal defect
    - pectoralis major myocutaneous flap
    - myocutaneous free flap – need bulk

Post-operative speech therapy – speech regained by all patients

Natural history and patterns of recurrence of tongue tumours

Haddadin. *Br J Plast Surg* 2000

Retrospective study of 226 patients over 17 years with tongue SCC (Canniesburn Hospital, Glasgow)

Management principles

- Complete surgical excision of the tumour wherever possible
- Therapeutic cervical LND for palpable disease
- Elective cervical LND for 'high risk' tumours or where the neck is opened for access/reconstruction
- Post-operative radiotherapy indicated for:
    - large tumours
    - infiltrating tumours
    - narrow excision margins
    - positive cervical nodes

Commonest presentation

- ulcer (52%)
- tongue mass (19%)
- neck mass (4%)
- anterior 2/3 : posterior 1/3 ratio 1.8 : 1
- clinically negative neck in 156 patients (69%)

Stage at presentation

- T_1 (23%)
- T_2 (50%)
- T_3 or T_4 (27%)

110 patients underwent cervical LND

- 58 ELND
- 52 TLND
- 70 (64%) proved positive histologically
  - 36% of clinically negative necks upstaged
  - 7.7% of clinically positive necks downstaged

5-year survival:

- pT_1 9%
- pT_2 52%
- $pT_{3/4}$ 35%
- no improvement in overall survival could be demonstrated with time during the 17-year period

Loco-regional failure

- Recurrence sites:
  - primary site (27 patients)
  - ipsilateral neck (34 patients)
  - contralateral neck (19 patients)
  - primary site and neck (42 patients)
  - second oral primary (22 patients)
  - systemic disease (18 patients)
- Disease-related deaths (108 patients) due to:
  - advanced local disease (80 patients)
  - systemic spread (18 patients)

Oropharynx

Access to the posterior pharyngeal wall and the base of the tongue may be gained by a midline mandibular osteotomy and midline glossotomy. Defects on the posterior pharyngeal wall may be left to granulate

Principles of excision

- Posterior pharyngeal wall tumours are excised at the level of the prevertebral fascia
- Tumours are generally larger than they appear clinically

Impact on the structures involved in swallowing:

- bolus preparation
- transport – tongue contacts hard palate
- oropharyngeal component
  - tongue base moves posteriorly
  - velopharynx closes off
  - hyoid moves anteriorly elevating the larynx
  - cricopharyngeus relaxes

Reconstruction

- allow small defects to granulate
- primary closure
- flap closure
  - pectoralis major myocutaneous flap
  - temporalis muscle flap
  - temporoparietal fascial flap
  - free flap, e.g. radial forearm flap

Depth of invasion as a predictor of nodal disease in tongue carcinoma
Fukano. *Head and Neck* 1997

Depth of invasion <5 mm → ~6% incidence of nodal disease

Depth of invasion >5 mm → ~60% incidence of nodal disease

Clinically negative necks overall (N0 = stage I and II) had 30% incidence of occult disease

Recommend tumour excision and frozen section: if >5mm invasion → ELND

> **Self-assessment: How would you manage a patient presenting with a tumour on the side of the tongue?**

Take a history

Age (may not take on aggressive surgery if very old)

Smoker? (implications for pulmonary function but not predictive of flap success)

Alcohol? (implications in hospital – heminevrin, etc.)

General health/fitness (implications for complexity of procedure)

Examination

Tumour size → T status

Site

Involvement across the midline?

Tongue fixed to floor of mouth?

Hypoglossal nerve palsy?

Feel for neck nodes → N status

Investigations

Chest X-ray

FBC, U and Es, LFTs

MRI scan of tumour and neck if available or CT of tumour

LA biopsy → histology

Treatment

TisN0 – CO_2 laser

T1N0

- tumour: local excision and SSG or direct closure (could argue for radiotherapy only)
- neck: observe

T2N0

- tumour: local excision, RFF
- neck: ipsilateral functional ELND. 60% occult nodes >5 mm invasion (Fukano. *Head and Neck* 1997); upstaging of clinically negative neck in 36% of patients (Haddadin. *BJPS* 2000).
- radiotherapy

T3N1

- tumour: excision adequate to gain tumour clearance, pectoralis major for bulk or other flap (including free)

- neck: ipsilateral functional TLND (types 1–3) wherever possible, if not then radical
- radiotherapy

Contralateral neck dissection for T2 tip of tongue tumours or N2c disease

> **Self-assessment: How would you manage a patient presenting with a tumour on the floor of the mouth?**

Take a history

Age (may not take on aggressive surgery if very old)

Smoker? (implications for pulmonary function but not predictive of flap success)

Alcohol? (implications in hospital – heminevrin, etc.)

General health/fitness (implications for complexity of procedure)

Examination

Site – adjacent to mandible?

Size → T status

Fixity to tongue, mandible, floor of mouth, trismus?

Dentate or edentulous? (implications for mandibular involvement and need for osseo-integrated implants)

Feel the neck → N status

Investigations

Chest X-ray

FBC, U and Es, LFTs

MRI scan of tumour and neck if available or CT of tumour

LA biopsy → histology

Treatment

T1N0

- tumour: local excision, NL flap **or radiotherapy only**
- neck: observe – 20% risk of occult disease; Hicks. *Head and Neck* 1997

T2–3N0

- tumour: excision, RFF
- neck: functional ELND
- radiotherapy

T4N1

- tumour: excision and reconstruction with skin paddle from RFF, skin paddle from FF
- mandible
  - abutting → rim resection
  - invading or previous radiotherapy → segmental resection
  - reconstruction:
  - large defect or need osseo-integration → FF
  - small defect, no need for osseo-integration → RFF
- neck: ipsilateral functional (types 1–3) or radical TLND
- radiotherapy

Pharyngeal reconstruction using free jejunal flaps

First reported by Seidenberg in 1959

Flexible and self-lubricating

Preservation of near normal swallowing

Technique

- open or laparoscopic approach; Gherardini. *PRS* 1998
- isolate the second or third jejunal loop (or 40 cm) beyond the ligament of Treitz on a 'V'-shaped mesentry containing an artery and a vein
- anastomose the cut small bowel but leave the raised jejunal flap *in situ* until ready to transfer (short ischaemic time)
- inset the jejunal flap, proximal anastomosis first, in an isoperistaltic direction
  - tack the posterior surface to the prevertebral fascia
  - upper end may be too narrow to anastomose to the distal pharyngeal stump: reverse L end–side anastomosis or jejunal expansion with a patch flap may be considered; Yoshida. *BJPS* 1998
- then perform the microvascular anastomosis – superior thyroid artery and external jugular vein ideal recipients. Average donor vessel diameters: artery 1.2 mm, vein 3.0 mm – a single pedicle allows perfusion of a segment of jejunum up to 40 cm in length; Huang. *Ann Plast Surg* 1998

Flap monitoring

- achieved by exteriorizing a minor segment of the flap (~2 cm) to observe colour, secretion and peristalsis; Katsaros. *BJPS* 1985
  - a 4–5 cm segment produces initially ~100 ml/24 h, decreasing to ~10 ml/24 h at 2 weeks, collected in a stoma bag; Giovanoli. *Microsurgery* 1996
  - exteriorized segment excised ~5 days under local anaesthesia
- alternatively, a window can be created in the neck skin flap to expose the serosa of the underlying jejunal flap – this serosal layer is tacked to the skin and covered with a thin SSG; Baftis. *PRS* 1989
- fibreoptic examination of the major segment may be necessary

Gastrograffin swallow performed on day 7 to define any leaks and then oral intake is reinstated

Postoperative radiotherapy can be commenced ~5 weeks post-reconstruction

Success rates generally ~95%

- if one flap fails and another is harvested, avoid leaving a segment of jejunum between two donor sites as denervation of this segment leads to motility disorders
- most anastomotic thromboses occur within the first 24 h

Can also be opened out as a 'patch' for reconstruction of intra-oral mucosal defects – opened along antemesenteric border

A separate de-mucosalized and skin grafted segment, based on the same pedicle, can also be used to reconstitute overlying soft tissue defects; Carlson. *PRS* 1996

Tumours of the paranasal sinuses

Nasal polyps

2% malignant potential

Transnasal biopsy

If positive → WLE via lateral rhinotomy and radiotherapy

Treatment results in epiphora due to blocked nasolacrimal duct

Ethmoidectomy is achieved by piecemeal excision

Paranasal sinus tumours

Needle biopsy directly through medial wall of the sinus

Mainly SCC (80%), also adenocarcinoma

Present in >60-year age group

Commonest in Japan and Uganda

Maxillary antrum most commonly affected

Maxillectomy first claimed by Dupuytren

Lymph node metastases are rare (except for tumours of the maxillary sinus which involve buccal mucosa)

MRI and CT useful for definition of soft tissue and bony involvement

Most tumours treated by surgery and post-operative (brachy) radiotherapy

Exceptions:

- sarcomas – chemotherapy then surgery
- lymphomas – chemotherapy and radiotherapy

Maxillary sinus tumours

Maxillary sinus may be invaded by a palatal tumour

Primary maxillary sinus tumours present with tooth pain (first and second premolars) or cheek numbness (due to involvement of the infra-orbital nerve)

Hence, most present with advanced disease

Periosteum of the orbital floor is an effective barrier to tumour spread but anterior and posterior bony walls are thin and readily eroded

Penetration through the posterior wall into the pterygopalatine fossa can lead to surgically inoperable disease due to involvement of the maxillary nerve and artery

Maxillectomy via an intra-oral, paranasal lip-splitting (Weber–Fergusson $\pm$ subciliary Dieffenbach extension) or craniofacial approach

Extensive maxillectomy should be accompanied by ipsilateral insertion of grommets to prevent secretory otitis media

Prevention of postoperative trismus is by excision of the coronoid process

Prefabrication of an obturator to close oronasal fistula or close off space with a muscle flap, e.g. free rectus

Alternatively reconstruct palate using a free bone flap, e.g. DCIA

Staging:

- T_1 – mucosal involvement only
- T_2 – inferomedial spread (hard palate, nasal cavity)
- T_3 – superolateral spread (orbit, anterior ethmoidal sinuses), posterior wall of maxillary sinus, skin involvement
- T_4 – invasion of peri-orbita, pterygomaxillary and infratemporal fossae, skull base including cribriform plate, posterior ethmoid sinuses

Ohngren's line is a **plane** that lies diagonally connecting the inner canthus with the angle of the mandible. Maxillary sinus tumours invading above this line carry a worse prognosis

Ethmoid sinus tumours

Labyrinth situated above and lateral to the level of the maxillary sinuses, between the orbits, with its roof the cribriform plate

Surgical access via a lateral rhinotomy or craniofacial approach

Sphenoid sinus tumours

Sinuses lie below the optic chiasma and the pituitary fossa within the body of the sphenoid bone

Treated mainly by radiotherapy alone

Frontal sinus tumours

Sinuses located within the frontal bone

4% of individuals do not have a frontal sinus

Surgery via a craniofacial approach followed by radiotherapy

Malignant tumours of maxillary complex: 18-year review

Stavrianos. *BJPS* 1998

Rare tumours ~1/100 000 in USA

Presentation

- facial symptoms
  - facial swelling
  - pain
  - cheek paraesthesia
- dental symptoms
  - gingival or palatal mass
  - tooth pain or unhealed extraction socket
- nasal symptoms
  - epistaxis
  - nasal discharge
  - nasal obstruction
- ocular symptoms
  - proptosis
  - impaired vision
  - pain

Investigations

- EUA and biopsy
- OPT
- CT or MRI

Distribution of paranasal sinus tumours

- 55% maxillary antrum
- 35% nasal cavity
- 9% ethmoid sinuses
- 1% sphenoid and frontal sinuses

>80% are SCC, remainder adenocarcinomas

Surgery + post-operative radiotherapy:

- 5-year control 68%
- 5-year survival 64%

Radiotherapy alone:

- control 39%
- survival 40%

Surgery alone – survival 30%

> **Self-assessment: A patient sits before you with a facial swelling related to the maxillary antrum. What is your differential diagnosis and approach to management?**

Benign, e.g.

- dermoid cyst
- ossifying fibroma

Malignant, e.g.

- squamous cell carcinoma
- adenocarcinoma
- lymphoma

History:

- age, sex, occupation
- symptoms due to swelling itself (stage 1):
  - duration of swelling
  - rate of growth
  - facial numbness
  - facial pain
- symptoms related to inferomedial spread (stage 2):
  - tooth pain or numbness
  - loosening of teeth
  - epistaxis or nasal discharge
  - nasal airway obstruction
- symptoms related to superolateral spread (stage 3) above Ohngren's line:
  - ocular pain
  - ophthalmoplegia
  - impaired vision

Examination:

- **Look**
  - general facial symmetry
  - eyes – exophthalmos, extra-ocular movements
  - nose – intranasal swelling
  - cheek – swelling, extent
  - mouth – mass, loose teeth
- **Feel**
  - sensation V1,2,3
  - facial nerve function
  - test visual acuity
  - fixity to skin
- **Move** – occlusion

Investigations

- Facial X-rays, dental panoramic tomogram (DPT)
- CT scan

- biopsy via Caldwell Luc approach

Treatment

- malignant tumours treated by surgery then radiotherapy
- unlikely to involve nodes – poorly supplied by lymphatics, node disease rare
- excision via Weber–Fergusson lateral rhinotomy approach
- resect as much maxilla as is required to gain tumour clearance
- bone graft orbital floor or reconstruct with titanium plate
- free flap soft tissue cover, e.g. rectus or LD
- excise coronoid process to prevent trismus
- obturator to oronasal (palatal) defect then later close with a free DCIA flap

Orbital tumours

Secondary tumours

- more common
- invasion from paranasal sinuses

Primary malignant tumours include

- lymphosarcoma
- rhabdomyosarcoma
- meningioma
- glioma
- orbital malignant melanoma
  - extrascleral extension of posterior uveal melanoma – choroid or ciliary body
  - extension of adnexal melanoma – eyelid or conjunctival primary
  - primary orbital melanoma – melanocytosis of the meninges of the optic nerve
  - metastatic melanoma – haematogenous spread from a skin primary

Investigations

- plain X-ray, CT, MRI
- biopsy (division of lateral canthal ligament to access behind the globe)

Types of excision:

- evisceration
  - removal of all the contents that lie within the scleral shell
  - not indicated in tumour surgery
  - provokes sympathetic ophthalmia
- enucleation
  - removal of the globe from the orbit
  - intra-ocular malignancy, e.g. uveal tract melanoma without extrascleral spread
- total exenteration
  - removal of the entire contents of the orbit along with the eyelids and bony orbital walls
  - reserved for life-threatening malignancies within the orbit
  - extensive involvement of the orbit by paranasal tumours
  - involvement of globe or extra-ocular muscles
  - resection of the primary sinus en bloc with the orbit and its entire contents
- subtotal exenteration
  - slow growing eyelid malignancies
  - recurrent BCCs of the inner canthus invading the lacrimal sac

- tumours of the paranasal sinuses that have invaded into the orbit but not breaching the peri-orbita (periosteum/membranes of the orbit)
  - spare the globe and extra-ocular muscles but clear peri-orbita and fat
  - often results in enophthalmos, dystopia and diplopia
- limited exenteration
  - removal of sections of the bony wall of the orbit with the overlying peri-orbita and fat
  - localized invasion by paranasal sinus tumours

Reconstruction

- split skin grafts
  - used to cover exposed fat following subtotal exenteration
  - used to line the orbit following total exenteration including excision of the eyelids (can be applied directly to the bone)
  - does not mask recurrence
- temporalis muscle flap and SSG
  - also used to line the orbital after total exenteration without bony resection
  - tunnelled through a bony window created in the lateral orbital wall
  - socket maintained, accommodates prosthesis
  - but may mask recurrent tumour and leaves a temporal hollow
- pectoralis major
  - myocutaneous flap pedicled on the thoraco-acromial vessels only and tunnelled beneath the clavicle
  - used for large defects following maxillectomy
  - tunnelled through maxillary defect to provide lining to the exenterated orbit
  - risks tip necrosis – long way to travel
- free flaps
  - latissimus dorsi
  - rectus abdominis
  - provide skin and muscle bulk to fill the orbital defect

Reconstruction of the orbit
Spinelli. *Surg Oncol Clin N Am* 1997

Orbital septum forms a barrier to haemorrhage, infection, inflammation and neoplasia

Determine whether the tumour is likely to recur → skin grafts, allow to heal by secondary intention → allows for observation

If definitive surgery has been performed and do not need to observe closely → can perform reconstructive surgery

Allowing to heal by secondary intention:

- takes weeks – months
- not practical in irradiated tissues

Skin grafts

- take directly on to orbital bone
- heal quickly
- grafts inset on top of subgaleal fascial flaps allow for closure of sinus fistulae and dural defects

Dermis/fat grafts

- prone to resorption
- used for enucleated sockets
- extra-ocular muscles gain insertion on the dermis → movement of a prosthesis

Pedicled muscle flaps

- frontalis
- temporalis (above)
- pectoralis major – two-stage procedure exteriorizing pedicle, ligated at 2 weeks

Free muscle flaps:

- seal dural leaks
- good for an irradiated bed
- combat infections from, and seal off, sinus fistulae
- good fillers

Temporoparietal fascial flap:

- layer continuous with SMAS
- tunnelled subcutaneously into orbit
- BUT may → hair loss, VII N injury
- may be used as a free flap based on the superficial temporal vessels

Bony reconstruction:

- free split calvarial bone grafts
- bone composite free flaps
- alloplastic materials – titanium plates

Orbit in children:

- almost adult size by 2 years, fully adult size by 7 years
- children do not have sinuses
- teeth roots abut the infra-orbital rim
- cranium is thinner and more cancellous
  - do not attempt to split until >9 years of age
  - iliac crest and rim grafts are alternatives
  - do not use alloplastic material in children

Skull base tumours

Investigations:

- clinical examination
- nasendoscopy
- CT scan with and without contrast
- MRI scan
- MRI angiography – assess vascularity of tumour, may consider pre-operative embolization
- metastasis screen

Surgery may be combined with radiotherapy for some tumours (although BCC and SCC invading bone may become more aggressive if irradiated)

Access to the anterior skull base

- Weber–Fergusson (lateral rhinotomy) incision extended on to the forehead ('facial split') provides good access to the maxilla and anterior skull base

- bicoronal flap gives excellent exposure of the anterior skull base
  - subgaleal dissection to a point ~1.5 cm above the supra-orbital rim, then subperiosteal
  - good approach **even when the patient is bald** – scars heal well
  - may be used in combination with a facial split incision
- excision of the anterior cranial base required for resection of ethmoidal and sphenoidal sinuses – central craniotomy with osteotomy proceeding along the supra-orbital rim, through the medial orbital walls and linked by a nasal osteotomy
- exposure osteotomies (removing segments of the craniofacial skeleton and later replacement) – Le Fort III osteotomy – exposure of the posterior nasopharynx for resection of clivus tumours via a buccal approach

Access to the lateral skull base

- lateral temporal approach for access to the middle cranial fossa, the infratemporal fossa and the petrous temporal bone – facelift incision extended around the temporal region
- orbitotemporal exposure osteotomy
  - frontal and temporal craniotomies
  - removal of bone blocks, e.g. supra-orbital rim, orbital roof and lateral orbital wall

Complications of excisional surgery

- death
- blindness
  - raised intra-orbital pressure treated by
    - steroids
    - mannitol
    - lateral canthotomy
- severe haemorrhage
- infection (potentially leading to death) – due to a communication between the nasopharyngeal area and the intracranial space
- CSF leaks
  - dural tears closed by direct suture and with fibrin glue (but made from pooled serum hence infection risk)
  - defects reconstructed with free pericranial or fascial grafts
  - free fascial flaps for large defects

Principles of skull base reconstruction

- delay reconstruction until margins have been confirmed as clear and when there has been no early recurrence
- reconstruction of the bony skull base rarely required as brain herniation (encephalocoele) is uncommon
- soft tissue reconstruction required to obliterate dead space and close off intra- and extracranial communication
  - galea frontalis myofascial flap
    - based on supratrochlear and/or supra-orbital arteries at the supra-orbital rim
    - raised at a level just beneath the hair follicles down to the full-thickness of galea
    - turned down to close off the roof of the nasopharynx from the anterior cranial fossa and sutured through drill holes to the bony margins of the defect
  - temporal galeal flap
    - similar to the galea frontalis flap but based on the superficial temporal vessels
    - can reach to the frontal area to just beyond the midline
    - risks the frontal nerve if raised too low

- temporalis muscle flap
  - can be elevated down to its insertion on the coronoid process of the mandible
  - based on the superficial and deep temporal vessels
  - may be used to close off the roof of the orbit
- free tissue transfer
  - particularly useful in closing off dead space
  - free latissimus dorsi or omentum (long pedicle) – good blood supply to an area which has often been irradiated
- Branemark prosthesis

Petrosectomy for invasive tumours
Malata. *BJPS* 1996

60% of external auditory meatus and petromastoid tumours involve bone at presentation

50% present with established nerve palsy – often VII – a poor prognostic sign

Radical surgery offers the only hope for cure – achievable in ~20%

Petrosectomy sacrifices facial and vestibulocochlear nerves and occasionally IX–XII

Work-up includes 3D-CT and carotid angiography

Combined intra- and extracranial approach – need a neurosurgeon

Parotidectomy and neck dissection commonly performed synchronously

- neck dissection also allows dissection of the internal carotid A and internal jugular V as they enter the skull base
- metastatic parotid tumours are more difficult to treat with radiotherapy than involved neck nodes

Complications including injury to dural sinuses (haemorrhage), CSF leaks and meningitis

Defects reconstructed with free flaps including rectus as the flap of choice

Bone grafts to support the brain are unnecessary

Salvage petrosectomy following radiotherapy for recurrent disease is largely futile

Petrosectomy may be considered for palliation of pain and fungation

Salivary gland tumours

Serous versus mucous

- parotid mainly serous
- submandibular mainly mucous
- sublingual mainly mucous
- minor salivary glands entirely mucous

80% of all tumours are of the parotid

- 75% are pleomorphic adenomas
- 10% are adenolymphomas
- 3% mucoepidermoid carcinoma
- 3% adenoid cystic
- 9% other carcinoma including carcinoma ex-PSA

10% of tumours are submandibular

- 65% are pleomorphic adenomas

- 16% are adenoid cystic carcinoma
- 3% mucoepidermoid carcinoma
- 16% other carcinoma including carcinoma ex-PSA

10% are of the minor salivary glands – especially of the hard palate

The smaller the salivary gland the more likely that a tumour is malignant and the more likely that a malignant tumour will behave aggressively

Parotid gland

Enveloped by the parotid fascia – derived from the investing fascia

From superficial to deep pass:

- facial nerve, its upper and lower divisions and the pes anserinus
- retromandibular vein
- external carotid artery and its two terminal branches

Also within the gland are:

- pre-auricular lymph nodes
- filaments of the auriculotermporal nerve

Parotid duct (5 cm long) turns around the anterior border of masseter to pierce buccinator and open opposite the second upper molar

Nerve supply to the parotid:

- sensation – auriculotemporal nerve
  - branch of the mandibular N (V3)
  - emerges anterior to the tragus
  - also supplies the upper part of the pinna (rest supplied by the greater auricular N; posterior auricular N is the immediate branch of the VIIth N and is motor to occipitalis)
- secretomotor – preganglionic fibres from the inferior salivary nucleus/IXth N/tympanic branch of IX/lesser petrosal N/otic ganglion/postganglionic fibres in the auriculotemporal nerve – otic ganglion is closely applied to the mandibular nerve beneath the foramen ovale in the infratemporal fossa
- sensation to the parotid fascia – greater auricular N (C2,3)

Posterior belly of digastric is on the deep inferior surface of the gland and is a guide to where the facial nerve emerges from the stylomastoid foramen

Most parotid tumours are either superficial or deep to the plane of the facial nerve

Submandibular gland

Superficial and deep parts separated by the free border of mylohyoid

Submandibular lymph glands lie in contact with or within the gland

Superficial part grooved posteriorly by the facial artery

Deep part lies between the lingual N above and submandibular duct and the hypoglossal N below

No structures pass **through** the gland

Submandibular duct emerges from its superficial (inferior) surface, is also 5 cm long and passes deep to mylohyoid and geniohyoid to open in the mouth next to the frenulum

Nerve supply – preganglionic fibres in the superior salivary nucleus/nervus intermedius/ facial N/chorda tympani/via petrotympanic fissure to lingual nerve/submandibular ganglion/postganglionic fibres pass directly to the gland

Salivary gland tumours

Present as a localized painless nodule ± fixed

Pain usually suggestive of malignancy

May involve the facial nerve – weakness – strong indicator of malignancy

Biopsy is largely contraindicated in the major salivary glands unless the features of the lump and history are strongly suggestive of pathology other than pleomorphic adenoma

Biopsy of the minor salivary glands is much less hazardous because there is less likelihood that the lump will be a pleomorphic adenoma – more likely to be a carcinoma for which treatment based on the results of the biopsy may be instituted

Classification

Adenoma

- monomorphic (**adenolymphoma, Warthin tumour**)
  - uniform epithelial tissue, usually glandular
  - lymphoid stroma
  - mainly in males >50 years
  - benign tumour accounting for 10% of parotid tumours
  - may be multifocal or bilateral (15%)
  - 10% recurrence rate
- pleomorphic adenoma
  - different types of epithelial tissue
  - different types of stroma – chondroid, myxoid, mucoid
  - arises from duct epithelia
  - slow growth
  - incomplete excision or seeding leads to recurrence
- myoepithelioma
  - minor salivary gland tumour similar to pleomorphic adenoma
  - large intra-oral swelling
  - secondary middle ear obstruction → effusion (may require grommet)
  - slow growth over many years suggests the diagnosis → avoid biopsy
  - may require no treatment
  - MRI defines tissue planes and resectability
- Mucoepidermoid tumour
  - squamous and mucous metaplasia within ductal epithelium
  - low- to high-grade malignancy
  - tend to be low grade in the major glands, behaving much like pleomorphic adenomas
  - in the minor glands behave more like adenoid cystic carcinoma
  - rarely maintain a discrete capsule – excision commonly followed by recurrence
  - common parotid tumour

Carcinoma (epithelial tumours)

- adenoid cystic carcinoma
  - Swiss cheese pattern histologically
  - no capsule
  - marked perineural spread and infiltration of tissue planes without a lymphocytic response
  - skip lesions
  - slow rate of growth

- embolic spread to lymph nodes very rare but may be involved due to direct invasion
- haematogenous spread to the lungs more common
- excision followed by 'inevitable' recurrence
- the smaller the gland the more likely that a tumour might be adenoid cystic
- adenocarcinoma
- squamous carcinoma
- anaplastic carcinoma
  - (all of these show growth, local invasion and embolic spread to neck nodes)
- carcinoma in pleomorphic adenoma
  - carcinoma ex-PSA
  - sudden increase in rate of growth
  - development of fixity
  - swelling present for many years
  - facial nerve weakness or paralysis
  - behaves like anaplastic carcinoma with a poor prognosis

Lymphoid tumours
- malignant lymphomas
  - may occur in a gland affected by Sjogren's syndrome
  - in the otherwise normal gland there is a diffuse rapid swelling but **no facial nerve involvement**
  - diagnosis by biopsy
  - treated by chemotherapy rather than surgery

Management
- benign or low grade parotid tumours:
  - superficial lobe – superficial lobectomy (parotidectomy), e.g. mucoepidermoid
  - deep lobe – total parotidectomy preserving the facial nerve
- high-grade parotid malignancy:
  - radical parotidectomy sacrificing the facial nerve and surrounding involved structures including masseter and medial pterygoid medially and the styloid process + muscles and the posterior belly of digastric
  - may need to also sacrifice overlying skin
- benign or low-grade submandibular gland tumours – submandibular gland excision
- high-grade submandibular gland tumours – submandibular gland excision plus excision of surrounding structures including platysma, mylohyoid and hyoglossus muscles, hypoglossal and/or lingual nerves
- minor gland tumours – radical local excision
- neck dissection:
  - clinically positive necks including MRI-diagnosed disease (modified radical neck dissection)
  - recurrent tumours
  - high-grade malignancy
  - extensive involvement of the deep lobe of the parotid with a malignant tumour
- nerve grafts may be required where branches of the facial nerve have been sacrificed (can use greater auricular nerve)
- even where there is an extensive adenoid cystic or mucoepidermoid tumour for which surgery and reconstruction are only palliative, this should still be considered

because recurrent disease may take many months or years to become apparent and is often painless
- radiotherapy:
  - tend to respond poorly to radiotherapy
  - assume surgical resection is the only chance of cure
  - no place in the management of pleomorphic adenomas – should be properly excised and radiotherapy may increase risk of malignant change
  - neutron therapy may be of some benefit with adenoid cystic carcinoma

Parotidectomy

Identification of the facial nerve
- sites of identification
  - at the stylomastoid foramen
  - where a triangular projection of the tragal cartilage points to the nerve
  - where the buccal branches run alongside the parotid duct
  - where the marginal mandibular branch accompanies the retromandibular vein as it emerges from the inferior surface of the gland

Excision of the tumour
- superficial parotidectomy – mucoepidermoid tumours of the superficial lobe
- facial nerve-sparing total parotidectomy
  - superficial and deep lobes separately
  - external carotid artery and retromandibular vein ligated and excised with the specimen
  - may need to chase deep lobe tumour into the parapharyngeal space – may require dislocation of the TMJ or mandibular osteotomy
- radical parotidectomy
  - sacrifices the facial nerve
  - high-grade tumours

Complications

Intra-operative – facial nerve palsy

Early
- skin flap necrosis
- infection
- haematoma
- sialocoele or salivary fistula

Late
- Frey's syndrome
  - gustatory sweating
  - postganglionic PNS secretomotor fibres destined for the parotid hitch-hiking in the auriculotemporal nerve – sensory nerve to the ear and temple
  - trauma of parotidectomy divides PNS branches of the nerve which degenerate to the level of the cell bodies in the otic ganglion and regenerate along the auriculotemporal nerve
  - these link up with sweat glands in the absence of the parotid gland
  - subsequent eating (activating salivation nerves) induces sweating in the distribution of the auriculotemporal nerve

- incidence 10–40%
- treatment with antiperspirants, dermofat grafts, tympanic neurectomy

Malignant tumours of the parotid gland – a 12-year review Malata. *BJPS* 1997

Uncommon tumours about one-to-four cases/100 000 population in the UK

51 patients underwent parotidectomy, mean age 64 years

Just over one-half had T_3 or T_4 disease on presentation

88% sensitivity of FNA in diagnosing malignancy

MRI more useful than CT (especially for imaging neck nodes)

Radical parotidectomy was accompanied by immediate nerve grafting in five patients

Three-quarters of patients received postoperative radiotherapy (including all adenoid cystic)

Independent prognostic factors for a poorer outcome

- male sex
- incomplete excision
- pre-operative facial palsy

Carcinoma arising in pleomorphic adenoma was the most frequent parotid malignancy (transformation in up to 10%)

Fixed tumours without facial nerve palsy:

- total parotidectomy (sparing all or part of the nerve) and postoperative radiotherapy; or
- radical parotidectomy and facial nerve reconstruction

Free flap coverage of a fungating tumour acceptable for palliation

Metastatic tumours are usually located within nodes in the superficial lobe of the parotid and are suited to superficial parotidectomy

Neck dissection reserved for palpable disease or positive MRI findings or where the neck is entered for access purposes

Immediate temporary tarsorrhaphy indicated in palsied patients to prevent exposure keratitis

Nerve grafting did not contraindicate post-operative radiotherapy

Management of parotid haemangioma in children

Greene, Rogers, Mulliken. *Plast Reconstr Surg* 2004

- Retrospective review of 100 children with parotid haemangiomas treated at Boston Children's Hospital
- Female: ratio 4.5:1
- Deep (little/no skin involvement)
- Combined (skin and parotid involvement – 86%)
- 10% of children require drug treatment for complications of parotid haemangiomas including narrowing of obstruction of the auditory canal
  - Small haemangiomas may be managed by intralesional steroid injection
  - Systemic steroid recommended for larger lesions
  - Response rates to interferon up to 80% but potential for neurological complications limit its use
- Surgery for parotid haemangioma during the proliferative phase risks excessive blood loss and injury to the facial nerve
  - Patients with larger lesions were more likely to require surgery during the involutional phase later in childhood

- Resection of fibrofatty tissue overlying the parotid
- Facelift-type mobilisation and resection of affected skin

Imaging parotid malignancy

Raine. *Br J Plast Surg* 2003

Magnetic resonance imaging is capable of diagnosing malignant parotid disease with up to 93% sensitivity

- Key feature is a poorly defined tumour boundary with radiological evidence of local tumour invasion
- A useful tool in conjunction with the clinical history, examination findings and fine needle aspiration cytology for the diagnosis of malignant parotid lumps
- Also facilitates staging of the neck and defines the relationship of the tumour to the facial nerve

Malignant tumours of the submandibular salivary gland – 15-year review
Camilleri. *BJPS* 1998

70 patients, mean age 64 years

Average duration of symptoms 3 months

Main symptom – painless enlarged gland

Main tumour adenoid cystic then carcinoma in pleomorphic adenoma

Malignancy often diagnosed after removal of the enlarged gland (previously assumed to be due to duct obstruction)

FNA 90% sensitive

Primary surgery plus postoperative radiotherapy

Prognosis related to TMN status at presentation

Submandibular gland malignancy accounts for 8% of all salivary gland malignancy

Salivary duct carcinoma
Guzzo. *Head and Neck* 1997

Histologically resembles invasive ductal carcinoma of the breast

Aggressive tumour

Mainly affects the parotid duct

Presents with rapidly enlarging swelling, pain and facial nerve paralysis

Nodal and distant metastases are common

Surgery and postoperative radiotherapy is the treatment of choice

Local recurrence rate is high

Commonly fatal within 2 years

Some patients in whom ductal Ca has arisen in association with a pleomorphic adenoma, may present with a more indolent form of the disease

Hyperbaric oxygen therapy for wound complications after surgery in the irradiated head and neck
Neovius. *Head and Neck* 1997

Increases oxygen tension in hypoxic tissues following radiotherapy

2–3 bar, 100% oxygen, 75 min

30–40 daily treatments may be required

Increases fibroplasia and angiogenesis to aid wound healing

Facilitates oxygen-mediated phagocytic killing of pathogens to reduce infection

Bactericidal effect on anaerobes

Complications

- oxygen toxicity and seizures
- temporary myopia

No apparent effect on cancer cells

Indications

- radionecrosis of the mandible
- prophylactic pre-operative therapy (20 pre-operative sessions, 10 postoperation)
- postsurgical, postirradiation wounds and fistulae

Prediction of outcome in 150 patients undergoing free tissue transfers to the head and neck
Simpson and Batchelor. *BJPS* 1996

5% flap failure rate

- correlated with bronchodilator therapy and nitrate treatment for angina
  - GTN therapy predictive of thrombosis of the venous anastomosis – a reflection of generalized vascular disease?
  - bronchodilator therapy → higher ventilation pressures postoperation and coughing → higher blood pressure
- diuretic therapy predictive of thrombo-embolic problems (DVT, PE) – dehydration and decreased venous tone

20% re-exploration rate – increased with use of NSAID – antiplatelet activity → bleeding

Mortality rate = 4.7% – mortality and CVA commoner in patients with pre-existing vascular disease (especially previous MI) and steroid treatment (related to increased BP?)

Chest infection proportional to age and commoner in men

Patients taking bronchodilators had more hypoxaemia

Nutritional problems associated with low weight and opioid therapy

Donor site problems related to anaemia, previous radiotherapy and peripheral vascular disease

Donor and recipient site infections both related to hypertension – more bleeding and a reflection of vascular disease?

No correlation between flap failure and

- extremes of age
- gender
- ASA status
- smoking
- alcohol consumption
- previous radiotherapy or chemotherapy – recipient vessels unaffected by radiotherapy
- diabetes
- duration of surgery

Localized amyloidosis of the head and neck
Nandapalan. *Head and Neck* 1998

Rare and benign process

May be local or systemic

Primary amyloid

- AL (immunoglobulin light chains)
- mainly affects skin, nerves, heart, gut – diagnosed by biopsy of the rectum or gums

Secondary

- AA (protein A – precursor of a normal acute phase protein)
- inflammation, e.g. TB, RA
- neoplasia
- may be hereditary – usually AD (except Mediterranean fever – AR)
- mainly affects liver, kidneys, spleen

Amorphous fibrillar protein deposition or β-pleated sheet

Perivascular, connective tissue and smooth muscle deposition

Congo red stain $\rightarrow$ birefringence in polarized light

Affects the head and neck in 90% of patients with systemic amyloidosis

Affects mainly the larynx

No specific therapy for systemic amyloidosis – colchicine (AA) and melphalan (AL) have been advocated

---

Self-assessment: Outline the management of a patient attending with a lump overlying the parotid gland

---

History

- age (elderly men think monomorphic adenoma), occupation
- duration of the lump – longer duration suggestive of benignity
- growth of the lump – steady (benign) or rapid (malignant) or steady then rapid (carcinoma ex-PSA)
- any pain – pain suggestive of malignancy
- any sense of facial weakness or drooling – facial nerve involvement with a malignant tumour
- any discharge from the lump – differential diagnosis may be sebaceous cyst
- does the pain/swelling come and go before meals – suggestive of sialolithiasis (only if the whole gland is swollen)
- drug treatment, smoking, diabetes and health in general – **factors which predict a poor anaesthetic risk, intra-operative bleeding and postoperative wound healing problems**

Examination

- Look
  - symmetry in the face (facial nerve weakness)
  - sensation – particularly the ear as the auriculotemporal nerve may be involved
  - lump: site, shape, size, overlying skin
  - *Look at the other side – monomorphic adenomas are bilateral in 15%!*
- feel the lump:
  - hard/soft, smooth/craggy
  - fixed deep or mobile over the gland but within skin – think of sebaceous cyst (look for a punctum), possibly lipoma

- **feel the neck nodes**
- **feel other node basins – could be a lymphoma**
- move – test the facial nerve branches
- intra-oral examination:
  - look in the mouth – if there is intra-oral swelling may be deep lobe tumour or a parapharyngeal tumour – Schwannoma
  - bimanual palpation of the lump
  - ask the patient to stick out the tongue – testing for hypoglossal nerve weakness/wasting

Investigations
- if the lump is thought to be separate from the parotid gland (e.g. sebaceous cyst) then USS to confirm and deal with as appropriate (excise)
- sialography if thought to be sialolithiasis
- if the lump is truly a parotid swelling then FNA to obtain a tissue diagnosis
- MRI to determine the extent of the tumour: superficial or deep lobes or both and to assess the neck nodes
- CXR as a pre-operative work-up but also to look for metastatic spread if malignant

Treatment
- malignant
  - **Parotid**: parotidectomy (sparing a working facial nerve if possible) and removing sufficient surrounding structures to gain clearance
  - superficial parotidectomy for a superficial lobe mucoepidermoid tumour
  - **Neck**: if N0 and no nodes negative on MRI then observe. Node positive neck (unusual) or highly aggressive tumour → synchronous lymphadenectomy. Also if the parotid tumour is a metastasis from a face/scalp primary → lymphadenectomy
  - **Adjuvant**: post-operative radiotherapy to the parotid area
  - if nerve sacrificed immediate nerve grafting and temporary lateral tarsorrhaphy
  - may need pectoralis major, DP flap or a free flap (RFF) for skin
- benign – superficial (usually) parotidectomy only
- lymphoma – refer to an oncologist for chemotherapy
- Frey's
  - antiperspirants
  - dermofat grafts beneath the skin
  - tympanic neurectomy via an endonasal approach

Adenoid cystic carcinoma of the head and neck

Chummun. *Br J Plast Surg* 2001
- Typically a protracted disease prone to local recurrence (especially where there is perineural invasion) and late metastatic potential
- Presents most commonly in the fifth decade
- Histological subtypes:
  - Solid (worst prognosis)
  - Cribiform
  - Tubular (best prognosis)
- Series of 45 patients reviewed
  - Commonest sites were nose and paranasal sinuses and parotid and submandibular salivary glands
  - Most patients treated by combined surgery and radiotherapy

- Incomplete resection in 20 out of 35 patients undergoing surgery
  - Bone invasion frequent with maxillary sinus tumours
- Local recurrence in 7 out of 35 patients
- Commonest site for distant recurrence was the lungs
- Overall survival 65% at 5 years

Neurofibromatosis

Neurofibromatosis-1 (NF-1)

AD

1 in 3000

Multiple cutaneous neurofibromas (proliferating Schwann cells and fibroblasts)

Café au lait patches (more than five is abnormal)

Axillary freckles

Iris hamartomas (Lisch nodules)

Associated features

- Neural
  - optic nerve glioma
  - meningioma
  - plexiform neurofibroma
  - phaeochromocytoma
  - neurofibromas may undergo sarcomatous change
  - mental retardation
- Cardiovascular
  - orbital haemangioma
  - renal artery stenosis
  - obstructive cardiomyopathy
  - also pulmonary fibrosis
- bony:
  - scoliosis
  - fibrous dysplasia

May present with skin lesions for excision or with large facial mass and facial asymmetry

Most individuals with NF-1 lead healthy and productive lives

Gene for NF-1 has been identified

Neurofibromatosis-2 (NF-2)

Less common

Separate gene defect

Also AD

Associated with acoustic neuroma

Self-assessment: Discuss the problems with which a patient with neurofibromatosis might present to a plastic surgeon

Two types of neurofibromatosis

- Type 1 – AD, 1 in 3000
  - cutaneous neurofibromas (Schwann cells plus fibroblasts) **may be irritating and need to be excised**
  - café au lait patches – **undiagnosed skin pigmentation**
  - axillary freckles
  - Lisch nodules (iris hamartomas)
  - plus neural, cardiovascular and bony problems:
  - neural:

    plexiform neurofibroma with **facial asymmetry and need for debulking surgery**

    sensorineural deafness

    optic nerve glioma

    meningioma

    phaeochromocytoma

    sarcomatous change of neurofibromas – **management of sarcoma**
  - cardiovascular:

    cardiomyopathy

    pulmonary fibrosis

    renal artery stenosis

    orbital haemangioma – **management of orbital haemangioma – steroids, etc**.
  - bony:

    fibrous dysplasia – **bone reconstruction problem**

    scoliosis
- Type 2
  - different gene, less common, still AD
  - more commonly associated with acoustic neuroma – excision → **need for reanimation surgery for facial palsy**

Tuberous sclerosis

AD inheritance

Sebaceous adenomas

- nodules on cheeks and around the mouth
- treated by CO_2 laser

Epilepsy

Severe mental retardation

Torticollis

Congenital – vertical orbital dystopia (craniosynostoses, facial clefts, hemifacial microsomia).

Child holds head on one side to compensate and attain stereoscopic vision

Acquired – idiopathic cervical dystonia – ICD

- previously thought to be a psychiatric illness, now viewed as a neurological illness
- 10–20% of patients may experience remission, but nearly all patients relapse within 5 years and are left with persistent disease

- aetiology of ICD is unknown but may follow trauma
- botulinum toxin is the most effective treatment – development of neutralizing antibodies occurs in at least 5–10% of patients
- anticholinergics and baclofen may also help
- SCM myoplasty reserved for after failed conservative management
- selective denervation of the muscles responsible for the abnormal movement or posture

Musculoskeletal, ophthalmologic, infectious, neurologic and neoplastic conditions may present early with only torticollis

First step in evaluation is always a careful and complete physical examination

Congenital muscular torticollis and associated craniofacial changes

Hollier. *Plast Reconstr Surg* 2000

Torticollis: *tortus* (twisted) *collum* (neck)

Adult onset (paroxysmal) torticollis most commonly spasmodic

- 25–60 years of age
- may be associated with psychiatric disorder
- drug therapy including botox

In most children congenital torticollis

- Due to a primary fibrosis of sternocleidomastoid
- May have a palpable mass within the substance of the muscle
- Associated with possible birth trauma in up to 60% of cases and a muscle specific compartment syndrome?

Other potential causes:

- Cervical spine abnormalities
- Ocular abnormalities (e.g. congenital nystagmus)
- Posterior fossa tumours
- Infections (e.g. parapharyngeal abscess)
- Trauma (e.g. brachial plexus palsy)

16 patients assessed for associated craniofacial abnormalities

- Left side affected in 13/16
- All patients initially managed by physiotherapy
- Surgical release or resection of sternocleidomastoid undertaken in 4 patients
  - Myoplasty incorporates step-lengthening of the muscle
- Associated abnormalities included:
  - Displacement of the ipsilateral ear (backwards and downwards)
  - Recession of the ipsilateral zygoma
  - Mandibular displacement (chin points to affected side)
  - Ipsilateral eye inferiorly displaced
  - Deviation of the nasal tip to the affected side

Facial reanimation

Aims

Symmetry at rest and with voluntary and involuntary motion

Control of the ocular, oral, and nasal sphincters (may need temporary tarsorrhaphy)

Aetiology – four sites

Facial nerve nucleus

Usually infarction (stroke) → UMN signs with contralateral weakness sparing the brow (cross-innervation), i.e. no brow ptosis

Pons and cerebellopontine angle

Tumours: acoustic neuroma, glioma

Vascular abnormalities

Central nervous system degenerative diseases including MND

Congenital abnormalities and agenesis including Moebius syndrome

Trauma

Within the petrous temporal bone

Tumours (including cholesteatoma)

Trauma (including iatrogenic)

Bacterial and viral infections

- *Bell's palsy*: viral infection, swelling of the facial nerve within the petrous temporal bone, 15% have permanent palsy, rarely bilateral, most recover within 12 months
- *Ramsey–Hunt syndrome*: herpes zoster infection of the geniculate ganglion (chorda tympani/taste relay station in the petrous temporal bone)

Extracranial

Tumours (parotid tumours)

Trauma (including iatrogenic)

Moebius syndrome

Rare congenital anomaly

Multiple cranial nerve palsies – VII nerve palsy associated with other cranial nerve palsies, most often of the VI

Facial vessels often abnormal

Limb anomalies

Abnormal facies

Drooling of saliva

Missing primary and permanent teeth

Almost always of normal intelligence

High incidence of congenital cardiac disease, spinal anomalies, corneal abrasions and peripheral neuropathies, microglossia

Aetiology is unknown – genetic or embryopathic (hypoxia, infection or toxic)

Pathogenesis is also unclear – nervous or muscular aplasia or dysgenesis of the two first branchial arches

Children present for:

- correction of strabismus
- improvement of limb function
- facial reanimation

- Harrison uses latissimus dorsi free flap with a pedicle long enough to reach down into the neck
- nerve coaption to one of the nerves to masseter (Zucker)

Techniques

Direct nerve repair
Facial nerve grafting
Cross facial nerve grafting
Nerve crossovers
Muscle transfers
Static suspension

Direct nerve repair

Usually possible for traumatic or iatrogenic injury to the nerve

Facial nerve grafting

Best performed within 3 weeks–1 year of injury
Some good results as late as 2–3 years post-injury
Immediate grafting after ablative surgery (up to 95% response)
Branches of the cervical plexus or sural nerve
Expect 20% shrinkage of the graft – hence, no tension
Epineural repair comparable if not superior to fascicular repair
6–24-month interval to return of facial movement

Cross-facial nerve grafting

Cross-innervation from the non-paralysed side
Appropriate coordination of contraction
Depends upon overlap in the innervation of muscles from other nerve trunks on the donor side
Graft from distal branches of the donor nerve to the recipient nerve at a site distal to the level of injury
Alternatively, allow axons to grow across (9–12 months) before coapting to the recipient nerve
Reversal of the sural nerve graft may help reduce axonal escape
May graft from branches of temporal, zygomatic, buccal and mandibular nerves
Only 15% success with temporal and mandibular grafts
Axonal regeneration 1–3 mm/day
Only 20–50% of axons cross the nerve graft

Nerve crossovers

Glossopharyngeal, accessory, phrenic, and hypoglossal nerves
Used when direct suture or grafting is not feasible, e.g. facial paralysis resulting from intracranial lesions or disorders of the temporal bone
But movement is uncoordinated (synkinesis) and there is loss of function in the donor nerve

- synkinesis can be palliated by injections of botulinum toxin around the orbicularis oculi muscle
- this reduces involuntary closure of the eye when attempting to smile

Hypoglossal nerve crossover leads to >50% moderate and 25% severe tongue atrophy

Most suited to immediate reconstruction of the facial nerve trunk as part of the primary ablative surgery

Can also be used to baby-sit the facial musculature awaiting the regeneration of fibres along a XFNG

Muscle transfers

Local muscle transfers

- temporalis
  - turnover flap originally described by Gilles
  - alternatively detach the tendinous insertion by an osteotomy of the mandibular coronoid process, pass a strip of fascia lata through the detached bony insertion and anchor distal end to nasolabial fold and upper/lower lips
- masseter
- sternocleidomastoid – too bulky, pull in wrong direction
- platysma – too delicate, not enough power
- impulse for movement originates in the trigeminal nerve – not physiological
- also suffer from synkinesis

Free muscle transfer

- requires one of
  - ipsilateral nerve coaption to the stump of the facial nerve on the affected side:
    - ~5% of patients have a proximal nerve stump
    - faster nerve regeneration into the donor nerve
    - can also coapt to a nerve other than the facial nerve if this is unavailable and a two-stage operation is to be avoided, e.g. hypoglossal nerve (but → synkinesis)
  - preliminary cross facial nerve grafting
    - long-standing paralysis
    - nerve stump unavailable
    - wait 6–12 months before second stage
  - cross-face vascularized nerve coaption in a single stage (below)
- most commonly used:
  - **pectoralis minor** (described by Manktelow)
  - **gracilis** (described by Harii) – single-stage free tissue transfer made possible by coaption of the nerve to gracilis (anterior division of the obturator nerve) across the philtrum to the buccal branch of the intact contralateral facial nerve and **avoids the need for a XFNG**; Kumar, *BJPS* 1995. But disadvantaged by the loss of motor end plates on the donor muscle while awaiting regeneration of axons across the face
    - pedicle on deep surface to allow for thinning
    - acts as a vascularized nerve graft
    - simultaneous harvesting and preparation in the cheek
  - **latissimus dorsi**
    - single-stage reconstruction also possible: the thoracodorsal nerve reaches over to the other side of the face
    - muscle trimmed to the required size *in situ* – pedicle placed on the deep rather than superficial surface to facilitate further secondary thinning

- serratus, rectus abdominis and platysma also used
- bank the XFNG at the tragus and perform free muscle transfer 6 months later according to progress as per Tinel's sign
- XFNG in a retrograde direction reduces axonal escape
- fascicular nerve stimulation of the donor muscle to determine which fascicle supplies which strips of muscle
- **zygomaticus major alone nearly produces a normal smile** – all surgical efforts are directed at reproducing this action
- normal facial muscles have ~25 muscle fibres innervated by one axon, whereas gracilis and pectoralis minor muscles have ~150–200 muscle fibres to each axon

Static suspension

Fascia lata slings

Superficial temporal fascia suspension

Gold weight to upper lids

Botulinum toxin to weaken contralateral (normal) side – effect lasts up to 6 months, ACh inhibition

Facelift

Pectoralis minor vascularized muscle graft for the treatment of unilateral facial palsy

Harrison. *Plast Reconstr Surg* 1985

Muscle transfer should receive impulses from the uninjured facial nerve if a natural smiling response is to be provided

XFNG has a role in young patients and early palsy

More long-standing palsies – >1 year – suffer from muscle atrophy

Hence, palsies >1 year require importation of fresh muscle

Must expect a considerable loss of muscle power following transplantation

Gracilis has a long NV bundle but is rather bulky

XFNG (sural) from the buccal branch of the VIIth nerve overlying the parotid duct, over the upper lip to a banked position at the contralateral tragus

Six months later (when Tinel's sign is positive at the distal end of the graft) → free pectoralis minor muscle flap

- raised on medial and lateral pectoral nerves and a direct arterial branch from the axillary artery
- anastomosed to facial vessels on the paralysed side, nerve coapted to the XFNG
- muscle is inserted into the alar base and the upper and lower lips with a point of origin at the zygoma (with the pedicle superficial to aid microsurgery)
- lagophthalmos is addressed by insertion of gold weights

Good donor site scar (anterior axillary fold) with no adverse functional sequelae

20–50% of axons reach the other side by 6 months

But:

- only provides the lip elevation part of a smile – lacks depressor function and lateral pull normally achieved by buccinator
- some axons are lost as they attempt to innervate pectoralis major passing through medial and lateral pectoral nerves

Irreversible contracture after ipsilateral nerve coaption

Chuang *et al. BJPS* 1995

Four patients underwent free gracilis transfer with nerve coaption to the ipsilateral facial nerve

Irreversible muscle contracture developed with onset between 6 and 12 months

Postulate that over-re-innervation $\rightarrow$ over-stimulation $\rightarrow$ contracture

Over re-innervation due to coaption to the ipsilateral facial nerve stump is potentially avoided by XFNG

But later correspondence suggests that contracture may occur after both techniques and may be related more to muscle fibrosis before re-innervation

Free muscle transfer for Romberg's disease (hemifacial atrophy) rather than facial palsy may result in direct neurotization of the muscle which also leads to contracture

Recovery of facial palsy after cross-facial nerve grafts

Iñigo. *BJPS* 1994

Best chance for restoring spontaneous facial expression is direct nerve repair or interpositional graft – but this may not be possible, e.g. following excision of an acoustic neuroma

Patients >40 years or facial palsy >10 years were excluded

Eight patients had nerve palsy due to hemifacial microsomia

- performed within the first year
- in these patients the XFNG was coapted to facial muscle (neurotization)
- excellent results with this approach

Otherwise the XFNG was coapted to the distal stump of the contralateral facial nerve

Patients referred within 1 year of onset of palsy are suitable for XFNG

- worst results in patients undergoing surgery 4–10 years later

Treatment of drooling by parotid duct ligation and submandibular duct diversion

Varma *et al. BJPS* 1991

Opening of one parotid duct is cannulated and the distal part of the duct dissected out for ligation

Other parotid duct is left intact

Openings of both submandibular ducts are similarly cannulated next to the frenulum

Duct is dissected out with a surrounding cuff of mucosa and re-routed backwards in the mouth towards the anterior fauces

Suitable for cerebral palsy patients with excessive and troublesome drooling

Transient swelling of the (ligated) parotid and both submandibular glands common postoperation

Submandibular duct obstruction is complicated by sialolithiasis due to the higher calcium and phosphate content of mucous secretions and antigravity drainage

---

Self-assessment: Outline the management approach to the patient with a facial palsy

History
- congenital or acquired
- if acquired was this a:

- spontaneous palsy (Bell's)
- post-traumatic (facial laceration, head injury)
- secondary to tumour excision (parotid, acoustic neuroma, glioma)?
- **hence what is the level of the palsy** – intracranial, intratemporal, facial?
- what is the duration of the palsy? – longer duration → wasting of ipsilateral muscles making re-innervation impossible: need to import muscle

Examination

- temporal (frontal branch) → brow ptosis, lack of wrinkling
- zygomatic branch → orbicularis problems → lagophthalmos, corneal exposure
- buccal branch → lip weakness, lack of a smile
- marginal mandibular branch → drooling, droopy lip

Investigation – MRI and NCS?

Treatment

- intracranial and intratemporal: no **proximal** stump
  - <1 year → XFNG to distal nerve stump or directly into muscle
  - >1 year
  - younger patient (nerve regeneration and fit for free flap) – XFNG and pectoralis minor or gracilis
  - older patient (poor nerve regeneration, unfit for major surgery)
    muscle transfer: temporalis turnover
    static suspension: facelift, fascia lata sling
    nerve transfer: IX, XI, XII
    Henderson correction of drooling
    Gold weight into upper lid
- first line approach to extratemporal division: **proximal and distal** stumps
  - <1 year → direct repair or primary nerve graft
  - >1 year → pectoralis minor coapted to ipsilateral nerve stump

Temporalis transfer vs. microneurovascular transfer for facial reanimation

Erni. *Br J Plast Surg* 1999

Evaluation of McLaughlin's technique for temporalis tendon transfer (ten patients) vs. two-stage free tissue transfer using latissimus dorsi and gracilis (three patients each) and pectoralis minor (one patient)

Temporalis transfer:

- Facelift incision
- Masseter splitting approach to coronoid process of mandible
- Apex of coronoid process detached with an osteotome
- 6 mm drill hole through detached segment threaded with a strip of fascia lata
- fascia lata sling then re-routed to the corner of the mouth and anchored to previously inserted conchal cartilage grafts

Microsurgical reanimations:

- Resulted in significantly better measurements of excursion during smiling while static symmetry was similar to temporalis transfer
- Only patients under 50 years of age were offered microsurgical reanimation
- Swelling of the cheek soft tissues and skin tethering was more problematic compared with temporalis transfer

Marginal mandibular nerve palsy

Restoration of the dynamic depressor mechanism

Terzis. *Plast Reconstr Surg* 2000

Lower lip is animated by:

- orbicularis oris
- depressor labii inferioris
- depressor anguli oris
- mentalis
- platysma

Injury to the marginal mandibular nerve causes:

- inability to form a natural smile
- drooling
- elevation of the lower lip at rest

Reanimation options:

- palsy <12 months (EMG evidence of depressor activity): direct neurotisation of depressors using a cross-facial nerve graft
- palsy 12–24 months (EMG still some depressor activity) or failure of the above: mini XII transfer to VII or direct neurotisation (incorporates 20–30% of the nerve trunk)
- longstanding palsy: platysma transfer (if functional) or transfer of the anterior belly of digastric
  - supplied by the mandibular division of V
  - tendon divided and mobilized to corner of mouth
  - insertion on mandible then divided and inset to reproduce smile vector
  - in young patients re-education successful in reproducing a physiological smile
  - older patients required coaption to a cross-facial nerve graft

Paralysis of the marginal mandibular nerve: treatment options

Tulley. *Br J Plast Surg* 2000

Marginal mandibular nerve vulnerable to trauma in the submandibular fossa, lying deep to platysma below the body of the mandible

Paralysis of depressor anguli oris and depressor labii inferioris results in asymmetry of smile, the lower lip on the affected side unable to move downwards or laterally or to evert

Treatment options include:

- Botulinum toxin injection of contralateral depressors
  - temporary symmetrization
  - alternative to contralateral depressor myectomy
- Anterior belly of digastric transfer (ABDT)
  - Innervated by the nerve to mylohyoid (branch of inferior alveolar N from V^3)
  - Anterior belly left attached to mandible, posterior belly/central tendon divided and re-routed to the corner of the mouth
  - Simple and very effective one stage procedure
  - But generates a scar in the submandibular fossa
- Two-stage microsurgical transfer of extensor digitorum brevis
  - complex microsurgical procedure
  - greater donor and recipient site scarring
  - useful when ABD is absent due to surgical trauma of complex facial hypoplastic syndromes

Depressor labii inferioris resction for marginal mandibular nerve paralysis

Hussain. *Br J Plast Surg* 2004

- Careful assessment of the surface marking of depressor labii inferioris on the unparalysed side is undertaken by palpation of the vermillion border while the patient attempts to show the lower teeth
- A muscle block is undertaken by intramuscular injection of local aneasthetic to simulate the effect of myectomy (alternatively botulinum toxin can be used and lasts 3–4 months)
- Muscle is exposed from an intraoral incision 0.5cm above the buccal sulcus, retracting the orbicularis oris fibres
- A segment of muscle is then resected across its entire width
- Improvements in appearance, oral continence and lip biting reported

Maxillofacial trauma

Features in the history

degree of force
direction of force
previous eyesight
previous occlusion

General evaluation

ABC
- maxillofacial injuries picked up as part of the primary or secondary survey:
  - segmental mandibular symphyseal fractures may be pulled backwards into the oropharynx along with the tongue due to the unopposed action of geniohyoid and digastric muscles and cause airway obstruction
  - also haemorrhage from the internal carotid A into the tonsillar fossa

All fractures → bruising, swelling and tenderness ± loss of function

Upper face
- forehead sensation
- crepitus indicating frontal sinus fracture
- CSF rhinorrhoea (anterior cranial fossa fracture)

Mid-face
- Orbits
  - ocular dystopia, restricted eye movement (e.g. down and out)
  - tenderness/depression of orbital walls
  - exorbitism or enophthalmos
  - pupil size and reactivity
  - diplopia/field defects
  - racoon eyes (anterior cranial fossa fracture)
- Zygoma
  - fractures often present with orbital signs
  - malar flattening when viewed from above

- palpable step
- trismus
- Nasal bones
  - palpable deformity and tenderness
  - check for septal deviation and haematoma
- Maxilla
  - infra-orbital nerve numbness on the cheek and upper lip
  - malar flattening
  - intra-oral lacerations/bleeding
  - increased maxillary mobility
    - maxillary alveolus moves but nasofrontal area does not → Le Fort I
    - maxillary alveolus AND nasofrontal area move → Le Fort II
    - entire mid-face moves → Le Fort III
    - but fracture may be impacted → no movement

Lower face
- mandible:
  - malocclusion
  - trismus
  - lower lip numbness due to inferior alveolar N injury
- laryngotracheal injuries – cricoid/thyroid cartilage fracture
- Ears
  - haemotympanum
  - signs of middle cranial fossa fracture:
    - CSF otorrhoea
    - Battle's sign
  - conductive or sensorineural hearing deficit
- soft tissue injuries:
  - examine for facial N injury
  - parotid duct division

Investigations

CT scan is the investigation of choice for all maxillofacial trauma except perhaps for isolated mandibular injuries
- AP mandible open and closed
- OPT
- reversed Towne's view for the condyles
- OM views for mid-facial injury

Medial orbital wall fractures are virtually undetectable on plain X-ray
Anterior orbital floor fractures may → teardrop sign but many of these can be treated conservatively – only the posterior floor fractures need treatment for enophthalmos
Endoscopic evaluation is of current interest

Principles of surgical management

Early one-stage repair
Access to all fracture fragments

Rigid fixation

Immediate bone graft

Definitive soft tissue cover

Frontal sinus fractures

Severe force to the glabellar area

Swelling, bruising, crepitus

Late complications include sinusitis, mucocoeles and meningitis

Give antibiotics

Anterior wall

- not depressed → no treatment
- depressed, not comminuted → elevate and plate/wire
- depressed and comminuted → may need cranial bone graft

Posterior wall

- CSF rhinorrhoea and pneumocephalus
- injury to both nasofrontal ducts → impaired drainage → mucocoeles, sinusitis and meningitis – hence, need to cranialize the sinus
- injury to one nasofrontal duct → remove midline septum

Orbital fractures

Consultation by ophthalmologist within 24 h is essential

General symptoms and signs:

- diplopia
- peri-orbital oedema and bruising
- ptosis
- exophthalmos/exorbitism
  - exophthalmos is the result of increased ocular tissue but normal orbital volume
  - exorbitism (→ proptosis) is the result of normal ocular tissue but decreased orbital volume – decreased orbital volume may be due to retrobulbar haemorrhage, tumour, blow-in fracture
  - enophthalmos is due to a discrepancy between ocular tissue and orbital volume causing the globe to sink in, e.g. blow-out fracture
- ophthalmoplegia (decreased movement), e.g. inferior rectus tethering
- subconjunctival haemorrhage
- dystopia
  - orbital dystopia – bony obits either do not lie on the same horizontal plane (vertical dystopia) or are too close together (hypotelorism) or far apart (hypertelorism) – orbital dystopia is usually the result of craniofacial developmental anomalies
  - ocular dystopia refers to the position of the globe
    - ocular dystopia results more commonly from trauma
    - change in the volume of the orbit compared with the globe, e.g. enophthalmos
  - telecanthus – inner canthi are widely separated

Rupture

Vitreous and anterior chamber haemorrhage

Lens dislocation

25% of orbital fractures are associated with globe injury

Superior orbital fissure syndrome

- lacrimal (VI), frontal (VI), trochlear (IV), superior division III, nasociliary (VI), inferior division III, abducent (VI)
- III carries PNS fibres
- fracture, oedema or haemorrhage causes pressure within the muscular cone formed by the recti
- exorbitism, ophthalmoplegia, **dilated pupil** (loss of PNS constrictor tone – unopposed SNS dilator activity), ptosis (loss of SNS supply to Muller's muscle – travels with lacrimal branch), anaesthesia in VI territory

Orbital apex syndrome

- fracture through the optic canal with division of the optic nerve (II) at the apex of the orbit
- neuritis, papilloedema or blindness
- early steroid therapy also indicated

Blow-in fracture

- wall displaced towards the globe
- decreased orbital volume
- exorbitism
- impingement of recti – forced duction test – elicits inferior rectus muscle entrapment with orbital floor fracture

Blow-out fracture

- wall displaced away from the globe
- increased orbital volume
- enophthalmos (although haemorrhage and oedema may → exorbitism)
- fracture of the medially placed thin lamina papyracea of the ethmoid bone

Superior wall fractures – may also have anterior fossa, frontal sinus and frontal bone fractures

Lateral wall fractures – usually have an associated zygoma fracture

Medial wall fractures

- bone is thin
- often treated conservatively

Orbital floor fractures

- suspensory ligament and inferior rectus injury
- may require ORIF for enophthalmos, muscle entrapment or ocular dystopia
- access to the orbital floor:
  - subciliary
  - transconjunctival with lateral canthotomy

Indications for surgical treatment

- muscle entrapment
- increased orbital volume with enophthalmos

Insertion of a BIP pack into the maxillary antrum supports the orbital floor and can be left *in situ* for many months pending definitive floor reconstruction

Strategies for the management of enophthalmos

Grant. *Clin Plast Surg* 1997

Image the orbit to define bony abnormalities – a 5 mm displacement of the orbital rim can causes significant enophthalmos

Mobilize soft tissues over the fracture and slightly beyond

- multiple incisions may be required:
  - bicoronal → superior rim, roof, upper medial and lateral walls
  - conjunctival → floor, walls
  - gingivobuccal → inferior rim

Reposition the bony fragments

- reposition the rim first then internal walls
- orbital roof and floor are the most amenable to fixation
- medial and lateral walls may be onlay grafted with split calvarial (less resorption) or split rib grafts (alloplastic materials also used)
- restore soft tissue attachments, close periosteal layers to avoid periosteal 'slippage' and resultant soft tissue deformity

Maxillary fractures

Anatomy

- Four main processes of the maxilla
  - alveolar (becomes resorbed in the edentulous patient)
  - frontal – supports the nasal bones
  - zygomatic – articulates with the zygoma
  - palatine – articulates with vertical/horizontal plates of palatine bone
- Body of the maxilla
  - contains the maxillary sinus (fully formed by 15 years)
  - posterior wall including maxillary tuberosity is the anterior border of the pterygopalatine fossa
  - superior wall forms the infra-orbital rim

Consider the four vertical pillars of the face – these transmit forces from the maxilla to the skull base:

- nasomaxillary (canine) buttress – alveolar process of maxilla (opposite canine) to the frontal process of the maxilla and nasal bones – medial to the orbit
- zygomatic buttress – alveolar process of the maxilla (opposite first molar tooth) to the zygomatic process of the frontal bone – lateral to the orbit
- pterygomaxillary buttress – posterior body of the maxilla to the skull base via the sphenoid (including the pterygoid plates)
- mandibular buttress – ascending ramus to the skull base via the TMJ

And the five horizontal buttresses:

- supra-orbital bar
- infra-orbital rim
- zygomatic arch
- palate
- body of the mandible

Fractures present with malocclusion – but consider **pretraumatic** class II or III malocclusion

Also malar flattening with loss of height

Cracked tea-cup sign: percussion of an upper tooth

Look for a mid-palatal fracture

Mid-face fractures are commonly comminuted

Lift floating segment forwards to restore the airway

About one-third of Le Fort II and III fractures are complicated by CSF rhinorrhoea:

- fractures of the naso-ethmoid area (cribriform plate)
- 95% resolve within 3 weeks
- antibiotic prophylaxis of meningitis
- persistent leaks may need repair of the dural tear – craniofacial approach

Le Fort classification

I

- **horizontal** fracture
- separates the alveolar and palatine processes from the body of the maxilla

II

- **pyramidal** fracture
- similar to I but fracture line passes through the maxillary antrum and the orbital floor and across the nasofrontal area
  - incorporates the nasal skeleton – nasal bones and bony septum (perpendicular plate of the ethmoid and the lower half of the vomer) – and the infra-orbital foramen
  - disruption of the medial canthal ligament – attached to the frontal process of the maxilla → telecanthus
- maxillary segment displaces backwards and up → anterior open bite
- transient or permanent infra-orbital nerve injury
- lacrimal duct injury

III

- **transverse** fracture
- fracture line passes through frontomaxillary junction, orbit and frontozygomatic junction to separate off the whole of the maxilla and mid-face from the skull base (craniofacial disjunction)
- 'free-floating' maxilla
- anterior open bite as for II
- anaesthesia of maxillary teeth usually resolves

Aims of treatment

Nasotracheal intubation or tracheostomy – allows access to mid-face and teeth
Re-establish bite and correct facial deformity

- dental wiring and arch bars (use the patient's dentures if edentulous) used to reduce fractures
- fracture immobilization
  - intermaxillary fixation
  - intra-osseous wires
  - plates/screws
  - external fixation used for mid-face fractures:
    - requiring anterior traction
    - concomitant fracture/dislocation both condyles
    - severe comminution
- uninjured or healthy teeth in the fracture line need not be removed – fracture line usually passes through or around the tooth socket
- soft tissue closure

Le Fort I
- mandible is the key so **fix this first if fractured**
- Rowe or Tessier disimpaction forceps
- beware haemorrhage from descending palatine As
- maxillomandibular dental wiring alone is usually sufficient
- miniplate fixation reduces duration of interdental wiring – positioned to reconstruct the injured buttresses
- Le Fort I fractures in the edentulous patient may need no treatment

Le Fort II
- reduce by interdental wiring as above
- fixation using miniplates/screws or intra-osseous wires

Le Fort III – as for II

Zygomatic (malar) fractures

Look
- swelling, bruising
- conjunctival haemorrhage lateral to the limbus
- malar flattening when viewed from above
- may have enophthalmos with an associated blow-out fracture

Feel
- tenderness
- fracture mobility

Move – trismus
- vast majority of zygomatic fractures do need plating to avoid late recurrence of deformity – malar flattening
- usually unstable due to the pull of masseter

X-rays
- submentovertex
- occipitomental views at 0, 15, 30 and 45

Classification – Knight and North
- undisplaced
- arch fracture
- depressed body fracture
- depressed body fracture with medial rotation
- depressed body fracture with lateral rotation
- comminuted fracture

Access to the zygoma
- upper lid incision to access the temporal process and supra-orbital rim
- subciliary incision to access the sphenoid process (infra-orbital rim) and arch
- buccal incision to access the maxillary process
  - may cause numbness in the distribution of zygomaticotemporal and zygomaticofacial Ns
  - undisplaced fractures may be treated conservatively but need regular re-evaluation

Gilles lift
- arch fractures
- incision through the scalp to deep temporal fascia
  - splits to encircle the zygoma hence need to be beneath this fascial layer

- superficial temporal fascia (temporoparietal fascia) is continuous inferiorly with SMAS and superiorly with galea
- Bristow or Kilner elevator inserted and tunnelled deep to the zygomatic arch
- lifting action to reduce fracture while the head is stabilized

Zygoma contributes to the lateral orbital rim at its articulations with the sphenoid and frontal bones

Also contributes to the orbital floor where it articulates with the maxilla

- hence, the zygoma is fractured in blow-out or -in fractures of the orbit
- wiring or plating of more complex zygomatic fractures may be indicated
- **zygomaticofrontal** suture is the strongest and the last to fracture completely – if this is disrupted open reduction and internal fixation is usually indicated

ORIF complications

Early

- diplopia (usually resolved within 24 h)
- bleeding including retro-orbital haematoma
- nerve injury

Late

- plate infection, extrusion, migration
- scars and cicatricial ectropion
- union problems – delayed, malunion, non-union
- sinus problems

Mandibular fractures

Fractured in at least one-half of all facial fractures

Only nasal bone fractures are more common

Most are open into the mouth – cover against *Staphylococcus aureus* and anaerobes – fractures near the root of a tooth are considered open

Look for:

- pain
- swelling
- trismus
- mental N numbness
- **intra-oral (sublingual) haematoma**
- chin deviating towards the side of a fractured condyle

X-rays:

- reversed Towne's view shows the condyles well
- also need OPT and PA mandible

Classified according to anatomical location of the fracture

At the thin condylar neck

At the angle where the root of the wisdom tooth represents a weak area

Parasymphysis where the long canine root is lined up with the mental foramen

- order of frequency of mandibular fractures:
  - C – condyle

- A – angle
- B – body

Look for the contra-coup fracture

Muscle action on the mandible

Parasymphyseal fragment is:

- pulled down by geniohyoids
- pulled down and laterally by the digastrics
- pulled backwards by genioglossus

Body of the mandible is:

- pulled up by masseter
- pulled up and backwards by temporalis
- pulled backwards by the pterygoids

Unfavourable fractures are those which become displaced due to muscle action

Most fractures require some form of reduction and immobilization

Fractures that can be treated conservatively (soft diet):

- undisplaced fractures including the condyle
- greenstick fractures
- normal occlusion
- minimal trismus

Restore occlusion and reduce the fracture by dental wiring (intermaxillary fixation) **first** – then plate:

- unicortical fixation
  - intra-oral approach
  - two plates anterior to the mental foramen to stabilize against complex muscle pull
  - one plate at the angle – must be on the upper border since this is the tension side of the fracture that pulls open
- caution in children – screws may disrupt tooth buds

Angle fractures approached via a submandibular incision:

- 2 cm inferior to the lower border of the mandible to preserve the marginal mandibular N
- dissect over the submandibular gland at the level of the investing fascia (i.e. much the same as a neck dissection)
- may need percutaneous placement of screws

Isolated coronoid process fractures are rare and are treated conservatively unless displaced:

- maintain dental wires for 2 weeks
  - liquid/blended diet
  - malocclusion is the main complication

Indications for ORIF of condylar fractures

High fractures of the condyle or ramus are approached via a Risdon incision combined with a pre-auricular incision

Failure of IMF to correct occlusion after 2 weeks

Bilateral fractures (BF) – fix one side

BF, e.g. bullet

Head-injured patients/mental retardation → unable to tolerate IMF

Significant displacement – intracapsular fractures are usually stable

But difficult surgery and to be avoided if at all possible!

Undisplaced condylar fractures do not need treatment – soft diet for 2 weeks and mobilize

TMJ dislocation – usually bilateral – reduced by downward and backward pressure by thumbs placed on the posterior molar teeth under GA

Guardsman's fracture

Blow to the chin → bilateral condylar fractures ± parasymphyseal fracture

May cause retraction of the mandible → anterior open bite

Generally fix only one condylar fracture – IMF used to gain initial occlusion and left for 2 weeks to treat the other condylar fracture

IMF – Leonard buttons

Can be used alone to treat comminuted mandibular fractures or where there is contamination

If used alone then maintain for 6 weeks

IMF fitted to incisors over a long period (6 weeks) → loosening of teeth – choose molars if possible

When a secondary twist develops on the wire stop turning or will break!

Need to prestretch wires

Gunning splints used in the edentulous patient – held in with wires passed around the mandible and through the maxillary sinus

Teeth

'Mesial' describes the position of a tooth towards the central incisors in the midline

'Distal' describes a position away from the midline

Surfaces of a tooth:

- buccal vs. lingual
- occlusal vs. apical

Indications for dental extraction:

- carious tooth
- fractured tooth
- wisdom tooth in the line of the fracture (interferes with plate positioning)

Mandibular fractures in children

IMF is precarious during mixed dentition (6–11 years) – loose

plates can damage the permanent tooth roots

Do not use bone grafts or alloplastic materials

Imperfect restoration of occlusion will self-correct over ~2 years

Nasal and naso-ethmoid fractures

Nasal bones usually fracture in their lower half where the bone is thinner

Numbness at the tip of the nose indicates anterior ethmoidal nerve injury

Nasoethmoid fractures

- telecanthus as medial canthal ligaments displace laterally – bowstring test
- restore drainage or obliterate the sinus
- often need ORIF and bone grafting

Nasal packs:

- splint fracture fragments

- splint the septum
- control bleeding and septal haematoma – septal haematoma requires drainage

Nasal POP used to maintain position after reduction of a widely displaced fracture

Stranc classification

- upper – bone, bony septum
- middle – upper lateral cartilage, cartilaginous septum
- lower – lower lateral cartilage, cartilaginous septum

MUA at 2 weeks

- Ash forceps for correction of septal deviation
- in or out fracture of bone

Late correction by post-traumatic rhinoplasty

Look for telecanthus

- rupture of medial canthal ligament
- normal intercanthal distances:
  - male 28 ± 4 mm
  - female 25 ± 3 mm

Maxillofacial and ocular injuries in motor vehicle crashes

Brookes. *Ann Roy Coll Surg Engl* 2004

Drivers' airbags introduced in USA in 1986 and have been responsible for a 30% reduction in fatalaties in frontal crashes when used in combination with a lap–shoulder belt

- Marked reduction in maxillofacial trauma from impact upon steering wheel

But small stature occupants and those sitting close to the steering wheel or improperly restrained (i.e. out of position) are at risk from injury due to the deployment of the airbag itself

- Airbag deploys within 50 milliseconds at 160–320 km/h
- Spike of force up to 20 kN during the 10 ms 'punch-out' phase
- Injuries include cardiac tamponade, traumatic amputation of digits, upper limb fractures and maxillofacial fractures
- Ocular injuries also reported due to the shock wave transmitted through the globe
  - At less than 30 mph include ocular rupture and retinal tears or detachment
  - At speeds over 30 mph include vitreous haemorrhage and retinal detachment

Treatment of mandibular fractures using bioabsorbable plates

Kim & Kim. *Plast Reconstr Surg* 2002

- Rigid internal fixation of mandibular fractures reduces the need for intermaxillary fixation
- Titanium plates may be complicated by infection, localized long term tissue damage and may be palpable
- Bioabsorbable plates (without compression) used in 49 patients to treat 69 mandibular fractures
  - Single plate fixation of angle or body fractures
  - Two-plate fixation of symphyseal fractures
  - Six patients experienced complcations
    - infection (4)
      - one patient developed osteomyelitis following compound symphyseal fracture
    - premature occlusal contact

- TMJ disorder
- No mal or non-unions
- Poly-L/DL-lactide plates:
  - Bending modulus close to that of bone
  - Slowly transfer stress forces to healing bone as they absorb (helps to prevent bone atrophy)
  - Potential complications:
    - Screw holes visible radiologically due to osteolysis
    - Inflammatory reactions
    - Partial resorption
    - Bulky
    - Expensive
    - Not suited to comminuted fractures or patients with poor oral hygiene

Craniofacial surgery

Craniofacial growth

Enlow's principles of facial growth:
- mid-face and mandible are proportionately very small in the neonate
- growth by:
  - displacement – whole bone mass moves
  - remodelling – occurs behind the wave of displacement
Mediated by pull of muscle attachments – Moss' functional matrix principle

Encephalomeningocoele

Congenital midline swelling
Herniation of meninges/brain tissue from the anterior cranial fossa via the foramen caecum
Association with metopic synostosis and hypertelorism
Investigate by skull X-ray and CT/MRI
Intra-/extra-cranial approach via bicoronal incision with the assistance of a neurosurgeon
Herniation is only glial tissue – ?can be safely excised
Bone defect reconstructed with diploic bone graft

Craniosynostosis

Premature fusion of one or more sutures
Growth retarded in the plane perpendicular to the suture
Syndromic
- Crouzon's
- acrocephalosyndactyly syndromes; Prevel. *J Craniofac Surg* 1997
  - Apert's
  - Pfeiffer's

- Saethre–Chotzen
- Carpenter's
- Goldenhar's
  - craniofacial microsomia
    - microtia
    - mandibular hypoplasia – aplasia of lateral pterygoid
  - epibulbar dermoids
  - pre-auricular appendages and sinuses
  - abnormalities of cervical vertebrae
  - elevated scapula (Sprengel deformity)
  - rib abnormalities
  - basilar impression – deformity of the skull base around the foramen magnum, e.g. occipitalization of the atlas
- In general
  - AD inheritance ± variable penetrance – Carpenter's = **AR**
  - >90 reported syndromes
  - most have associated limb and cardiac abnormalities
  - all have mid-face hypoplasia
  - turribrachycephaly (turret-like) due to bicoronal synostosis

Non-syndromic

- gestational influences
- toxic influences
- sporadic congenital finding
- 0.6/1000

Aetiology

- mutations in FGFR genes
  - encode tyrosine kinase receptors
  - FGFR1 – Pfeiffer's
  - FGFR2 – Pfeiffer's, Apert's, Crouzon's
- dura mater communicates with overlying cranial suture via paracrine activity of growth factors to regulate suture fusion

Craniosynostoses

- metopic (between the frontal bones) synostosis → trigonocephaly
- sagittal synostosis → scaphocephaly
- unilateral coronal synostosis → plagiocephaly
- bilateral coronal synostosis → brachycephaly
- unilateral lambdoidal synostosis → plagiocephaly
- positional (deformational) plagiocephaly of the occiput – non-synostotic deformity, self-correcting

  'plagiocephaly without synostosis' (PWS)

Raised intracranial pressure

- disparity between brain growth and remodelling of overlying bone due to premature fusion of sutures
- raised ICP commoner in **multiple** fused sutures – raised ICP → thumb printing, copper beating or a wormian appearance on the skull X-ray
- uncommon where only one suture is fused
- leads to optic atrophy

Intracranial pressure in single suture synostosis

Cohen. *Cleft Palate Craniofac J* 1998

Single suture synostosis includes unilateral coronal synostosis, unilateral lambdoidal synostosis, metopic synostosis, sagittal synostosis

Elevated ICP diagnosed when pressure is >15–20 mmHg under unstressed conditions

Raised ICP commoner with **multiple** suture synostoses

The higher the ICP the lower the IQ

Clinical indications of raised ICP

- developmental delay
- headaches
- other neurological symptoms – fits, seizures
- bulging fontanelle
- papilloedema
- hydrocephalus on CT

In patients resigned to undergoing corrective surgery ICP monitoring is unnecessary

In patients showing clinical signs of raised ICP but unwilling to undergo surgery then ICP monitoring may be performed

In patients without signs and unwilling to undergo surgery → close F/U

Hydrocephalus

- commoner in syndromic craniosynostosis
- uncommon in non-syndromic craniosynostosis
- increased venous pressure in the sagittal sinus?

Mental retardation

- more common where ICP is raised (multiple suture synostosis)
- also more common with hydrocephalus (syndromic synostosis)
- effect of surgery on single suture synostosis and mental development remains controversial

Mental development/single suture synostoses

Kapp–Simon. *Cleft Palate Craniofac J* 1998

Children with unilateral coronal synostosis are more likely to suffer from learning disabilities than the general population

But early surgery did not seem to prevent learning disability in the long-term

Investigations

- **all craniofacial patients should be assessed, investigated, planned for and treated within a multidisciplinary team environment**
- plain skull X-ray, CT, MRI – CT may help differentiate between deformational plagiocephaly and lambdoid synostosis

Modern principles of treatment of craniofacial surgery

- access
- rigid fixation
- bone graft
- pericranial/galeal flaps

Timing of surgery

- ~3 months, or sooner if raised ICP supervenes
- skull bones are malleable and large bony defects can be reconstituted with new bone in children <2 years
- brain triples in size during the first year of life

- skull and brain growth are ~85% complete by 3 years of age
- brain continues to grow until 6–7 years of age, modelling overlying bone
- globe triples in size between birth–adolescence: 90% of adult volume by 7 years

Complications of surgery

- death due to:
  - uncontrolled intra-operative haemorrhage (disruption of dural sinuses)
  - air embolus
  - inadequate blood volume replacement
  - cerebral oedema
  - respiratory infection
  - meningitis – use of antibiotics which cross the BBB
  - respiratory obstruction
- other complications:
  - optic nerve injury if bicoronal flap is reflected over the eyes for too long
  - persistent CSF leak
  - seizures

Metopic synostosis

Metopic suture fuses ~2 years of age

Metopic synostosis → trigonocephaly

<10% of non-syndromic synostosis

~4% have raised ICP and mental retardation

Hypotelorism and anti-Mongoloid slant

Flattening of the frontal bones

Flaring of the parietal bones

Surgery aimed at correcting orbital rim hypoplasia

Most occur spontaneously, AD inheritance has been reported

Surgical treatment:

- frontoparietal advancement and remodelling with radial barrel stave osteotomies
- supra-orbital bar advancement
- hypotelorism is then self-correcting without the need for orbital translocation and interorbital bone grafts

Sagittal synostosis

Most common craniosynostosis

Skull is long and narrow, scaphocephaly

Frontal and occipital bossing

May affect anterior or posterior areas unequally

Usually sporadic

2% have a genetic inheritance

Males 4 × more common than females

Treatment:

- surgery aims to reduce AP length and increase skull width
- sagittal strip craniectomy
- frontal, parietal and orbital bone remodelling (barrel stave)

Unilateral coronal synostosis

Uncommon (1 in 10 000)

Plagiocephaly (Greek oblique skull) – torticollis occurs in two-thirds of children with deformational plagiocephaly

Retarded growth in an AP direction on the affected side – anterior cranial fossa becomes shorter

Ipsilateral frontal flattening

Contralateral parietal bossing

Compensatory growth:

- upwards → long forehead
- downwards → distortion of the sphenoid → loss of height of the lateral wall of the orbit → 'harlequin orbit' on X-ray (pathognomonic of coronal synostosis) and proptosis of the globe. Harlequin orbit – 'devil's eye' – slanted upwards with deficient lateral wall

Corneal exposure, ulceration and ultimately blindness

Surgery restores the supra-orbital rim by advancing this segment (bilateral fronto-orbital advancement) along with frontal remodelling as above

Surgery for unilateral coronal synostosis (plagiocephaly): unilateral or bilateral correction?

Sgouros. *J Craniofac Surg* 1996

Unilateral frontal craniotomy and supra-orbital bar advancement may give unsatisfactory results

Bilateral frontal craniotomy and supra-orbital bar was shown to give a superior appearance

Bilateral coronal synostosis

Growth retardation in an AP direction → brachycephaly – shortened skull

Turribrachycephaly – shortened and tower-shaped skull

Compensatory growth **upwards** and laterally – hence **turri**brachycephaly

Bilateral harlequin orbits may be present on X-ray

Frontal flattening and hypoplasia of the supra-orbital rims

Surgery:

- frontal advancement within the first year
  - 'floating' advancement of the frontal bone
  - releases the synostosed suture
  - advances the supra-orbital bar to protect the globe
- mid-face advancement by Le Fort III osteotomy ~9–12 years of age at which time mid-face growth is complete and the patient is less likely to require secondary surgery
  - originally performed by Gilles, later by Tessier
  - alternatively the whole frontal advancement and Le Fort III advancement can be done as a **monobloc** – Monasterio – but communications between nasal and cranial cavities leads to a high infection risk and need bone graft
- secondary Le Fort I osteotomy may later be required to correct occlusal problems and possibly also mandibular osteotomy ~18 years of age – but beware causing VPI (velopharyngeal incompetence) with significant advancement – **pertinent also to correcting malar hypoplasia associated with cleft palate**

Resorbable plates:
- vicryl or dexon
- can persist due to variable degradation rates
- also can be palpable and are mobile (but migration does not necessarily do harm)
- need to tap screw holes

Effect of supra-orbital bar advancement on the frontal sinus and frontal growth

Marchac. *PRS* 1995

Supra-orbital bar advancement may inhibit growth of the frontal sinus which then affects the projection of the glabellar region – a theoretical complication not borne out by this series

Lambdoid synostosis

Least common synostosis

Synostotic plagiocephaly

Occipital flattening on the affected side but no ipsilateral frontal bossing

Ear displaced inferiorly and **posteriorly**

Foramen magnum deviated towards the fused suture on X-ray

Severe progressive deformity

Surgery usually advocated – occipital remodelling

Deformational plagiocephaly (plagiocephaly without synostosis – PWS)

Up to 1 in 300 births including very minor plagiocephaly

Parallelogram head – occipital flattening with ipsilateral frontal bossing; contralateral frontal flattening and occipital bossing

No radiographic synostosis and foramen magnum in the midline

5% have mental retardation

Self-correcting in most cases

Occipital flattening more common on the right side due to decubitis position of the foetus

Also due to moulding in the birth canal – resolves within 6 weeks

Ear is positioned **anteriorly** on the side of occipital flattening

Related to restricted movement *in utero*

Must be distinguished from plagiocephaly due to unilateral coronal or lambdoidal synostosis – 3D-CT reconstruction helpful

Treat by repositioning lie of baby at sleep

Dynamic orthotic cranioplasty – acrylic mould allowing a space into which the head can grow

Occipital plagiocephaly

David. *Br J Plast Surg* 2000

Initial cranial asymmetry excerbated by infant's preference for lying on the flattened side

Occipital plagiocephaly may be due to lamboidal synostosis or may be non-synostotic (PWS)
- PWS (majority of cases) can be managed by conservative means
  - Head positioning
  - Physiotherapy in patients with torticollis
- True lamboidal synostosis (or PWS failing to respond to conservative treatment) requires operative intervention to release (resection of) the fused suture

- True lamboidal synostosis is rare – most resected sutures show sclerosis rather than true fusion histologically
- Morphological differences can be used to differentiate between unilateral lamboidal synostosis and PWS
  - Synostosis associated with
    - ipsilateral inferior posterior skull tilt
    - ipsilateral occipitomastoid skull bossing
    - contralateral parietal bossinganetroinferior ear displacement
  - Plain films (or CT if unclear) also used to help identify true synostosis

Crouzon's syndrome

Crouzon 1912

1 in 25 000 live births

AD inheritance

Mid-face hypoplasia:

- Class III malocclusion
- high arched palate
- shallow orbits – ocular proptosis
- conductive hearing impairment

Multiple synostoses including:

- turribrachycephaly
- scaphocephaly
- trigonocephaly
- clover-leaf skull

Raised ICP in two-thirds of patients

Others have about normal intelligence

Usually have no digital abnormalities

Development often normal

FGFR2 mutation

Apert's syndrome

Apert 1906

1 in 160 000 live births

Most cases are **sporadic** (but AD inheritance has been reported) – advanced paternal age a risk factor for the sporadic type

Symmetrical syndactyly of hands and feet

- type I – 'spade hand' – **mid-digital hand mass**
- type II – 'mitten hand' – thumb joined to mid-digital mass by a simple syndactyly
- type III – 'hoof hand' – complete osseous fusion between thumb–ring with simple syndactyly in the fourth web space
- atypical type of Apert's does not have a mid-digital hand mass

Perinychial abscesses during infancy

Most commonly turribrachycephaly due to bicoronal synostosis

May have *kleeblattschädel* (clover leaf skull) → poor prognosis with profound mental retardation

Raised ICP in ∼43% – but mental retardation common in even the absence of raised ICP due to primary brain abnormality

Mid-face hypoplasia

- orbital proptosis (exorbitism)
- class III malocclusion
- may have a cleft palate

Anti-Mongoloid slant and hypertelorism

Low set ears

Beaked nose

Vertebral fusions C5–6

Mild–severe mental retardation in ~50%

- hydrocephalus
- agenesis of the corpus callosum
- some have normal intelligence

Polycystic kidneys and cardiopulmonary abnormalities

FGFR2 mutation

Pfeiffer's syndrome

Pfeiffer 1964

AD and sporadic inheritance (defect on chromosome 8)

Raised ICP

Type I

- craniosynostosis especially turribrachycephaly
- **broad thumbs and great toes**
- **incomplete** syndactyly of second web space
- mid-face hypoplasia
- intelligence more likely to be normal

Type II

- as above but with ankylosis of elbows and *kleeblattschädel*
- mental retardation

Type III

- ankylosis of elbows but no *kleeblattschädel*
- mental retardation

FGFR1 and FGFR2 mutations

Saethre–Chotzen syndrome

Saethre in 1931, Chotzen in 1932

AD inheritance, incomplete penetrance – deletion or mutation of the TWIST gene

Mainly turribrachycephaly due to bicoronal synostosis

Low set hairline

Ptosis of the eyelids

Short stature

Facial asymmetry with deviation of the nasal septum

Incomplete syndactyly, mainly second web space

Mid-face hypoplasia as above including cleft palate

Mild mental retardation and schizophrenia have been reported

Carpenter's syndrome

Carpenter 1901

Short hands, symbrachydactyly and **polydactyly of the feet**

Acrocephalosyndactyly

Autosomal **recessive**

Sagittal synostosis → scaphocephaly, also lambdoid synostosis

Nearly all have mental retardation

Short stature and decreased hip mobility

Timing of treatment for craniosynostosis

Marchac. *BJPS* 1994

Brachycephaly → frontal advancement: 2–4 months

Other craniosynostoses → correction between 6 and 9 months

Between 2 and 5 years supra-orbital bar advancement is complicated by the development of the frontal sinus – in these patients the frontal sinus is cranialized and will usually redevelop

Frontofacial monobloc advancement only indicated for severe exorbitism in infancy

- infection risk due to dead space and intracranial communication with the nasal airway → loss of most of the forehead
- major surgery with risk of blood loss
- if performed <5 years of age can → recurrent deformity
- prefer a two-stage approach to craniosynostosis with mid-face hypoplasia (Apert's, Crouzon's):
  - frontal advancement first – then facial advancement 6–12 years (Le Fort III)
  - Le Fort I advancement may ultimately be required for final correction of bite at 12–18 years

Facial bipartition for the hypertelorism associated with Apert's accompanies facial advancement

Although ICP may not be raised in Apert's (wide open fontanelle) frontal advancement → better intellectual development in Marchac's series

Beware use of miniplates during infancy: bone resorption → intracranial migration – absorbable sutures may be used

Parents reluctant to accept craniofacial surgery → measure ICP: if borderline or raised → stronger argument for surgery

While cosmesis is important, mental development is paramount

Fronto-orbital re-operation

Wall. *BJPS* 1994

Significant increase in re-operation rates when fronto-orbital advancement is performed before, compared with after, 9 months

Suggests that unless there is raised ICP or severe exorbitism surgery should be delayed beyond 12 months

Self assessment: Outline the management of a baby with an abnormally shaped skull

History

- any family history of craniosynostoses?
- any problems during pregnancy, e.g. abnormal USS showing cardiac abnormalities, twin pregnancy (deformational), – or delivery (assisted)?
- drug history
- condition at birth (Apgar scores)
- positional preference during sleep?

- any known cardiac problems?
- developmental milestones?

Examination

- turribrachycephaly, scaphocephaly, trigonocephaly?
- malar hypoplasia:
  - anti-Mongoloid slant
  - hypertelorism
  - Class III malocclusion
  - anterior open bite
  - shallow orbits with proptosis
- parallelogram shaped?
- obvious hydrocephalus?
- any hand abnormalities?
- any lower limb abnormalities?
- developmental examination

Investigations

- skull X-ray – shape and thumb printing
- paediatric consult including echocardiogram
- anaesthetic consult
- ICP measurement if reluctant to undergo surgery?
- 3-D-CT reconstruction

Determine whether this is:

- true craniosynostosis
- deformational synostosis

Possible diagnoses

- turribrachycephaly plus:
  - no hand abnormality → Crouzon's
  - spade, mitten or hoof hand → Apert's
  - broad thumbs ± ankylosis of elbow → Pfeiffer's
  - low forehead, ptosis, short stature → Saethre–Chotzen
  - dry frizzy hair, grooved nails, bifid nasal tip → craniofrontonasal dysplasia
- scaphocephaly → Carpenter's

Treatment plan

- deformational → observe
- syndromal synostosis:
  - advise corrective surgery to avoid increased ICP and facilitate remodelling
  - timing of first surgery – Marchac's protocol (*BJPS* 1994):
    - <3 months for severely elevated ICP or exorbitism (often due to turribrachycephaly)
    - 6–9 months for other synostoses – but may → increased re-operation rates compared with surgery >9 months; Wall. *BJPS* 1994

Paediatric transcranial surgery

Kirkpatrick. *Br J Plast Surg* 2002

Craniofacial surgery:

A procedure combining neurosurgical and plastic surgical expertise to access the craniofacial area by craniotomy

Abnormality	Deformity	Operation no. 1	Other operations
Bicoronal synostosis Most syndromal synostoses including Crouzon's Apter's, Pfeiffer's	Turribrachycephaly	Floating fronto-parietal advancement and remodelling with supra-orbital bar advancement: if raised ICP/exorbitism perform early (3 months) Alternative monobloc advancement	• Palatal cleft surgery ~6 months • Surgery to hands <2 years • Le Fort III advancement aged 6–12 years • Le Fort I advancement 12–18 years
Unilateral coronal synostosis	Plagiocephaly	Bilateral supraorbital bar advancement with frontoparietal remodelling aged 6–9 months	
Sagittal synostosis Carpenter's syndrome	Scaphocephaly	Sagittal strip craniectomy and frontoparietal remodelling aged 6–9 months	
Unilateral lambdoidal synostosis	Plagiocephaly	Occipital remodelling aged 6–9 months	
Metopic synostosis	Trigonocephaly	Supra-orbital bar advancement and frontal remodelling aged 6–9 months	No need to correct hypotelorism

Potential major complications following transcranial surgery for complex syndromal synostoses include:

- Death
- Loss of vision
- Life-threatening blood loss intra-operatively or post-operative haematoma
- Cerebral oedema
- Cerebral abscess
- Meningitis
- Post-operative seizures
  - Previous transcranial surgery or head injury increases seizure risk
  - Consider prophylactic anticonvulsants in these patients
    - Routinely prescribed in some units for all patients

Review of 114 consecutive craniofacial procedures in 110 patients over 8 years:

- Major complications included:
  - Major intra-operative haemorrhage (two patients)
  - Post-operative infection (two patients)

- Tracheostomy thought to increase infection risk
- Minor complications included:
  - Isolated convulsion in one patient
  - Prolonged conjunctival chemosis and facial swelling (12 patients)
    - Triamcinolone now added to the bupivicaine/adrenaline and hyaluronidase solution for infiltration of the surgical field in the subgaleal plane

Craniofrontonasal dysplasia
Orr. *BJPS* 1997

Combination of coronal synostosis with frontonasal dysplasia
- mainly unilateral coronal synostosis
  - unilateral coronal synostosis → plagiocephaly
  - bilateral coronal synostosis → brachycephaly
- frontonasal dysplasia → hypertelorism, bifid nasal tip and a broad nasal bridge
- **also have dry frizzy hair and long grooved nails** – disordered deposition of large keratin filaments

Ten patients treated by the Oxford craniofacial unit, all females

Treatment of the synostosis was forehead advancement and remodelling – within the first year

Treatment of hypertelorism was by facial bipartition and excision of paramedian bone and ethmoid sinuses – between 4 and 9 years (cosmetic, so can wait)
- skin allowed to re-drape
- need for medial canthoplasty 12 months later to remove any residual excess skin/epicanthic folds (Mustardé canthoplasty – jumping man)
- in this age group children may understand the deformity and the need for surgery
- no subsequent impairment of mid-facial growth

Binder's syndrome

Maxillonasal dysostosis

Unknown aetiology

15% familial

Maxillonasal dysostosis → hypoplastic mid-face

Short, flat nose

Decreased vertical height of maxilla

Short columella

Convex upper lip

Wide, shallow philtrum

90° nasolabial groove

Vertebral abnormalities in 50%

Normal intelligence

Nasal augmentation and Le Fort II advancement osteotomy

Patau syndrome

Patau 1960

Trisomy 13

A single defect during the first 3 weeks of development of the prechordal mesoderm can lead to morphologic defects of the mid-face, eyes and forebrain

- microcephaly with sloping forehead
- wide sagittal sutures and fontanelles
- aplasia cutis congenita
- eyes – microphthalmia or anophthalmia
  - colobomata of iris (congenital fissure or gap)
  - retinal dysplasia
- mouth – cleft lip (60–80%) ± palate
- ears – abnormal helices ± low set ears
  - deafness (sensorineural, conductive)
  - recurrent otitis media
- hands
  - camptodactyly
  - polydactyly of hands ± feet
- CNS
  - holoprosencephaly (lack of septation of the forebrain – lack of a corpus callosum) with incomplete development of the forebrain and the olfactory and optic nerves – associated with facial cleft
  - severe mental retardation
- other features
  - coarctation, ASD, PDA, VSD, dextroposition
  - males: cryptorchidism, abnormal scrotum, ambiguous genitalia
  - females: bicornuate uterus
  - polycystic kidneys
- very poor prognosis with:
  - 45% dying by 1 month
  - 69% dying by 6 months
  - 72% dying by 12 months
- genetic counselling – recurrence rate depends on genotype

Beckwith–Wiedemann syndrome

Unknown aetiology
Gaping mouth, prognathism and macroglossia
Large body size and visceromegaly
Umbilical hernia or omphalocoele
Neonatal hypoglycaemia

Metopic synostosis
Large prominent eyes

Complications
Wilm's tumour (most common) or other malignancies, ~10%
Profound hypoglycaemia
Seizures, choking and aspiration pneumonia

Parry–Romberg disease (hemifacial atrophy)

Described by Parry, 1825, and Henoch and Romberg, 1846

Slowly progressive atrophy of the soft tissues of half the face

Onset <20 years of age

May be a form of localized scleroderma

Eventually burns itself out

Flap reconstruction includes omentum – popularized by Wallace, 1979

Facies

- slowly progressive hemifacial soft tissue atrophy
- localized facial bony depressions

Neuro

- contralateral Jacksonian epilepsy
- trigeminal neuralgia
- migraine-like headache

Skin

- hyperpigmentation
- vitiligo

Hair

- hair blanching
- alopecia

Mouth – hemi-atrophy of tongue and salivary gland

Teeth

- delayed dental eruption
- dental malocclusion

Eyes

- enophthalmos
- refractive error
- heterochromia iridis

Inheritance – ?autosomal dominant, variable penetrance

Free flap correction of hemifacial atrophy

Longaker. *PRS* 1995

Average duration of disease in this series was 6.7 years

Unilateral in 95%

Right = left

Female:male ratio 1.5:1

Affects skin and subcutaneous tissues early on, then later muscle and bone

Coup de sabre deformity – subcutaneous atrophy in a line from the chin to the malar area, eyebrow and forehead

Atrophic tissues show chronic inflammation and scarring

Treatment aims to restore facial contour

- in this series 13 parascapular free flaps and three superficial inferior epigastric flaps were used
- advantages of the parascapular flap:
  - long pedicle
  - large diameter pedicle

- good donor site scar
- fascial extension gained beyond de-epithelialized skin paddle while achieving primary closure – advancement of fascial extensions towards the midline 'feathers' the contour augmentation
- two-thirds of patients require revisional procedures, e.g. debulking/augmentation/recontouring – consider only after 6 months

Hemifacial microsomia

Number 7 cleft (see below)

Alternative name – craniofacial microsomia

Can be unilateral or bilateral

- bilateral in ~10%
- bilateral craniofacial microsomia must be distinguished from Treacher Collins (TC) syndrome:
  - in TC syndrome there is loss of the medial lower eyelashes
  - TC deformity is **symmetrical** but bilateral craniofacial microsomia is not
  - TC has a well-defined pattern of inheritance – AD – but bilateral craniofacial microsomia has no inheritance pattern

Affected structures are derived from the first and second arches and pharyngeal clefts

- first arch:
  - bones of the mid-face – maxilla, zygoma, palatine
  - mandible – especially the ascending ramus
  - contributions to inner ear bones
  - cleft abnormality – defects of external ear and tympanic membrane
  - trigeminal nerve – hypoplastic muscles of mastication
- second arch:
  - bones of the inner ear – malleus, incus, stapes
  - facial nerve

Also may lack pneumatization of the mastoid and vertebral defects

Commonly have pre-auricular skin tags or sinuses on the affected side

Parotid gland may be hypoplastic

Macrostomia

Frontal flattening

25% have a palatal cleft

Aetiology – theories

- 'mesodermal insufficiency'
- vascular insult to the arches (stapedial artery) – haemorrhage and haematoma

Spectrum of abnormality – includes simple isolated microtia

OMENS classification (Vento 1991)

- grading system of involved structures:
  - orbital dystopia (includes maxilla, zygomatic bone hypoplasia, etc.)
  - mandibular hypoplasia
  - ear defects
  - facial nerve deficits
  - soft tissue abnormalities

Surgical options during childhood
- excision of pre-auricular skin tags
- reconstruction of microtia
- commissuroplasty for macrostomia
- nerve grafting of palsied facial nerve
- fronto-orbital advancement for frontal flattening
- correction of orbital dystopia
- mandibular ramus distraction osteogenesis or reconstruction (if severely hypoplastic)
- Le Fort I maxillary advancement osteotomy used to restore bite
- Le Fort III osteotomy used to correct exorbitism
- complications:
  - airway compromise
  - haemorrhage
  - nerve injury
  - non/malunion
  - trauma to tooth roots
  - velopharyngeal incompetence
  - malocclusion
- becoming superseded by distraction osteogenesis techniques

Current concepts in the understanding and management of hemifacial microsomia

Cousley. *BJPS* 1997

Incidence ~1 in 5600 births

Facial asymmetry even in bilateral cases (hence distinguish from Treacher Collins syndrome)

Mandibular hypoplasia is the cornerstone – severity of this determines the severity of associated abnormalities

Time of mandibular distraction coincides with time of rapid maxillary growth ~6 years of age

Sural nerve grafting most successful during the first year

Skeletal surgery should be allowed to settle before soft tissue reconstruction is contemplated

Treacher Collins syndrome (mandibulofacial dysostosis)

Described by Treacher Collins, 1900

AD inheritance

Gene on chromosome 5

- also on chromosome 5 – **cri du chat**:
  - hypertelorism
  - prominent ears
  - small stature
  - mental retardation

Males = females

1 in 25 000–50 000

Bird-like facies

- anti-Mongoloid slant

- wide hypertelorism
- absent lower lid lashes medially
- low set/hypoplastic ears
- micrognathia → anterior open bite
- cleft palate
- mid-face hypoplasia
- broad nasal dorsum
- choanal atresia or stenosis

Airway concern in neonates due to combination of micrognathia and choanal atresia

>95% have moderate conductive hearing loss due to stenosis of external auditory canal or ankylosis of inner ear ossicles

Deformities are non-progressive with age – do not worsen

Consortium of facial clefts 6, 7, 8

- contributions from numbers 6 and 8 clefts
  - lower lid colobomas (notches), hypertelorism and anti-Mongoloid slant
  - hypoplasia of lateral orbital wall
- contributions from number 7 cleft
  - macrostomia
  - external and internal ear defects

Surgical options

- mandibular reconstruction/distraction osteogenesis/sliding genioplasty
- Le Fort I maxillary advancement (mid-face hypoplasia) to restore bite to the advanced mandible
- zygomatic reconstruction with onlay split calvarial bone grafts
- rhinoplasty – dorsal hump reduction
- ear reconstruction and bone-anchored hearing device
- correction of colobomas (Tessier technique, Kuhnt–Symanowski blepharoplasty)

> **Self-assessment: You are faced with a patient with craniofacial asymmetry – differential diagnoses are?**

Congenital:
- hemifacial microsomia (unilateral or bilateral – still asymmetrical)
- unilateral coronal synostosis

Acquired:
- hemifacial atrophy
- lipodystrophy
- differential growth due to radiotherapy/surgery for childhood malignancy

What is the difference between bilateral hemifacial microsomia and Treacher Collins syndrome?

What is the management of TCS?

Hemifacial microsomia is the result of a Tessier number 7 facial cleft whereas TCS is a consortium of abnormalities associated with numbers 6, 7 and 8

Hemifacial microsomia plus features of a number 8 cleft (peribulbar dermoids, etc.) = Goldenhar syndrome

90% of hemifacial microsomia affects one side of the face only – in the 10% with bilateral involvement the face is still asymmetrical whereas TCS is always symmetrical

TCS has a genetic basis on chromosome 5 with AD inheritance whereas hemifacial microsomia has no inheritance pattern – sporadic (stapedial A thrombosis?)

Features of TCS:

- bird-like facies
- downward slant of supra-orbital ridge and anti-Mongoloid slant to eyes
- hypertelorism
- orbital walls hypoplastic inferolaterally
- absence of lower medial eyelashes
- colobomas of lower lid
- broad nasal bridge
- beaked nose
- macrostomia
- malar (zygomatic) hypoplasia
- maxillary hypoplasia
- mandibular hypoplasia
- palatal cleft
- external ear defects including microtia and skin tags
- sensorineural hearing impairment

Treatment plan for TCS

- Should be conducted within a multidisciplinary team environment, e.g. speech therapist and audiologist – external bone conduction hearing device with a head band – orthodontist
- Variability of expression demands that treatment be tailored to the individual patient
- Coloboma correction by Tessier Z-plasty or K–Z-plasty – only performed once zygomas reconstructed
- Tessier treatment timing:

0 months	Airway: may need a tracheostomy
6 months	Palate: cleft palate repair
5–6 years	Split calvarial onlay grafts to inferolateral orbit and zygomas – may need repeated grafts due to resorption
6 years	Soft tissue correction: 1, correction of colobomas; 2, ear reconstruction; 3, commissuroplasty for macrostomia (reposition muscle); 4, sideburns set back
6–12 years	Orthodontics and jaw surgery: cephalometric assessment and planning, Le Fort III maxillary advancement and mandibular ramus sagittal split osteotomy and advancement or distraction
12–18 years	Le Fort I advancement to finalize bite, sliding genioplasty
18 years	Rhinoplasty to broad nasal bridge

Similar treatment plan for hemifacial microsomia

- O – fronto-orbital advancement for frontal flattening; cleft palate correction; Le Fort III and I
- M – mandibular advancement or distraction – may need to be asymmetric
- E – hearing device; excision of accessory auricles; microtia reconstruction
- N – facial nerve and muscles of facial expression show variable degrees of agenesis – hence, need to import muscle and nerve → two-stage facial reanimation
- S – commissuroplasty

Craniofacial clefts
Tessier. *J Maxillofac Surg* 1976

Numbered 0–14

Facial clefts extend to cranial clefts

- facial cleft number plus cranial cleft number = 14
- for example 0–14, 1–13, 2–12 3–11, etc.

Cleft 0
- **midline facial cleft**
- median cleft lip (**absent prolabium**), bifid nose, bifid tongue, maxillary midline cleft
- extends to cleft 14 – holoprosencephaly deformities (including cyclopia) and frontonasal encephalocoele may be present

Cleft 1
- soft tissue cleft from Cupid's bow through alar dome
- bony cleft passes between central and lateral incisors
- extends to cleft 13 – passes medial to the inner limit of the eyebrow, hypertelorism

Cleft 2
- rare
- soft tissue cleft from cupid's bow but lateral to alar dome
- maxillary alveolar cleft lateral to the lateral incisor
- no. 12 cleft passes through medial third of eyebrow

Cleft 3
- **oblique facial cleft**
- from cupid's bow to lacrimal punctum, medial canthal ligament agenesis
- bony cleft begins between lateral incisor and canine, passes along the nasomaxillary groove (nasolacrimal duct disruption) into the orbit. Absent medial wall of maxillary sinus → confluent cavity formed from the mouth, nose, maxillary sinus, and orbit
- involves the secondary hard palate – posterior to the incisive foramen
- surgery directed at cleft lip and palate repair, nasal correction, bony reconstruction of orbital floor and maxilla and transnasal medial canthopexy
- cleft 11 passes through the medial third of the upper lid and eyebrow, bony cleft lateral to the ethmoid, producing hypertelorism

Cleft 4
- similar to a number 3 cleft but begins just lateral to cupid's bow and passes more towards the eye
- bony cleft passes medial to the infra-orbital foramen
- may have **microphthalmos or anophthalmia**
- number 10 cleft continues through the middle third of the supra-orbital rim – fronto-orbital encephalocoele displaces the eye inferolaterally → hypertelorism

Cleft 5
- rare
- soft tissue cleft from around the lateral commissure to the middle third of the lower lid – **draws lip and lid together**
- bony cleft from the premolars passing lateral to the infra-orbital foramen to involve the orbit in its middle third – eye herniates into maxillary sinus

- cleft 9 is the rarest of all craniofacial clefts – passes from the supra-orbital rim into the forehead as the continuation of a number 5 cleft

Cleft 6

- bony cleft centred on the **zygomaticomaxillary** suture and lateral third of infra-orbital rim
- soft tissue abnormality includes lower lateral lid colobomas, hypertelorism and anti-Mongoloid slant
- cleft numbers 6, 7 and 8 → **Treacher Collins** syndrome
- cleft number 8 → disruption of the **lateral canthus** (incomplete closure) – component of **Goldenhar** syndrome

Cleft 7

- cleft number 7 → **hemifacial microsomia**
- may be bilateral
- centred on the line between the oral commissure and the ear
- affects structures around this line (see above):
  - soft tissue structures: macrostomia; ear defects; facial N; parotid
  - bony structures: ascending ramus of mandible; maxilla, etc.

Lateral clefts → more severe bony abnormalities

Medial clefts → more severe soft tissue abnormalities

Clefts do not pass through bony foraminae, the site of neurovascular structures

Bilateral clefts do not have to be equally severe

Facial clefts can be combined with craniosynostoses

Concept of 'time zones' – but facial clefts do not have to extend as cranial clefts

Fibrous dysplasia

Monostotic, polyostotic

Painless bony swellings in <30-year age group

Craniosclerosis → deafness

Albright's disease – FD plus patchy skin pigmentation and precocious puberty

0.5% osteosarcoma

Treat by curettage (20–30% recurrence) or excision and reconstruction

Other papers and considerations

Amniotic band syndrome – facial clefts and limb ring constrictions

Coady. *PRS* 1998

Facial clefts with limb ring constrictions are paramedian type (2–12, 3–11, 4–10)

May also have truncal defects

Theories:

- mechanical disruption due to amniotic bands
- disorders of fetal blood supply
- genetic programming error
- disorder of tissue morphogenesis

Maxillary distraction osteogenesis in Pfeiffer's syndrome

Britto. *BJPS* 1998

Coordinated augmentation of facial skeleton and soft tissues

Advanced at 1 mm/day, increased to 2 mm/day after the first week

Case report illustrating distraction following Le Fort III osteotomy as an adjunct to
supra-orbital bar advancement in the management of ocular proptosis

Also useful for mandibular distraction in TCS and Pierre Robin

Gradual advancement avoids creating a dead space with the resultant danger of infection

Le Fort III distraction using internal devices

Chin. *PRS* 1997

Gradual distraction in craniosynostotic patients (Crouzon's, Apert's, Pfeiffer's) between
4 and 13 years of age

'Substantial' advancement gap (~10 mm) created by Le Fort III osteotomy before distraction
tolerated well in **children** → no non-union and increased advancement compared with
bone–plate fixation alone – eliminates latency period

Nasal-frontal osteotomy was grafted with cancellous bone

Accelerated distraction rate was **guided by the resistance created in the soft tissues**

- torque wrench used to guide advancement
- conventionally only 1 mm of advancement per day is observed
- this technique increased advancement to ~2 mm/day for ~5 days
- device left in place for 6 months

Distraction devices custom made using computer-aided design based on cephalometric
assessment in each patient

Improvement in exorbitism, class III malocclusion and obstructive sleep apnoea
postoperatively

Discussion points

Goals of distraction osteogenesis:

- to establish a fibrovascular bridge which becomes ossified by tension forces into new bone
- to stretch out soft tissues
- to decrease the need for bone graft

Rate of distraction:

- too slow → premature fusion
- too fast → non-union

Infections in craniofacial surgery

Fearon. *PRS* 1997

2.5% infection rate in 567 intracranial procedures

No patients <13 months developed an infection – ?rapid brain growth obliterates dead space

Infection rates higher in secondary surgery:

- longer operating times
- scarring → decreased vascularity → increased infection
- older patients with more sinus development

Cephalosporin prophylaxis of meningitis may have contributed to incidence of *Candida* and
Pseudomonas infection

Shaving hair does not influence infection rates

Half of all infections related to fronto-facial monobloc surgery

Drainage and irrigation of soft tissues

Extensive bony debridement is unnecessary

Management of obstructive sleep apnoea in Down's syndrome

Lefaivre. *PRS* 1997

Presentation:

- daytime somnolence
- poor school performance
- developmental delay
- failure to thrive
- snoring
- enuresis

Aetiology in Down's syndrome:

- increased upper airway secretions and infections
- tonsillar and adenoid hyperplasia
- mandibular and maxillary hypoplasia
- macroglossia or disproportionately sized tongue (small oral cavity)
- hypotonia

Treatment:

- CPAP at night
- tonsillectomy and adenoidectomy
- uvulopalatopharyngoplasty
- septal surgery to correct deviation and inferior turbinectomy
- maxillary advancement (Le Fort I or III) or distraction – over-advancement can precipitate VPI
- Genioplasty
- Central tongue reduction

Vertical orbital dystopia

Tan. *PRS* 1996

Orbits lie on unequal horizontal planes

Associations

- **craniofaciocervical scoliosis complex**
  - hemifacial microsomia
  - torticollis
  - cervical abnormalities
- Goldenhar syndrome
- unilateral coronal synostosis
- asymmetric bilateral coronal synostosis
- craniofacial clefts
- trauma
- fibrous dysplasia

Eye on the affected side may be blind or amblyopic

Requires orbital translocation – translocation of the orbit containing the only seeing eye is contraindicated

Degree of movement planned according to where the medial and lateral canthi needed to end up

Bicoronal approach

Osteotomies around the orbit to allow rotation in the coronal plane to bring the lateral orbital wall up or down as required

- easier to elevate the lower orbit
- lowering an orbit requires subjacent wedge resection

Medial canthal ligament and lacrimal apparatus left attached – if this proved impossible, then transnasal canthopexy was indicated

If the frontal sinus was inadvertently opened it was cranialized and the frontonasal duct plugged with diploic bone

Pre-operative diplopia improved

In patients with normal vision pre-operatively, transient diplopia may occur postoperation

Scaphocephaly secondary to ventricular shunting

Shuster. *PRS* 1995

Premature fusion of the sagittal suture may be precipitated by the insertion of a VP shunt (secondary synostosis)

- acutely reduces intracranial volume
- overriding of sutures
- ?synostosis may be related to the primary pathology which caused the hydrocephalus

Affects mainly children <6 months of age

Excision of the fused suture (sagittal strip craniectomy) and occipital remodelling ± frontal remodelling

Management of orbitofacial dermoids in children

Bartlett. *PRS* 1993

Most are subcutaneous, a minority have deeper extension

84 patients retrospectively reviewed

Three anatomical locations:

- frontotemporal – outer eyebrow area – 65%
  - slow growing
  - soft
  - non-fixed
  - asymptomatic
  - subperiosteal excision, splitting orbicularis oculi
  - need no work-up
- orbital – 25%
  - females twice as common as males
  - may adhere to frontozygomatic or medial sutures
  - easily dissected free
  - no transosseous extensions – rarely need work-up
- nasoglabellar – 10%
  - mass ± punctum (fine hair growth or sebaceous debris from punctum)
  - may have splitting of the nasal bones
  - midline glabellar lesions had no deep extensions

- dorsal nasal lesions have associated occult nasoethmoid and cranial base abnormalities on the CT
- these need radiological work-up and may need bicoronal approach

Classification of dermoid cysts:

- congenital
  - teratoma type
  - inclusion type (at sites of embryonic fusion plates)
- acquired – implantation type (insect bite, minor trauma, etc.)

Facial clefts and encephaloceles

Hunt and Hobar. *Plast Reconstr Surg* 2003

Embryology

- Majority of craniofacial anomalies arise during the first 12 weeks of embryological development
- By the end of week 8 the face is recognizably human
- Derived from 5 facial prominences – the frontonasal process and maxillary and mandibular processes
- Fusion of facial prominences occurs around day 46–47
  - Failure of fusion leads to facial clefting
  - Mesodermal penetration theory postulates that clefting occurs due to failure of migration of mesoderm into a bilaminar ectodermal membrane resulting in loss of support to the overlying epithelial seam

Potential factors contributing to craniofacial anomalies

- Genetic (e.g. FGF receptor mutations)
- Radiation (associated with microcephaly)
- Maternal infection during pregnancy (toxoplasmosis, rubella, CMV) or other health problems (PKU, diabetes, vitamin deficiency, smoking)

Facial clefts

- Commonest facial cleft is cleft lip/palate followed by isolated cleft palate
  - Other facial clefts are rare (up to 5 cases per 100 000 live births)
- Tissue deficiency: failure of cleavage of prosencephalon leading to failure of longitudinal separation of cerebral hemispheres
  - Arhinencephaly
  - Holoprosencephaly
    - A hypoplastic Tessier 14 cleft
    - Usually associated with severe malformations of the brain incompatible with life
- Tissue excess: failure of complete tissue development
  - Most severe form represented by extreme hypertelorism
  - Tessier classification (anatomical)
  - Van der Meulen classification (embryological)
- Aims and principles of reconstruction
  - Functional and aesthetic correction of
    - Macrostomia
    - Eyelids (to prevent corneal exposure)
    - Separation of confluent oral, nasal and orbital cavities
  - Achieved by
    - Excision of cleft scar tissue

- Layered soft tissue closure
- Delayed skeletal reconstruction

Encephaloceles

- Worldwide incidence 1 in 5000 births
  - Anterior encephaloceles more common in Russia and south east Asia
  - Back-of-the-head encephaloceles predominate in Western Europe, North America, Australia and Japan
- Herniation of cranial contents through a defect in the skull
  - Meninges (meningocele)
  - Meninges and brain (meningoencephalocele)
  - Meninges, brain and ventricle (meningoencephalocystocele)
- Anatomical classificaton
  - Basal
  - Sincipital
    - Frontoethmoidal
      - Arise due to failure of regression of a dural diverticulum projecting through developing nasal and frontal bones
      - Nasofrontal
      - Nasoethmoidal
      - Naso-orbital
    - Interfrontal
    - Associated with clefts
  - Convexity
- Principles of management
  - Urgent closure of open skin defects
  - Incision of sac
  - Amputation of excess tissue beyond the limits of the skull
  - Dural closure
  - Soft tissue and bone reconstruction

Prenatal sonographic diagnosis of major craniofacial anomalies

Wong, Mulliken, Benacerraff. *Plast Reconstr Surg* 2001

Craniosynostosis

- Ultrasound imaging of cranial sutures possible from week 13
- Head measurements indicate pattern of suture fusion (e.g. scaphocephaly vs. brachycephaly)
- Measurement of interorbital distance to diagnose hypertelorism
- Imaging of hydrocephalus, encephalocoele and spinal defects
- Timing of synostotic suture fusion variable from late trimester to the early post-natal period
- Detection of single or multiple suture fusions possible from week 16 hence an early normal scan may does not exclude later synostosis
- Ultrasound findings should be comined with available genetic/molecular information
- Syndromic synostoses identifiable from associated limb abnormalities
  - Transvaginal ultrasound useful for demonstrating hand abnormalities

Pharyngeal and oromandibular abnormalities

- Imaging of the fetal maxillofacial skeleton possible from week 10
- Craniofacial abnormalities associated with hemifacial microsomia diagnosed from week 29

- Extracranial skeletal abnormalities (hemivertebrae, rib abnormalities, etc.)
- Cardiac, renal and pulmonary abnormalities
- Tracheo-oesophageal fistula diagnosed by absence of fluid in the stomach and polyhydramnios
- Treacher Collins syndrome
  - Diagnosis possible from 15 weeks
  - Canted palpebrae
  - Microtia and microphthalmia
  - Hypertelorism
  - Micrognathia
    - Also consider Robin sequence and Stickler syndrome
  - Symmetrical growth restriction
  - Nager syndrome: Treacher Collins phenotype with preaxial limb abnormalities
    - Proximal radioulnar synostosis
    - Thumb hypoplasia or aplasia

Final points

Thumb printing and copper beating of the skull on X-ray is indicative of raised ICP

Virchow's law relates to growth retardation in the direction perpendicular to the fused suture

Oxycephaly = pointed skull, forehead paralleling the plane of the nasal dorsum, due to multiple suture synostoses

Crouzon's syndrome patients usually have normal mental development (<5% retarded), Apert's rarely

Hypotelorism is associated with metopic synostosis, Down's and Binder's syndromes – most other CF syndromes → hypertelorism

Syndromal synostosis accounts for ~20% of all synostoses – sporadic synostoses tend to be single suture type

Commonest CF cleft is a number 7 at 1 in 3000

First facial bone to form embryologically is the sphenoid

Environmental factors thought to contribute to facial clefts include influenza A2 virus and toxoplasmosis infection, also drugs such as anticonvulsants, steroids and tranquillizers

In complete TCS the zygomas are absent

Principles in the reconstruction of CF clefts:

- remove abnormal bone elements and reconstruct defect with neighbouring bone or bone grafts
- reinsert muscles of facial expression to reanimate the face and stimulate growth
- provide skin cover with local skin flaps

Number 30 cleft: midline cleft involving the mandible, the hyoid bone and sternum

Hemifacial microsomia – risk of an affected parent having an affected child = 3%

9 Cosmetic surgery (lasers, facelift, chemical peel, dermabrasion, liposuction, abdominoplasty, rhinoplasty, botulinum toxin)

Laser surgery
Chemical peel and dermabrasion
Facelift
Blepharoplasty
Rhinoplasty
Liposuction
Abdominoplasty

Aesthetic breast surgery (see Chapter 7)

Laser surgery

Grabb and Smith, *Lasers in Plastic Surgery*; Achauer. *PRS* 1997

1916 – Einsteins's theory of stimulated emission of radiation

1950s – Schawlow and Townes: microwave amplification by stimulation emission of radiation (MASER)

1957 – Maiman: light amplification by stimulated emission of radiation (LASER) using a synthetic ruby crystal

Helium neon laser, Nd:YAG, CO_2 and argon lasers all developed in the early 1960s

Components of a laser:

- energy source
  - electricity (argon laser)
  - flashlamp (pulsed dye laser)
  - another laser (CO_2 laser)
- laser medium – solid or gas
- laser cavity (resonator)

Laser medium is energized to excite electrons into a higher energy state (unstable orbit around the nucleus, 'singlet state')

As electrons move back into a stable orbit (via a 'metastable state') a photon of light is emitted, i.e. **spontaneous emission**

Generation of photons then perpetuates the movement of electrons of other atoms back into a stable orbit → more photons, i.e. **stimulated emission**

Photons move randomly in the resonator but emerge through a pair of mirrors (one partially reflective) to become a parallel or collimated laser beam with all the same wavelength

Longer wavelength → better penetration

Energy (J) ∝ number of photons

Power = energy s^{-1}, i.e. rate of delivery of energy (W)

- $1\,W = 1\,J\,s^{-1}$
- rate of **input** of energy to create the laser beam

Irradiance = power per unit area (W/cm^2)

Fluence = energy cm^{-2} (J cm^{-2})

Gaussian distribution of heat within the spot – 10% overlap is not harmful

Absorption coefficient of tissues also determines penetration

Continuous wave lasers may be broken intermittently by a mechanical shutter to form a pulsed wave (pulsed-dye laser)

Flashlamp also → pulsed wave – high energy and high peak temperature

When the laser beam contacts the target:

- reflected
- transmitted – passes through unchanged
- refracted – passes through with a directional change
- scattered – by dermis (collagen)
- absorbed – maximal clinical effect
  - in tissues the laser is absorbed by 'chromophores' such as haemoglobin, melanin, tattoo pigments and water
  - different chromophores maximally absorb light at different wavelengths
  - destruction due to the absorption of energy as heat

The shorter the wavelength → increased scatter and reflectance

Depth of penetration proportional to:

- degree of scatter
- absorption by chromophores
- energy delivered
- wavelength of the laser beam

Selective photothermolysis – Anderson and Parrish 1983

- targeting tissues with:
  - a **wavelength** of laser light specific to chromophores of that tissue
  - a **pulse width** to maximize destruction of chromophores without collateral damage:
    - **pulse width < thermal relaxation time (T_r) → limited thermal diffusion minimizing unwanted collateral damage**
    - vessel diameter determines thermal relaxation time
  - a **fluence** above threshold for destruction of that chromophore
- for example:
  - argon laser → haemoglobin (coagulation)
  - if used vs. vascular malformations → depigmentation because melanin also absorbs this wavelength
  - pulse width (exposure time) – matched to the thermal relaxation time of the target tissue – T_r = time to cool to 50% of initial temperature achieved
  - pulsed delivery of laser light → higher energy

- Q-switching: electromagnetic switch → ultrashort pulse duration (ns range)

Goggles for each wavelength of laser available for safety – not interchangeable between lasers

Chromophore absorption peaks and T_r:

- melanin (500–600 nm) – 1μs
- haemoglobin (577–585 nm)

The darker a patient's skin colour, the more likely that there will be pigmentation changes after laser treatment

Laser plume can contain viable bacteria and viruses including HPV, HIV HBV – need suction and masks

Indications for different lasers in clinical situations overlap

Greatest heat concentration is below the skin surface

First pass causes coagulation and changes the optical properties of the tissue

Hence, second pass achieves only 50% coagulation compared with first

Individual lasers

UV	Visible spectrum		Infrared
(400 nm)	500 nm	600 nm	(>700 nm)
X-rays	Argon 488 (blue–green)		Television, radio and microwaves
γ-rays	Pulsed-dye 510 (green)		
	Nd:YAG 532 (green–yellow)		
	Pulsed-dye 585 (yellow)		
		Ruby 694 (red)	
			Alexandrite 755 (red)
			Nd:YAG 1064
			Erbium:YAG 2940
			CO_2 10 600

Argon laser

457–514 nm blue–green light

Continuous wave and mechanical shutter

Chromophores are haemoglobin and melanin

Shallow penetration depth ~1 mm

- increased energy required
- increased risk of scarring

Effective against PWS

Pulsed-dye laser

Fluorescent dye absorbed in water or alcohol

Flashlamp → dye → emission of light

Tuned between 400 and 1000 nm depending upon the dye used

Pulse duration very short

Penetration 1.2 mm at 585 nm

Good for vascular malformations with a high concentration of oxyhaemoglobin

Transient purple discoloration when used in the treatment of PWS

Nd: YAG laser

Laser media are the YAG crystals in which neodymium is an impurity

Poorly absorbed by haemoglobin, melanin, water → greater penetration

YAG crystals can also be grown in erbium

Haemangiomas and vascular malformations at 532 nm

1064 nm (double wavelength) laser more useful for pigmented lesions

Ruby laser

Flash lamp stimulation

Tattoos, hair removal

CO_2 laser

Continuous wave or pulsed by mechanical shutters

Gas mixture includes helium and nitrogen – helium → targeting beam as for laser pointers

Spot focused at 0.1–2.0 mm – measuring arm ensures that the hand set is at the appropriate distance from the patient as variation changes the focal length and affects fluence levels

Used as a surgical scalpel in neurosurgery and ENT surgery

Vascular lesions

Pulsed-dye laser (yellow light, 585 nm) for vascular malformations including PWS and haemangioma (strawberry naevus)

Local or topical anaesthesia in adults

Argon laser (blue–green light, 488 nm) good for PWS

Small vessels 30–40 µm – PWS – argon, pulsed-dye laser

Medium sized 100–400 µm – haemangioma – KTP or $CuBr_2$ (1–50 ms)

Large vessels >400 µm – venous malform – Nd:YAG (>100ms)

Try a test patch with different lasers and different fluences before attempting definitive treatment

Pulsed dye laser treatment of childhood haemangiomas

Batta. *Lancet* 2002

- Haemangiomas most common soft tissue tumours of infancy (<30% present at birth, 90% appear within first 4 weeks of life)
- Pulsed dye laser penetrates skin to approximately 1.2 mm
- 121 infants (<14 weeks) randomized to pulsed dye laser treatment (topical local anaesthesia) or observation only
- superficial early haemangiomas in the preproliferative or early proliferative growth phase
- 93% of treated lesions <1 mm in height, 46% face/scalp
- large, deep or complicated (obstructing vital structures) lesions excluded
- follow-up at 1 year showed no difference between observational and laser treated groups in terms of clearance of haemangioma
- skin atrophy and hypopigmentation rates higher in the treatment group

Tattoos

May undergo colour shifts following laser treatment (Peach. *BJPS* 1999)

Need different lasers for different pigments

- blue/green – Q-switched ruby laser (red light, 694 nm)
- red/orange – pulsed-dye (510 and 585 nm)
  - conversion of ferric oxide (Fe_2O_3) to ferrous oxide (FeO) in red pigments may $\rightarrow$ darkening of the tattoo
  - try a test area first
  - mainly a problem using Q-switched lasers
- black – Nd:YAG (1064 nm)

Initial tattoo $\rightarrow$ inflammatory response $\rightarrow$ fibrosis

Laser $\rightarrow$ fragmentation of tattoo pigment $\rightarrow$ facilitates phagocytosis

Hypopigmentation 10%

Red and black easiest to remove, green and purple more difficult

Amateur tattoos are generally easier to remove – less ink and more black pigment

Hair removal

Ruby laser

Success of 50% reduction at best

Dark hair more easy to remove than light hair

Individual follicles targeted therefore must not shave for 6 weeks pretreatment

Scars

Pulsed-dye laser for hypertrophic scars $\rightarrow$ flattening and less red

See Chapter 2

Pulsed-dye laser treatment of hypertrophic burn scars

Alster. *PRS* 1998

40 hypertrophic scars

- half due to thermal injury
- half following CO_2 laser resurfacing

Symptomatic relief after only one treatment

Decreased redness, softer and more pliable after 2.5 treatments

Pigmented lesions (blue–black)

Naevus of Ota, naevus of Ito, blue naevus

Q-switched ruby laser or Q-switched Nd:YAG

Treatment of benign naevi $\rightarrow$ two-thirds respond

Dysplastic naevi should not be treated by laser

Congenital naevi may be treated by laser but the malignant potential still exists

Predicting outcome in the laser treatment of pigmented lesions

Grover. *BJPS*, 1998

Some lesions are known to respond well to laser, e.g. café au lait

Response of others is first observed in a test patch

This study used 2 mm punch biopsy and immunohistochemistry to predict outcome following laser treatment

Unfavourable indicators were depth of melanocytes >0.3 mm and significant amelanocytosis (>20%) – amelanotic melanocytes are refractory to treatment but following treatment may form melanin and be a cause of hyperpigmentation

Treatment of congenital naevus with a carbon dioxide laser

Kay. *BJPS* 1998

Pulsed CO_2 laser used to treat a giant congenital hairy naevus which was unsuccessfully treated by curettage

Relies upon vaporization of superficial cells rather than selective photothermolysis directed at melanin

- the larger the naevus the more likely that deeper structures will be involved
- incidence of naevi >10 cm diameter ~1 in 20 000
- lifetime malignant potential ~4%
- complete eradication of risk may require disfiguring surgery
- no reports of melanoma at sites of successfully curetted naevi
  - but curettage is not always successful
  - may be difficult in the perineum, etc.
  - leads to blood loss
  - leads to scarring

44 days old at time of treatment

Immediate reduction in superficial pigmentation with four–six passes with the pattern generator head

Residual pigmentation treated by a single pass using a 3 mm collimated hand piece

Postoperative colloid resuscitation – plasma loss observed during treatment

Near-full healing by 2 weeks

Conclusion:
- good alternative to curettage
- area treated may be limited by plasma loss
- close F/U mandatory

Combined use of normal and q switched ruby laser in the management of congenital melanocytic naevi

Kono. *Br j plast surg* 2001

Two case reports illustrating a normal mode ruby laser follwed by a Q-switched ruby laser to produce lightening of pigmented lesions

NMRL used first to remove the epidermis and facilitate greater penetration of the QSRL

Short pulse duration of the QSRL prevents thermal injury to neighbouring dermis

High energery of the QSRL effectively destroys naevus nests

Leukoplakia, warts

No pigmentation, superficial cutaneous or mucosal lesions → CO_2 laser (10 600 nm)

Laser resurfacing

Fitzpatrick skin types

Skin type	Skin colour	UV sensitivity	Sunburn history
I	White	Very	Always burns, never tans
II	White	Very	Always burns, sometimes tans
III	White	Sensitive	Burns sometimes, tans gradually
IV	Light brown	Moderately	Burns minimally, tans well
V	Brown	Minimally	Never burns, tans to dark brown
VI	Black	Insensitive	Never burns, deeply tans

General points

Facial resurfacing – CO_2 laser as an alternative to dermabrasion or chemical peel (35% trichloroacetic acid or 50% Baker–Gordon phenol)

Laser resurfacing more controlled and predictable than chemical peels

Deep phenol peels remove deep wrinkles but result in permanent lightening of the skin

CO_2 laser $\rightarrow$ absorbed by water $\rightarrow$ superficial layers of skin (vaporization)

Typical energy $= 300$–500 mJ

Phenomenon of collagen shrinkage (by 10–30%) at 55–60°C

Magnitude of shrinkage decreases with successive passes

May also get remodelling and laying down of new shorter collagen over several months post-treatment

Patient should be encouraged strongly to give up smoking

Indications – removes fine wrinkles but not suited to loose facial skin and deep nasolabial folds

Skin preconditioning

Vitamin A (below) with glycolic acid preconditioning regimens are often used before laser resurfacing or chemical peel

These agents increase the metabolism of the skin, accelerate cellular division, boost collagen synthesis and reduce the thickness of the stratum corneum

In doing so subsequent therapy is more effective

Retinoic acid

Tretinoin 0.05% (**Retinova**) – photodamaged skin and mottled pigmentation

Tretinoin 0.025% (**Retin-A**) – used for acne treatment

Isotretinoin capsules 5 mg (**Roaccutane**) – used for acne treatment, isomer of tretinoin

- pretreatment with retinoids:
  - may help to reduce post-treatment hyperpigmentation
  - but may contribute to postoperative erythema
  - has a rejuvenating effect partially due to generating dermal oedema
  - overall not proven as a worthwhile pretreatment

- is also contraindicated during early pregnancy → teratogen
- Retinova is an excellent treatment for solar-induced lentigines on the dorsum of the hands
- **isotretinoin** → delayed healing and atypical scarring
  - if used it should probably be stopped 6 months before laser therapy
  - inhibits re-epithelialization from adnexal structures

Complications

Pigment changes – hypo- (3%) or hyperpigmentation (7%)

- hyperpigmentation especially in darker skinned individuals (Fitzpatrick types 4–6) although initially hypopigmented
- hyperpigmentation in dark-skinned patients avoided by pretreatment bleaching with **hydroquinone**
- hydroquinone may also be used post-operatively for the treatment of hyperpigmentation

Prolonged erythema >10 weeks (6%) – warn patients of erythema postoperation which gets redder when the patient blushes

Hypertrophic scarring (1%)

Infection (bacterial 7%, viral 2% overall)

Ectropion

Under-correction of rhytids

Acne and milia

- greater production of sebum
- avoid use of paraffin jelly
- retinoic acid, glycolic acid and hydroquinone at night → comedolysis – hydroquinone is toxic to melanocytes and inhibits tyrosinase
- may need oral tetracycline

Postoperative regimens

Two passes at 500 mJ → healing at 7–10 days

Antibiotics postoperatively

Sunscreens postoperatively

Topical steroids (1% hydrocortisone twice daily for 6 weeks) → decreased erythema

Acyclovir treatment for all patients pre- and post-operatively: laser resurfacing provokes herpes infection in individuals with or without a history of herpes in the past (12 and 6%, respectively, despite prophylaxis)

Open vs closed

- postoperative petroleum jelly or semipermeable dressings, e.g. omniderm
- dressing → decreased pain and faster re-epithelialization
- closed technique now unpopular as → infection
- open technique allows patient to shower/wash 3–4 × daily for 4 days then apply moisturizer (but dressing for first 24 h)

Nasal Bactroban (mupirocin) topically reduces infection rates

Hydrocortisone used mainly in USA and hydroquinone not licensed for use in UK

Post-resurfacing care

Weinstein. *PRS* 1997

Fair skin (I–III)	Dark skin (IV–VI)
Acyclovir 24 h pre-operation	Acyclovir 24 h pre-operation
Wash face twice a day	Plus:
Acyclovir until re-epithelialized (HSV)	hydroquinone 2.5% twice daily
Broad-spectrum antibiotics (bacterial infection)	retinoic acid 0.05% twice daily
Hydrocortisone 1% twice daily (erythema)	
Oil-free moisturiser (avoid milia)	
Sunscreen (hyperpigmentation)	
Glycolic acid 15% twice daily (hyperpigmentation)	

Facial rejuvenation with the carbon dioxide laser

Grover. *BJPS* 1998

Light energy $\rightarrow$ heat $\rightarrow$ vaporization of water in epidermal cells

Short pulse duration <1 ms $\rightarrow$ minimizes conduction of heat to neighbouring dermis cells $\rightarrow$ minimizes dermal scarring

Silicone cast made pre-operatively to measure depth of wrinkles (rhytids) by electron or light microscopy

Laser treatment:

- Silktouch CO_2 laser
- 200 μm spot scanned >3 mm diameter area for 0.2 s
- power 7–14 W
- yellow discoloration indicated penetration into the reticular dermis
- oral amoxycillin and chloromycetin ointment 48 h postoperatively, then aloe vera until skin had re-epithelialized
- patients told to avoid sunlight for 3 months and to apply sun block daily

Compared with postoperative mould $>91\%$ reduction in wrinkle depth at 6 weeks

Erythema lasted for ~2 months

Histological changes in the skin following CO_2 laser resurfacing

Stuzin. *PRS* 1997; Collawn. *PRS* 1998

Untreated skin:

- actinic damage
- epidermal atrophy
- increased number and size of melanocytes in the basal layer of the epidermis – uneven distribution of melanin
- dermal elastosis – thickened, curled elastin fibres

After one pass:

- epidermis totally removed
- little compaction of collagen
- elastin degradation in papillary and reticular dermis
- fibroblast necrosis in papillary and reticular dermis

After second and third passes:

- sequential and graded compaction of collagen
  - collagen loses its striations
  - widening of fibrils
- loss of extracellular GAG matrix
- visible skin tightening

7–10 days – re-epithelialization completed from adnexal structures

3 months post-treatment:

- epidermal atypia corrected, polarity restored
- melanocyte numbers back to normal – even distribution of melanin
- neocollagen formation
- elimination of elastoses
- decreased GAG ground substance

6 months post-treatment:

- resolution of inflammatory changes
- hypertrophic fibroblasts

Similar histological changes in pigmented and Caucasian skin

Cutaneous resurfacing with CO_2 and erbium: YAG lasers

Alster. *PRS* 1998

Pulsed and scanning CO_2 lasers introduced in the 1990s with a shorter pulse duration than traditional continuous wave lasers

- 10 600 nm wavelength is in the infrared spectrum
- wavelength strongly absorbed by water (most abundant chromophore in the skin)
- vaporizes the entire epidermis with the first pass – remove whitish eschar with a damp swab or will act as a heat sink causing further thermal damage
- dermal collagen shrinkage begins with subsequent passes
  - eyelid skin – two passes only
  - rest of face – three–four passes

Pulsed erbium:YAG laser introduced in 1996

- also in the infrared spectrum – wavelength 2940 nm
- closer to the peak absorption for water hence absorbed 12–18 × more efficiently than CO_2
- penetration depth 2–5 μm (compared with 20–30 μm for CO_2) – hence more precise with less collateral tissue damage
- hence faster recovery and fewer side-effects (erythema 2–4 weeks only)
- but less coagulative → more intra-operative bleeding and less collagen shrinkage – hence effects shorter-lasting
- indicated for milder forms of photodamage, rhytids and dyspigmentation

Contraindications to laser therapy

- absolute
  - **isotretinoin** use within the last 2 years (used in the treatment of acne)
  - infection (bacterial, HSV)
  - ectropion – lower lid laser
- relative
  - collagen, vascular or immune disorder
  - keloid tendency
  - perpetual UV light exposure

CO_2 resurfacing – long-term results

Schwartz. *PRS* 1999

Rhytids ablated at 3 and 6 months post-treatment

Some recurrence at 1 year – predominantly in dynamic areas

- peri-orbital – 56% improvement, cf. pre-operatively
- circumoral – 59%
- forehead – 61%
- cheeks – 77%

No data beyond 1 year

Simultaneous facelift and CO_2 resurfacing
Fulton, *PRS* 1998

Resurfacing techniques included CO_2 laser or superficial TCA peel (20–30%)

Then liposuction and SMAS facelift were performed

Ancillary procedures (brow lift, blepharoplasty, platysma band surgery, etc.) were also performed under the same anaesthetic

'Dramatic' rejuvenation

Convalescence and complications no greater than for facelift alone

Phenol peels do, however → thin skin flap so do not combine this with facelift or will risk flap necrosis

Preconditioning with glycolic acid and vitamin A is recommended

Tumescent low pressure liposuction before raising the skin flaps reduces bleeding and defines the appropriate plane more clearly

Combined erbium: yag laser resurfacing and face lifting

Weinstein. *PRS* 2000

- **Skin necrosis previously a concern in patients undergoing face lifting with CO_2 resurfacing**
- **Series of 257 patients undergoing combined treatment using the erbium:YAG laser (more efficiently absorbed by water so produces less thermal injury than CO_2)**
- **Range of face lift techniques used, most were subcutaneous lifts with SMAS repositioning (133)**
- **Laser fluence reduced over lateral cheek areas**
- **Complications were uncommon (skin slough two patients – both smokers, temporary ectropion in two patients, lower eyelid synechia in five patients)**
- **Good to excellent results in 98% of patients**

Chemical peel and dermabrasion

Including Rejuvenation of the skin surface: chemical peel and dermabrasion; Branham and Thomas. *Facial Plastic Surgery*, 1996.

Trichloroacetic acid peel

Depth of peel is proportional to the anatomical site which affects skin thickness and the concentration of the TCA

Concentrations ~10–25% → superficial peel (epidermis only)

Concentrations ~30–40% → medium depth peel (papillary dermis) but higher risk of scarring

Medium depth peel indicated for moderately photo-aged skin and field change early actinic damage

Better to repeat the treatment than overdo the concentration of TCA

No systemic toxicity reported using TCA

Pretreatment with Retin-A or glycolic acid is recommended to rejuvenate the skin and make the stratum corneum (horny dead layer) thinner

Remove oily secretions from the skin before applying the TCA with acetone (also helps to remove stratum corneum)

Stretch the skin to flatten wrinkles

Avoid contact with the eyes

Apply with cotton gauze in even strokes in cosmetic units and wait for frosting before removal with a dry gauze – and repeat

Must expect some darkening of the skin afterwards and peeling (as for sunburn)

Phenol peel

Baker–Gordon formula (first described in 1960s)

Used for field change actinic damage including actinic keratoses, superficial BCCs and solar lentigos

Also used for moderate rhytids and acne scarring

- acne scarring – ice pick scars best excised individually then proceed to CO_2 laser resurfacing – often need three-to-four treatments spaced 1 year apart
- risk of scarring following laser resurfacing <1%

Penetrates into reticular dermis – deep peel

Monitor for **cardiotoxicity** especially full-face peels – contraindicated in patients with a history of **cardiac disease**

80% is excreted unchanged in the kidney

- hence also contraindicated in **renal disease** because cardiotoxic levels may develop
- make sure that the patient is well hydrated before treatment

Ideally skin types I–III as will bleach darker skin

More painful than TCA therefore need anaesthesia/analgesia

Contact with the eyes → severe corneal burn

Apply slowly in cosmetic units after acetone degreasing – wait 15 min between cosmetic units to allow for renal excretion

Some advocate creating a mask with overlying tape (occlusive technique) left on for 24 h but increases depth of peel and removal of the mask is painful

Erythema may persist for some months

Glycolic acid peel

α-Hydroxy acids include:
- glycolic acid from sugar cane
- lactic acid from soured milk
- citric acid from citrus fruits

- tartaric acid from grapes
- malic acid from apples

Found in many cosmetics in low concentration

May be used as a primer for chemical peel or laser resurfacing (low concentration)

Achieves a chemical peel at concentrations of 30–70%

Rejuvenates the stratum corneum similar to vitamin A

Depth of penetration related to concentration and duration of treatment – usually a superficial peel

Initially get erythema, then areas of white eschar (epidermolysis) – do not wait for full frosting as for TCA peel – indicates dermal destruction

When the time is up, dilute with water or neutralize with $NaHCO_3$

Post-treatment management

Emollients help accelerate healing (up to 2 weeks)

Avoid sun exposure post-treatment

Consider topical antibiotics and acyclovir

Do not pull off crusts

When re-epithelialization is complete, α-hydroxy acids, retinoic acid and hydroquinone may be reinstated

Make-up can also be applied at this point

Complications

Hypopigmentation proportional to increasing depth of peel – invariable after phenol peel

Hyperpigmentation – inflammatory melanocyte response

Viral and bacterial infection

Scarring

TCA-based blue peel

Obagi. *Dermatol Surg* 1999

Variable results from chemical peel due to lack of control over depth of peel

Blue peel facilitates treatment of the papillary and immediate reticular dermis (junction of reticular and papillary dermis)

Shallow rhytids that disappear on light stretching respond to a 'skin tightening' (more superficial) peel whereas those that do not disappear require a 'skin levelling' (deeper) peel

The TCA Blue Peel:

- Formed by adding TCA at fixed concentration (15 or 20%) and volume with the Blue Peel Base
  - Contains glycerin, saponins and a non-ionic blue colour base
  - Forms a homogeneous TCA–oil–water solution for slow penetration and even coating
- Depth signs as an end-point of the peel easily recognizable
  - Depth dependent upon concentration and volume of TCA

- One coat of a 15% Blue Peel solution (30% TCA diluted by an equal volume of blue peel base) exfoliates stratum corneum
  - Four coats reaches the papillary dermis
- Two coats of 20% Blue Peel solution reaches the papillary dermis
  - more discomfort compared with the 15% solution and may require sedation to administer
- No systemic side effects or toxicity
- Acts by protein denaturation and coagulation
- Even blue colour confirms eveness of application

Frosting:

- Occurs as a results of protein denaturation
- Pink frost develops as the papillary dermis is reached, becoming white as the peel acts at a deeper level, ie the immediate reticular dermis – maximum recommended depth of peel

Period of relative resistance

- Time taken for the Blue Peel solution to begin exerting its action due to initial acid neutralization by dermal protein (approximately 2 minutes)
  - Wait 2 minutes before repainting

Complications:

- Scarring and pigment changes possible with increasing depth of peel
- Erythema lasting 3–7 days
- Bacterial or viral infections

Post treatment re-epithelialisation complete by 7–10 days

2 or 3 Blue Peels, spaced at 6–8 weeks recommended for maximum effect

Dermabrasion

Using a diamond burr on a drill, scratch pad or sandpaper

Over-dermabrasion → hypertrophic scarring – do not extend through the reticular dermis

Worse scarring also in patients undergoing surgery for acne scarring who have taken Roaccutane (isotretinoin) within 2 months

Adjunctive treatment of rhinophyma

Prophylactic acyclovir

Effect of chemical peels and dermabrasion on dermal elastic tissue

Giese. *PRS* 1997

Effect of chemical peel and dermabrasion on collagen (homogenization) and melanin granules (depletion) is well defined, but the effect on elastin is not

Elastin production does not decrease significantly until after age 70 years

Elastosis – altered elastin – occurs in photodamaged skin

Single application of 25–50% TCA peel and dermabrasion in pigs → no change in dermal elastin at 6 months

Single application of Baker's phenol peel → decreased amount of elastin and morphological change (thinner, immature elastin → stiffer, weaker skin)

In the discussion: the effect on the elastin may just be due to a deeper peel rather than a specific reaction to individual chemicals

Facelift

Addresses the gravitational effects on the face – not a treatment for fine wrinkling

Deep wrinkles may be improved but not eliminated

Redistribution not removal of fat (e.g. removal of the buccal fat pad makes the patient look older)

'Sets the clock back but does not stop it ticking'

Histological changes with age

Changes in the collagen make-up of the dermis (loss of type III collagen)

Loss of elastin/elastosis – elastin production ceases > 70 years

Reduction in GAG matrix

Flattening of the dermo-epidermal junction

Depletion of Langerhans cells and melanocytes

Clinical changes with age

Skin thinner and more fragile

Less elastic

Immunologic changes due to reduced numbers of Langerhans cells

Onset of skin cancers

Brow and eyelid ptosis

Wrinkles (crow's foot, circumoral)

Jowls

Submental skin excess

Epidermal dysplasia and dermal elastosis.

Patients to avoid:

- collagen/connective tissue diseases
- hypertension
- drugs – aspirin, steroids, warfarin
- **smokers**
- facial features:
  - thick, glabrous skin with deep creases
  - poor skin quality/keratoses
- unrealistic expectations
- **previous facial surgery**
- pigmented skin

Subperiosteal facelift:

- addresses only the upper two-thirds of the face
- can correct deep nasolabial folds
- more suited to the young patient who accepts or desires a change in eye appearance to an 'almond' eye shape

Examination

Skin thickness, elasticity and skin laxity

Look for asymmetry

Check facial nerve and sensation

Forehead

- look at level of hairline and quality of hair
- ptosis
- wrinkles
- glabellar lines
  - contraction of corrugator supercilii and procerus muscles
  - supratrochlear N lies on the superficial surface of corrugator while the supra-orbital N lies deep

Mid-face

- jowls
- circumoral wrinkles
- ptosis of the malar fat pad

Jaw

- submental fat deposits
- platysma divarication

Pre-operative photographs essential

Anatomy

Five layers to the face (condensed over the zygomatic arch)

- skin
- subcutaneous fat
- SMAS
  - dissect in a plane deep to SMAS until zygomaticus major
  - at this point the facial nerve branches turn superficially to innervate these muscles
  - SMAS layer in the face continuous with the temporoparietal fascia in the temple
- facial nerve
  - innervates muscles of facial expression on their deep surface
  - main exception to this is buccinator – lies **deep** to the buccal branch
  - 70% of subjects have communicating branches between buccal and zygomatic branches
  - marginal mandibular nerve may lie above the inferior border of the mandible at its posterior extent
  - temporal branch runs beneath a line drawn from the tragus to a point 1.5 cm above the lateral margin of the eyebrow
  - lies beneath the temporoparietal (superficial temporal) fascia
- fascial layer (parotid fascia, cervical fascia)

Hence the fascial layers form a continuum:

- **Galea – temporoparietal fascia – SMAS**
- **Pericranium – deep temporal fascia – parotid fascia**

Forehead anatomy

Frontalis muscle → elevates eyebrows and causes transverse skin creases
Supplied by the temporal branch ('frontal' branch) of the facial nerve entering the muscle on its deep surface

- usually have two–five branches
- passes deep to SMAS over the zygomatic arch

Opposes action of corrugator supercilii, procerus and orbicularis

- corrugator arises from the supra-orbital rim and inserts into the medial eyebrow, pulling it downwards and inwards to create a scowling appearance and resulting in **vertical** creases
- procerus arises from the nasal bones and inserts into skin in the glabellar area to create **transverse** wrinkles across the bridge of the nose

Sensation to the forehead is by the supratrochlear and supra-orbital nerves (ophthalmic division of V)

- supratrochlear nerve is superficial to corrugator
- supra-orbital nerve is deep to corrugator

Brow height:

- males – level with the supra-orbital rim
- females – just above the supra-orbital rim

Technique

Local anaesthetic with adrenalin infiltrated for haemostasis (or adrenalin only if general anaesthesia without paralysis preferred)

Hypotensive anaesthesia not desired (may bleed post-operation)

Subcutaneous undermining:

- to within 1 cm of the lateral orbital rim
- across the malar area to the nasolabial folds
- to within 1 cm of the oral commissure
- inferiorly to the level of the thyroid cartilage

Superficial musculo-aponeurotic system (SMAS) lift:

- Skoog 1974
- 'L'-shaped incision, horizontally along the inferior border of the zygoma then vertically 0.5 cm anterior to the tragus
- use rolled SMAS for malar augmentation
- alternatively: SMAS plication or excision and closure

Key points for skin fixation:

- 1 cm above the ear
- at the apex of the postauricular incision

Excision and/or liposuction of 'witch's chin'

Midline platysma plication – in patients with an obtuse cervicomental angle platysma transection may be beneficial

Suction drains

Subperiosteal face lift
Heinrichs. *PRS* 1998

Review of 200 cases

Rejuvenates the face by lifting all of the facial soft tissue in relation to the bone

Subperiosteal brow lift first described by Tessier in 1979

Addresses the upper and middle thirds of the face

Gingivobuccal sulcus incision or subciliary incision for elevation of periosteum over the maxilla including peri-orbital areas and the anterior arch of the zygoma

Posterior arch was approached via a tunnel at the level of the tragus after elevating a small flap of SMAS – reduces risk of nerve injury

All patients underwent synchronous endoscopic brow lift and 13% also underwent upper lid blepharoplasty

Complications – 5%

- transient 'frontal' nerve weakness
- transient infra-orbital nerve numbness
- haematoma

Avoids extensive skin undermining

Superficial temporal fascia (temporoparietal fascia) is a continuation of the galea aponeurotica and extends below the zygomatic arch as SMAS

Frontal branches of the temporal nerve (VII) and the superficial temporal vessels cross the zygoma deep to this layer

Deep temporal fascia overlies temporalis and is continuous with the periosteum overlying the calvarium above

As the deep temporal fascia descends to the zygoma, it splits into two leaves, which pass superficial (innominate fascia) and deep (blends with the parotid fascia) to the zygoma

Elevation achieved by placing two fat stitches into fat below orbicularis oculi and anchoring these to deep temporal fascia overlying temporalis

Suitable for patients who have previously undergone facelift

Complications

Intra-operative – facial nerve injury

Early

- skin necrosis
  - 1–3%
  - 12 × higher risk in smokers
- sensory disturbance in facial skin for several months post-operation
  - injury to the greater auricular N → neuroma and earlobe dysaesthesia
  - nerve lies just posterior to the external jugular vein
- haematoma – commoner in males
- infection
- salivary fistula

Late

- alopecia 1–3%
- scarring
- pigmentation changes (hyperpigmentation)

Effect of steroids on swelling after facelift
Rapaport. *PRS* 1995; Owsley, *PRS* 1996

Both studies prospectively randomized double blind study assessing impact of steroids on facial swelling after SMAS facelift in a total of 80 patients

Neither study demonstrated any advantage related to steroid medication in terms of a reduction in immediate or early post-operative swelling

Parotid salivary fistula following rhytidectomy
McKinney. *PRS* 1996, Wolf, *PRS* 1996

Parotid duct at risk with extensive undermining of the SMAS layer
Parotid gland larger and fuller in younger patients
Subcutaneous salivary collections or pseudocysts
Management:

- aspirate and test fluid for amylase to confirm diagnosis and exclude haematoma – early aspiration helps prevent fistulation
- insertion of a suction drain
- antibiotics
- compressive dressing
- excision of a fistulous tract

Avoiding haematoma after rhytidectomy

Grover, Jones and Waterhouse. *Br J Plast Surg* 2001 and *Plast Reconstr Surg* 2004
Haematoma is the commonest complication of facelift surgery

- Minor haematomas are amenable to percutaneous aspiration while major haematomas require a return to the operating theatre for formal drainage
- Haematoma risk increased by:
  - Anterior platysmaplasty
  - High pre-operative systolic blood pressure > 150 mm Hg
  - Male sex
  - Non-steroidal medication
  - Smoking
- Late haematoma >5 days post-op due to bleeding from the superficial temporal vessels and associated with physical exertion

678 patients reviewed initially

- Incidence of major haematoma was 4.4% (30 patients)
- No significant difference was observed with or without:
  - Use of tumescent solution (229 patients)
    - 25 ml 0.25% bupivicaine with 1:200 000 adrenalin
    - 25 ml 1% lignocaine with 1:200 000 adrenalin
    - 0.5 ml 1:1000 adrenalin
    - 1.25 ml 40 mg/ml triamcinolone
    - 1 ml hyaluronidase
    - 500 ml Ringers lactate
    - 200 ml infiltrated to each side
      - patients who did not receive tumescent solution did have local anaesthetic with adrenalin infiltrated along incision lines
  - Use of fibrin glue sealant
  - Use of suction drains
    - Four concertina suction drains used

Subsequent 232 patients reviewed

- All patients received tumescent solution as above but without adrenalin
- Comparison made with previous 229 patients who received tumescent solution with adrenalin
  - Significant decrease in haematoma formation amongst patients who did **not** receive adrenalin
    - 11 major and 6 minor haematomas in the adrenalin group
    - 0 major and 1 minor haematoma in the non-adrenalin group

DVT and PE after facelift

Reinisch. *Plast Reconstr Surg* 2001

5% of operative deaths in hospital

> 1500 deaths per year in USA due to PE

- Mostly elderly, immobilized or trauma victims

Abdominoplasty probably most high-risk aesthetic procedure for thromboembolic complications (Grazer, *PRS* 1977)

- DVT 1.2%
- PE 0.8%

Survey of 273 plastic surgeons in US undertaking aesthetic facial surgery

- Total of 9937 facelifts during the 12-month study period
- Average number of facelifts per surgeon 36.5
- Mean patient age 54.8 years
- 89.8% women

Thromboembolic complications (DVT/PE) reported by 31 surgeons

- 35 patients developed a DVT (0.35%)
- 14 patients developed a PE (0.14%)
  - 1 patient died

Thromboembolic prophylaxis protocols:

- none (60.7% of surgeons)
- pressure stocking (19.6%)
  - slightly higher (but not significant) risk of DVT/PE
- intermittent compression devices (19.7%)
  - only intermittant compression devices significantly decreased risk of thomboembolic complications
  - prevent venous stasis
  - induce fibrinolytic activity in veins
  - stimulate release of anti-platelet aggregation factor from vascular endothelial cells
- general anaesthesia significantly increases risk compared with local anaesthesia
- operative time longer in patients developing DVT / PE (5.11 hours compared with 4.75 hours)

A plastic surgeon could expect a thromboembolic complication once in every 200 facelift cases

Brow lift

Normal eyebrow position:

- male – at the level of the supra-orbital rim
- female – just above the level of the supra-orbital rim

Normal eyebrow shape:

- medial limit forms a line joining the inner canthus with the lateral alar groove
- lateral limit forms a line joining the outer canthus with the lateral alar groove
- medial and lateral limits lie on the same horizontal plane
- highest part of the eyebrow lies directly above the outer limbus of the iris
  - more lateral – cross appearance
  - more medial – sad appearance

Indicated for brow ptosis and transverse furrows

Also as a prelude to upper lid blepharoplasty

Coronal incision or endoscopic approach

- if a coronal approach is taken make the incision 7–9 cm behind the anterior hairline – anterior hairline incision if the brow is high
- bevel the incision parallel to hair follicles
- facial palsied patients may benefit from melon-slice skin excision above the eyebrow (supraciliary lift)

Elevate flap in a subgaleal (or subperiosteal) plane

Identify supra-orbital nerves deep to corrugator

Tease fibres of corrugator to identify supratrochlear nerves then resect muscle to reduce vertical creases

Pull back the forehead flap and excise any excess before closure

Complications:

- haematoma
- alopecia
- frontalis paralysis – rare – recovery within 12 months
- injury to sensory nerves → forehead numbness – posterior to the skin incision numbness is to be expected

Endoscopic brow lift dissection is in the subperiosteal plane

Galea pulled up and anchored to the calvarium via a Mitec bone anchor or suture passed through drill holes

Endoscopic brow lift

Chiu, Baker. *Plast Reconstr Surg* 2003

Survey of practice of 21 New York plastic surgeons practising endoscopic brow lift

- joint experience of 628 patients undergoing endoscopic brow lift over a 5-year period
- 618 women, 10 men
- age range 33–87 years

Observed complications:

- alopecia
- hairline distortion
- asymmetry
- prolonged forehead paraesthesia
- frontal branch paralysis
- implant infection

Progressive decline in number of endoscopic procedures carried out compared with open brow lift during this period

- 25% still practise endoscopic brow lift regularly
- 50% occasionally

- 25% no longer practise the endoscopic technique

Decline possibly due to:

- selection criteria becoming more limited
  - medial and lateral brow ptosis (half of respondents)
  - glabella and forehead creases (one-third of respondents)
- increased use of Botox
- endoscopic brow lift ineffective in a majority of patients

Endoscopic brow lift and fixation techniques

Jones, Grover. *Plast Reconstr Surg* 2004

Review of 538 endoscopic brow lifts

- > 80% of patients had a simultaneous facelift

Operative technique based upon that described by Ramirez, 1995

- Lift vector marked preoperatively
- Two parasagittal and two temporal incisions made
- Hydrodissection of the plane beneath the temporoparietal fascia with tumescent solution
- Surgical dissection with endoscopic elevators to 2 cm of the supraorbital rim
- Subgaleal fascial flap raised from the temporal incisions
- Fascia at the temporal crease divided and dissection extended subperiosteally along the zygomatic process of the frontal bone
- At the supraorbital rim, supraorbital and supratrochlear nerves are indentified
- Corrugator supercilli and procerus muscles debulked
- Brow then elevated and secured

Fixation:

- First 189 patients: fibrin glue
- Remaining 349 patients: sutures passed through drill hole bone tunnels

Results:

- Patients who underwent fixation with sutures/drill holes maintained their change in pupil–brow height better compared with those who underwent glue fixation

Management of platysmal bands

Mckinney. *Plast Reconstr Surg* 1996 and 2002

Bands are approached via a submental incision

- this may increase the local wound complication rate
  - haematoma
  - infection
  - 'leather neck' appearance

Aufricht retractor during skin undermining to expose medial edges

Bands are due to lateral laxity in the muscle rather than prominent free medial edges

- Lack of midline stabilisation may result in excessive lateral shift of medal borders of muscle during SMAS lift
- Bands then shift from vertical to oblique
- Author prefers to undertake midline stabilisation prior to lateral SMAS lift
  - But care to avoid dehiscence of the midline sutures

Subplatysmal fat best treated by liposuction

- Care to avoid treated area from becoming displaced laterally by subsequent SMAS lift

Blepharoplasty

General

History:

- age
- smoking
- diabetes
- sicca syndrome
- glaucoma
- aspirin treatment or coagulopathy
- previous scars – quality?

Examination:

- compensated brow ptosis
- enophthalmos
- facial nerve function
- fat herniation – press on the globe

Counselling:

- pink scars
- time off work
- re-operation
- gritty/sticky eyes
- scleral show

Upper lid

Surgery almost invariably directed at dermatochalasis – redundancy of the skin of the lids and herniated orbital fat – blepharochalasis is a rare AD condition affecting young adults where there is atrophy of upper lid tissues following episodes of atopic eyelid oedema

Surgical planning

Examine for brow ptosis

- most patients have compensated brow ptosis – occurs when constant frontalis activity masks the ptosis
- following upper lid blepharoplasty and resolution of dermatochalasis, frontalis relaxes and the brow ptosis becomes apparent (medially → laterally)
- hence should consider the need for synchronous brow lift

Examine for upper lid ptosis and lagophthalmos

Examine for a Bell's phenomenon

Check vision in case of postoperative visual disturbance (need baseline)

Technique

Draw caudal incision line sparing the supratarsal fold with its connections to the levator mechanism

Pinch skin with Adson forceps to determine amount of skin to be removed at various points along the lid

Remove skin and underlying strip of orbicularis (up to 3 mm)

- do not remove too much skin – 30 mm must remain between the lashes and the lower margin of the eyebrow
- if too much skin is removed **and then** brow ptosis is corrected lagophthalmos will result
- conservative skin/muscle excisions are often best performed in combination with (following) a brow lift and corrugator excision
  - bicoronal lift
  - melon-slice lift above the eyebrows
  - endoscopic lift
- invaginating suture techniques reserved for very thin lids with little/no fat excess (e.g. Orientals)

Gentle pressure on the globe accentuates fat herniation from medial and lateral upper lid compartments through incisions in the orbital septum → removed with bipolar cautery

- keep resected fat to compare with the other side
- prolapse of fat far laterally is likely to be the lacrimal gland
- bipolar → avoidance of retrobulbar haematoma

Complications

Infection

Inadequate correction

Ptosis due to injury to levator

Most commonly damaged extra-ocular muscle is the inferior oblique → diplopia looking up and out

Contact lens wearers – warn may be difficult to resume postoperation

Retrobulbar haematoma and blindness

Lower lid

Tear trough deformity

Palpebral bags – fat herniation, less commonly muscle festoons – muscle festoons excised or imbricated or tightened laterally as a sling

Distinguish **palpebral** bags from **malar** bags – latter are rarely corrected by blepharoplasty – chronic regional oedema of unknown aetiology

Lower lid laxity – correction is lid elevation rather than skin excision

Scars heal best just below the lashes

Surgical planning

Examine for lower lid tone (should snap back after being pulled away from the globe)

If unduly lax may benefit from lateral canthoplasty – see Chapter 8 for lateral canthoplasty techniques – or lid shortening (wedge resection)

Nearly all patients have some lower lid laxity and benefit from synchronous canthoplasty

Beware excessive scleral show and perform a Schirmer's test

Palpate the infra-orbital rim to ensure that a prominent bony margin is not mistaken for fat herniation

Technique

Elevation of a skin–muscle flap with the skin incision extended laterally just below the lashes beyond the lateral canthus – initially skin only to leave a cuff of muscle (overlying the tarsus)

Excision of a triangular piece of skin/muscle – determined by draping the flap without tension over the lash line

Excision of fat from each of the three lower lid compartments as above

- avoid over-excision which gives a 'hollowed out' appearance to the eyes
- fat may be transplanted to fill out a tear trough deformity
- bony tear trough deformities corrected with an alloplastic implant

Fat may be removed via a **transconjunctival approach** if there is no need for skin excision

- avoids postoperative lower lid retraction
- more suited to patients with little or no excess skin – often the younger age group
- may be combined with laser resurfacing
- incision in the conjunctiva dissecting between this and the tarsal plate
  (skin + orbicularis = anterior lamella; conjunctiva + tarsal plate = posterior lamella; tarsal plates contribute to the orbital septum)
- hence retroseptal approach which preserves the orbital septum
- useful as a secondary procedure for patients with inadequately corrected palpebral bags

Complications

Excessive scleral show

Ectropion

- over-correction and lagophthalmos
- store the removed skin – you may need to put it back 1 week later!
- do not do a wedge resection even if there is a positive snap test: do not do a blepharoplasty at all or do it transconjunctivally

Blindness due to retrobulbar haematoma

- risk ∼1 in 40 000
- emergency treatment includes release of sutures, lateral canthotomy, mannitol

Aftercare:

- suture strips
- chloromycetin eye ointment or artificial tears

Management of post-blepharoplasty lid retraction
Patipa. *Plast Reconstr Surg* 2000

Lateral canthal anchoring
McCord. *Plast Reconstr Surg* 2003

Otoplasty

Otoplasty by open anterior scoring
Caoutte-Laberge. *Plast Reconstr Surg* 2000

Incidence up to 5% of the population

Transcartilaginous incision originally described by Lucket in 1910

Open anterior scoring to recreate an antehelical fold described by Chongchet in 1963 (*BJPS*)

Preoperative evaluation:

- Assess degree of unfolding of the antehelix
- Note Darwin's tubercle, posterior antehelical crura (Stahl's bar)
- Exclude a constricted (lop) ear deformity
- Depth of conchal fossa
- Prominence of lobe

500 patients underwent surgery during a 3-year period, post-operative evaluation at least 2 years from surgery

Age range 4–53 years (except for one patient aged 2.9 years)

95% bilateral

59% under local anaesthesia

Complications:

- Bleeding 2.6%
- Haematoma 0.4%
- Wound dehiscence 0.2%
- Infection nil
- Keloid scars 0.4%
- Inclusion cysts 0.6%
- Tender ears 5.7%
- Loss of ear sensation 3.9%
- Cosmetic outcome by patient questionnaire:
  - Asymmetry 18.4%
  - Residual deformity 4.4%
    - both commoner in younger age groups
    - Younger children (especially aged 4 years, $n = 108$) more likely to have general anaesthetic and hence dual operator technique
    - Local anaesthetic procedures undertaken by one surgeon only
    - Dual operator technique was significantly more likely to give rise to asymmetry in this series

Overall satisfaction (very satisfied or satisfied) 94.8%

Otoplasty by closed anterior scoring

Bulstrode. *Br J Plast Surg* 2003

Use of sutures to recreate the antehelical fold described by Mustardé in 1967 (*PRS*)

Percutaneous anterior scoring possible using a number of instruments including bent hypodermic needle, toothed forceps and endoscopic carpal tunnel instruments

- Mustardé technique used in combination with percutaneous anterior scoring using a hypodermic needle in 114 patients to achive prominent ear correction
- Mean follow up 3 years 11 months
  - Bilateral procedure in 100/114 patients
  - Age range 3–66 years
  - local anaesthetic in approximately 50%
- Complications:
  - Haematoma nil
  - Infection 3.5%
  - Hypertrophic scarring 1.8%
  - Residual deformity 5.3%

Rhinoplasty

History:

- previous trauma or surgery
- nosebleeds
- allergic rhinitis
- headaches
- olfactory disturbances

Examination:

- forehead
- nose
  - consider the dorsal hump, look at the width and the tip
  - examine for septal deviation, collapse of the internal valve and turbinate hypertrophy
    - columellar angle
      males – 90°
      females – 100°
- maxilla
  - short/long
  - prominence of the anterior nasal spine
  - maxilla loses height with age and tooth loss – cannot correct this
- mandible
  - check occlusion
  - look for micrognathia (makes nose look bigger – treatment by chin augmentation or genioplasty)
- skin quality – specifically telangiectasia (can get worse)

Complications of rhinoplasty include:

- numbness to the upper teeth
- under-correction (residual defomity)
- over-correcting (new deformity)
- palpable step at lateral maxillary osteotomy site
- persistent nasal tip oedema (up to 2 years) and numbness
- airway obstruction
- scars (inner canthi, columella)
- potential for secondary rhinoplasty at extra cost
- black eyes

Causes of secondary rhinoplasty:

- deviation
- valving
- residual deformity

Open rhinoplasty

- useful for tip work and the preferred routine approach for many surgeons
- cleft nose
- secondary rhinoplasty
- Bulbous tip – a wedge or dart excised from the remaining cartilage (and closed with catgut) will further narrow a bulbous tip

- bifid tip – medial crura are widely separated and in addition to tip reduction must be plicated in the midline
- hanging tip – result of a columella lacking adequate skeletal support (over resection of the caudal edge of the septum) – needs a 'T'-shaped cartilage graft from the septum

Internal nasal valve

Angle made by the caudal edge of the upper lateral cartilages with the septum – usually ~15°
Nose accounts for 50% of upper airway resistance
Lateral traction on the cheeks or sprung devices worn by athletes → opening of the internal nasal valve and reduced airway resistance
Spreader grafts during rhinoplasty have the same effect

Inferior turbinate

Undergoes a 3-hourly cycle of congestion and decongestion in 80% of the population
Decongestion may be induced by ephedrine spray (vasoconstriction)
Persistent congestion may warrant inferior turbinectomy

Basic open rhinoplasty

Exposure
- Local anaesthesia including nasal block and cocaine pack/spray
- Shave vibrissae
- Mark incision (step) across the columella
- Evert nostril with a double hook and make a curved rim incision in the nasal mucosa connecting the two sides with the columellar incision
- Lift up the columellar skin and nasal tip soft tissues off the cartilage framework
- Separate the lower lateral cartilages from each other and the septum
- Dissect the mucosa off the septum and create extramucosal tunnels beneath the upper lateral cartilages
- Divide, with scissors, the upper lateral cartilages from the septal cartilage
Identify and reduce the bony hump
- Trim the upper edges of upper lateral and septal cartilages
Use an osteotome to cleanly excise the bony hump – save in case of need for radix graft
Close the 'open roof'
- make a stab incison in the inner canthus
- use a periosteal elevator to dissect a subperiosteal tunnel down the side of the nasomaxillary angle for maxillary osteotomy
- introduce a 2 mm osteotomy and create a series of perforations along the osteotomy line
- in-fracture the nasal bones using digital pressure
- correct any irregularities after in-fracture by rasping
Return to the tip
- excise a portion of the cephallic edge of the lower lateral cartilages to refine the tip
- reduce the caudal edge of the septum as necessary
- approximate the lower lateral cartilages with 6/0 ethilon
Closure

- close mucos with 5/0 vicryl rapide
- close skin with 6/0 ethilon
- jelonet packs and dorsal Plaster of Paris

Postoperative care

- remove packs after 24–48 hours
- remove plaster and sutures after 1 week
- must not blow nose for 2 weeks
- need to keep quiet/relaxed, etc.

Alar base excision

Used in patients in whom the nostrils may appear flared
An oblique excision of the alar base helps to narrow the nostril aperture

Dressing

Suture strips applied to the skin
Remove one outer layer of a Telfa dressing and apply shiny side down before fitting a POP splint – the Telfa dressing makes removal of the POP easier
Jelonet gauze in a 'trouser' pattern, each limb inserted into a nostril

Septoplasty (SMR – submucous resection)

Vertical incision on the side of the deviation in front of the deformity
Subperichondrial dissection (Negus suction dissector) over the buckled cartilage
Incise through the septum to pick up the subperichondrial plane on the other side and develop this
Cartilage is excised with a Ballenger swivel knife
Mucosa closed

Secondary rhinoplasty

Saddle deformity

- excess removal of dorsal bone and cartilage
- need to restore contour with septal (or conchal) cartilage graft

Pinched tip deformity

- when the lateral crura have fractured resulting in loss of a dome-like projection
- need to restore the dome with an on-lay cartilage graft

Supra-tip deformity

- inadequate septal dorsal hump reduction $\rightarrow$ lower the septal hump
- inadequate correction of a bulbous tip $\rightarrow$ further tip work + fatty debulking
- over-reduction of the cartilaginous skeleton $\rightarrow$ dorsal onlay graft

Closed versus open rhinoplasty
Gunter and Sheen, PRS 1997

Greater exposure afforded by an open approach:

- makes diagnosis of deforming factors easier

- cartilaginous framework is repositioned and stabilized rather than resected
- grafts secured under direct vision including dorsal spreader grafts and onlay grafts to the dorsum and tip
- facilitates teaching
- secondary rhinoplasty easier

Disadvantage of the open approach is the transcolumellar scar and prolonged tip oedema

Airway obstruction and rhinoplasty
Constantian, *PRS* 1996

Four factors → airway obstruction:
- septal deviation (septoplasty)
- inferior turbinate hypertrophy (inferior turbinate resection/crush)
- internal valve problem (dorsal spreader graft)
- external valve problem (tip on-lay graft)

Narrowing the nose by dorsal resection, osteotomy and in-fracture may render the internal valve too narrow resulting in airway obstruction – treat by insertion of dorsal spreader grafts

Malposition or over-resection of the alar cartilages may similarly compromise the external valve mechanism – treat by insertion of tip grafts to stiffen the lower lateral cartilage

Nasal sensation after open rhinoplasty
Bafaqeeh. *BJPS* 1998

Nerve supply to the nasal skin from:
- infratrochlear nerve (V1, branch of nasociliary) – over nasal bones
- external nasal nerve (V1, terminal branch or anterior ethmoidal) – over upper lateral cartilages, tip and upper columella
- infra-orbital nerve (V2) – over lower lateral cartilages and columella

Following open rhinoplasty nasal sensation was tested at 3 weeks and 1 year

Altered sensation at the nasal tip and upper columella was recorded at 3 weeks, recovered by 1 year

External nasal nerve emerges between the nasal bones and the upper lateral cartilages and is at risk when elevating lateral nasal skin

Recovery may be by nerve regeneration or recruitment from adjacent areas

Rhinophyma: review and update

Rohrich. *Plast Reconstr Surg* 2001

Greek: *rhis* = nose; *phyma* = growth

A severe form of acne rosacea

Affects up to 10% of the population, male > female

May be related to androgens (higher 5α reductase activity in acne-prone skin)

Familial component in around half of patients

Celtic races

No aetiological link with alcohol but facial flushing following alcohol intake makes nose look more red (acne-prone skin may be more vaso-reactive to certain stimuli including alcohol and stress)

In its severest form:

- Skin is thickened (dermal hyperplasia), red-purple, pitted, fissured and scarred
- Sebaceous hyperplasia
- Pustules
- Underlying nasal skeleton unaffected
- Nasal tip affected more than rest of nose

Other areas may also be affected:

- Mentophyma
- Otophyma
- Zygophyma

Freeman classification (*PRS* 1970):

- Early vascular
- Moderate diffuse enlargement
- Localised 'tumour'
- Extensive diffuse enlargement
- Extensive diffuse enlargement plus localised tumour

Occult basal cell carcinoma reported in up to 10% of rhinophyma

Non-surgical treatment:

- Antibiotics
  - Metronidaole
  - Tetracycline
- Retinoids
  - Tretinoin
  - Isotretinoin (impairs re-epithelialization and concurrent surgery should be avoided)

Surgical treatment

- Excision of affected tissue ('sculpting') and healing by secondary intention
- Dermabrasion
- CO_2 and argon laser
- Combined techniques

Liposuction

Cellulite – fibrous septae in the superficial fat layer anchor the skin while fat hypertrophies and skin looses elasticity with age

Patients with skin laxity may not benefit from liposuction alone

Fat is sucked into the openings on the cannula tip then avulsed

Fibrous stroma surrounding NV bundles is relatively safe preserving blood supply and sensation to the overlying skin

Hence fascial network preserved while fat is removed

Conventional liposuction includes a blunt tip cannula attached to a vacuum pump

Ultrasonic-assisted liposuction

Pioneered by Zocchi 1980s

Ultrasound waves converted into mechanical vibration at titanium cannula tip

Vibrates at 20 000 cycles s^{-1}

Induces fragmentation and melting of fat

Liquid fat aspirated by vacuum pump

Leaves collagen network intact (less bleeding) and reduces energy expenditure

May also increase overall volume of fat removed

But may induce a burn at the deep surface of the overlying skin – must keep it moving but with slower strokes

Also needs a heat insulating sleeve at the entry site → larger incisions needed

Takes longer than conventional liposuction

Need to use conventional liposuction afterwards to remove any residual melted fat

Topographical markings outline areas of fat removal

Tumescent technique

Introduced by Klein 1986

Reduces pain and bleeding at the operative site

Blood loss 1–8% of aspirate volume compared with >40% without adrenalin

Adrenalin 1:1 million is effective

Marcain provides for long-lasting anaesthesia

Large doses of local anaesthetic but absorbed slowly and some is re-aspirated

- at least 70% of the total volume of tumescent fluid remains in the tissues and intravascular space at the end of the procedure

Also assists passage of the cannula

Fluid resuscitation (Pitman)

- tumescent solution volume > twice aspirate volume → no fluid resuscitation required
- tumescent solution volume < twice aspirate volume → give deficit
- beware infiltration of large volumes of tumescent solution in the elderly or patients with a propensity to CCF

Support garments to extremities for at least 2 weeks following procedure

Complications of liposuction

- infection
- bleeding
- residual contour irregularity requiring further liposuction
- injury to nerves, major blood vessels and overlying skin

Tumescent technique and absorption of lidocaine

Rubin. *PRS* 1999

In this study 7 mg/kg lidocaine was injected with or without 1:1 million adrenalin into healthy volunteers

Slower rise in serum lidocaine levels in adrenalin-treated solutions but peak concentration was the same with or without adrenalin

High- or low-pressure injection techniques did not influence absorption

During routine liposuction the safe dose of lignocaine injected is often exceeded

$4–5 \times (35\,\text{mg/kg})$

Lignocaine has a vasodilatory property which is surpassed by the vasoconstrictive effect of adrenalin

- dilution of both lignocaine and adrenalin in the tumescent solution → vasoconstriction – 1:1 million adrenalin has a biological effect whereas 0.1% lignocaine has little (i.e. 0.5% lignocaine in 1:200 000 adrenalin diluted fivefold)
- hence reduction in overall blood flow to the area inhibits absorption
- but dilution of adrenalin while maintaining lignocaine concentration constant → increased systemic absorption
- hence giving high total doses of lignocaine is safe because absorption is slow during which time tolerance develops

Fluid resuscitation following liposuction

Trott. *PRS* 1998

Resuscitation volumes should be assessed on an individual patient basis

Urine output is a useful given to volaemic status

2:1 ratio of infiltration:aspiration volumes suitable for small volume liposuction but for larger volume liposuction (e.g. 4 litres) a 1:4 ratio will prevent fluid overload and reduce lignocaine dose

Antibacterial effects of tumescent liposuction fluid

Craig. *PRS* 1999

Low incidence of infection post-liposuction (< 0.05%)

Lignocaine has bactericidal properties at concentrations of ∼1%

But no growth inhibiting activity at the dilutions used clinically

Other papers

Ultrasonic assisted liposuction – effect on peripheral nerves

Howard. *PRS* 1999

UAL selectively liquefies fat

Myelin sheaths have a high fat content and so potentially are at risk

However, no adverse sequelae demonstrated in a rat sciatic nerve model unless the probe made direct contact in which case reversible changes in ultrastructure and conductivity were seen

Liposuction and external ultrasound

Kinney. *PRS* 1999

External ultrasound used in the presence of tumescent fluid before liposuction

Heating and cavitation of fat

Constant motion of the ultrasound paddles and application of hydrogel required to prevent burn injury to the skin

Tissue temperatures during ultrasound-assisted lipoplasty

Ablaza. *PRS* 1998

Subcutaneous temperature probes were used to measure tissue temperatures during UAL

Infiltration of tumescent fluid at room temperature dropped tissue temperature to ∼24 °C but this rapidly recovered to ∼32 °C

Tumescent fluid at room temperature was thus felt to restrict elevation of peripheral tissue temperature during UAL but had no cooling effect on core temperature

During the procedure tissue temperatures remained stable except when treating the thighs when temperature rose to 41 °C but this did not result in a burn

Ultrasound-assisted lipoplasty: a clinical study of 250 consecutive patients

Maxwell. *PRS* 1998

Cavitation occurs 1–2 mm from the tip

Very little bruising

Effectively treats fibrous areas such as the male breast

Less physically demanding on the operator

Excellent results, few complications but

- must avoid aggressive superficial UAL (stay ~10 mm from the dermis)
- seromas more frequent with UAL

Series includes four UAL breast reductions

The effect of ultrasound assisted and conventional liposuction on the perforators of the abdominal wall

Blondeel. *Br J Plast Surg* 2003

Authors explored the theory that ultrasound assisted liposuction is less traumatic to perforating vessels perfusing an abdominal skin flap than conventional liposuction

Cadaveric study

- The territory of a lower abdominal skin flap marked out and each half subjected to the following procedures
  - Infiltration of tumescent solution plus UAL vs. control
  - Infiltration of tumescent solution plus UAL vs. infiltration
  - Infiltration of tumescent solution plus UAL vs. infiltration plus conventional liposuction
- After each experiment the abdominal flap was removed with the underlying rectus abdominis muscles and radio-opaque injection studies were undertaking by injection of the deep inferior epigastric arteries on each side
- A blinded panel of plastic surgeons was used to assess the severity vessel disruption

Human volunteer study:

- Infiltration of tumescent solution plus UAL vs. infiltration plus conventional liposuction prior to removing skin and fat as an abdominoplasty procedure

Results

- No significant difference was found in the degree of vessel disruption between UAL and conventional liposuction

Abdominoplasty

Fat anatomy:

- above Scarpa's fascia – compact, many fibrous septae
- below Scarpa's fascia – globular, fewer fibrous septae, determines secondary sexual characteristics

Examine the patient for skin excess and for musculo-aponeurotic laxity (divarication of the recti)

- above the arcuate line (half way between umbilicus and pubic symphysis) internal oblique aponeurosis splits to contribute to both anterior and posterior layers of the rectus sheath
- below the arcuate line contributes only to the anterior rectus sheath
- umbilicus lies in the midline half-way between the xiphisternum and the pubic symphysis, level with the anterior superior iliac spines

Mini abdominoplasty removes infra-umbilical skin excess without needing to reposition the umbilicus

Mostly abdominoplasty removes the entire abdominal skin excess to a point just above the umbilicus with undermining to the costal margin

Leaving flimsy fascia overlying the rectus sheath may help reduce seroma (fascia of Gallaudet)

Plication of the rectus sheath if there is any divarication – two continuous sutures – one above and one below the umbilicus to avoid umbilical strangulation

Urinary catheter and foot pumps/flowtron boots required

Technical tips

- subcutaneous infiltration of tumescent solution reduces blood loss
- lower incision within the pubic hair line 5–7 cm above the anterior vulval commisure
- bevel the upper skin flap edge
- partially anchor the umbilicus to the rectus sheath
- de-fatting in the midline below the umbilicus
- do not make over-tight – liberal use of micropore tape
- use fleur-de-lis technique for vertical skin excess

Complications

- early
  - umbilical necrosis
  - skin necrosis (especially in smokers)
  - wound dehiscence
  - wound infection
  - haematoma
  - seroma
  - death – PE
- late
  - scarring
  - altered sensation
  - revisional surgery to dog ears

Huger zones of blood supply to the anterior abdominal skin:

- Huger zone 1 – superior epigastric A
- Huger zone 2 – deep and superficial inferior epigastric A
- Huger zone 3 – intercostal arteries
- liposuction in zone 3 may theoretically interfere with perfusion to the upper skin flap

Matarasso classification:

Type	Features	Treatment
I	Excess fat only	Liposuction
II	Mild skin excess Infra-umbilical divarication	Mini abdominoplasty, infra-umbilical plication + liposuction
III	Moderate skin excess, divarication above and below umbilicus	Mini abdominoplasty, plication above and below umbilicus + liposuction
IV	Severe skin excess, rectus divarication	Standard abdominoplasty + sheath plication + liposuction

Majority of abdominoplasty procedures carried out are types IV

Pregnancy after abdominoplasty [letter]
Menz. *PRS* 1996

Pregnancy after abdominoplasty is possible but where midline rectus sheath plication has been performed the pregnancy should be closely monitored

Should diastasis recti be corrected?
Nahas. *Aesthetic Plast Surg* 1997

Position of recti assessed by CT 6 months post-operation
Muscles maintain corrected position

Fleur-de-lis abdominoplasty
Duff. *Br J Plast Surg* 2003
Fleur-de-lis component addresses excess tissue in the vertical plane
Suited to patients who have experienced significant weight loss
Retrospective review of 68 procedures
- 64 patients female
- mean BMI 29.3
- 40 patients had lost weight prior to surgery (mean loss 39 kg)

Emphasis on minimal undermining of skin flaps
Correction of rectus diastasis was undertaken as necessary but liposuction not performed in any patient
Mean operative time 2 hours 10 minutes
Mean length of stay 7.7 days
42/68 patients developed one or more complications postoperatively
- early wound dehiscence/infection in 9 patients
- delayed wound healing in 17 patients
- aesthetic complications in 12 patients
- no correlation between smoking and risk of a complication
- no correlation between BMI and wound breakdown in this series

> **Self-assessment: Discuss the management of a patient requesting a facelift**

History
- age, occupation
- what do you think is wrong?
- what do you want to achieve?
- what is your motivation?
- any previous facial surgery
- scar history
- drugs – aspirin, warfarin, steroids, roACcutaNE treatment for ACNE within the past year
- allergies – including retinoids
- medical problems – esp. connective tissue diseases, herpes simplex type I
- **smoker?**

Examination
- general examination for facial symmetry, scars, swellings, skin lesions, Fitzpatrick skin type, hair quality and distribution

- VII motor function
- V sensory function
- forehead: ptosis, frown lines and glabellar creases
- eyes – upper lid dermatochalasis, fat herniation, Bell's phenomenon, lagophthalmos, lower lid bags including muscle festoons, lower lid laxity (snap test) or ectropion, tear trough deformity, malar bags, eye movements and acuity, crow's feet
- cheeks – skin quality (glabrous?), nasolabial folds – depth, jowls, Marionette lines
- mouth – circumoral rhytids – depth, mandibular size and projection, dentate?
- chin – witch's chin, platysma divarication

Investigations

- routine pre-operative bloods, facial X-rays if suspecting significant maxillary collapse and mandibular resorption in an edentulous patient
- photographs

Discussion/counselling

- resurfacing options – chemical peel vs. laser – suited to patients with finer rhytids and solar damaged skin
- facelift ± ancillary procedures: brow lift with Botox injection to corrugator or corrugator excision, upper and lower lid blepharoplasty including canthoplasty, liposuction, correction of witch's chin, platysma band excision or plication

---

Self-assessment: Discuss how you would counsel a patient requesting rhinoplasty

History

- age, occupation
- what is wrong?
- what would you like done?
- why do you want to have it done?
- any trauma to the nose
- any surgery to the nose
- nosebleeds
- allergic rhinitis
- headaches
- olfactory disturbances
- drugs – aspirin, warfarin, steroids
- PMSH – diabetes, hypertension, etc.
- smoker?

Examination

- general shape and symmetry of the face
- scars/swellings on the face and nose
- vertical maxillary excess
- mandibular hypoplasia and malocclusion
- dorsum – deviation, width, hump
- upper laterals – deviation, hump, supra-tip deformity
- lower laterals/tip – width, size, hanging, pinched, valving (external valve) – one at a time
- columella – size, deviation, angle (men 90°, women 100°)
- internally – airway occlusion/septal deviation, valving (internal valve), prominence of the nasal spine

Investigations
- routine bloods
- nasal X-ray if there is a history of trauma
- photographs

Discussion/counselling
- surgery conducted under general anaesthesia
- sequelae:
  - painful nose
  - black eyes
  - POP for 1 week
  - nasal packs removed at 24 h
  - swollen initially but will settle
- complications:
  - intra-operative
    - cribriform plate fracture
    - excessive bleeding
  - early post-operative
    - infection
    - haematoma
    - nose bleeds (do not blow)
  - late postoperative
    - residual deformity – under-correction
    - new deformity – over-correction
    - scar at base of columella (open approach)
    - nasal tip swelling and numbness
    - palpable step at site of lateral maxillary osteotomy

Botulinum Toxin

Exotoxin of spore forming anaerobe *Clostridium botulinum*
Seven toxic serotypes have been isolated (A–G)
- similar structure to tetanus toxin
- 'A' most potent and commonly used sub-type

Mechanism of action:
- Binds presynaptic cholinergic receptors
- Becomes internalised within presynaptic neurone, entering lysosomes by endocytosis
- Undergoes cleavage to release a light chain component in to the presynaptic neurone cytoplasm
- Light chain catalyses proteolytic cleavage of membrane proteins responsible for exocytosis of acetylcholine
- Hence causes presynaptic inhibition of ACh release

Clinical effects:
- Dennervation of striated muscle (neurological disorders)
- Anhidrosis (useful for hyperhidrosis and Frey's syndrome)
- Onset of action 1–7 days
- Duration of action around 3 months
  - Action overcome by sprouting of motor axons and formation of new motor end plates

- Dose dependent activity
- Formation of neutralizing antibodies may gradually reduce efficacy

Manufactured as BoTox[®] (Allergan, 100 units per vial) or Dysport[®] (Ipsen, 500 units per vial)

- Manufactured in a small volume of human albumin solution
- Store as per manufacturers instructions and reconstitute with normal saline – keep refrigerated and use within around 4 hours of reconstitution
- Licensed for use in spasmodic torticolis, blepharospasm, and hemifacial spasm
- Avoid in pregnancy and patients with myaesthenia gravis, known allergy to human albumin solution or taking aminoglycoside antibiotics (potentiate clinical effect)
- Side effects:
    - pain, swelling, bruising and redness at injection sites
    - weakening of intrinsic muscles of the hand (palmar hyperhidrosis)
    - weakening of extraocular musculature (causing diplopia and ptosis)and dry eyes when treating periorbital rhytids
    - anaphylaxis not yet reported following cosmetic injection in humans (2 cases of severe reaction after injection for muscle spasticity)
    - maximum recommended dose in a 70 kg adult is 400u of BoTox
- Cosmetic doses around 25 μ Botox or 125 μ Dysport per patient

Areas commonly treated in cosmetic practice:

- glabellar lines
    - procerus and corrugator supercilii
- forehead creases
    - frontalis
- periorbital rhytids (crow's feet)
    - orbicularis oculi
- less commonly used to treat perioral rhytids and platysma bands

Technique

- avoid skin alcohol preparation (inactivates toxin)
- use small gauge needle
- inject in to muscle directly using anatomical knowledge of insertion points, demonstration by voluntary contraction and manual palpation
    - multiple injection points
- orientate injection away from the orbit to avoid inadvertant paralysis of extraocular muscles
- the greater the target muscle mass the higher the dose requirement

Further reading

Botulinum Toxin in Aesthetic Medicine. Sommer and Sattler (Eds). Blackwell Science 2001

Cosmetic Use of Botulinum Toxin. Rohrich. *Plast Reconstruc Surg* 2003

Miscellaneous (lower limb trauma, pressure sores, lymphoedema, VAC therapy, tissue expansion)

10

Lymphoedema
Tissue expansion
Lower limb trauma and reconstruction
Pressure sores
Necrotizing fasciitis
Vacuum-assisted closure

Lymphoedema

Accumulation of protein-rich interstitial fluid in subcutaneous tissues

Deep muscle compartments are uninvolved

Fascial involvement?

Thick brawny skin, fissuring and ulceration

- venous ulceration → thin skin and varicose eczema
- primary
  - lymphatic hypoplasia, lymphatic malformation, nodal fibrosis
  - at birth (Milroy's disease) or <14 years
    - genetically determined: sex linked
    - lymphatic aplasia
    - association with Turner's syndrome
  - adolescence – lymphoedema praecox (14–35 years) – 80% of all primary lymphoedema
  - later in life – lymphoedema tarda (>35 years)
- secondary
  - neoplastic – malignant nodes, extrinsic compression
  - infective – TB, *Wuchereria bancrofti*
  - iatrogenic – lymphadenectomy, radiotherapy

Women > men

Left leg > right leg

Lower limb > upper limb

Pathogenesis

Leakage of protein into the interstitium → raised tissue oncotic pressure → disruption of Starling's equilibrium

513

Increased interstitial protein and fluid → tissue hypoxia → cell death → chronic inflammatory response → fibrosis

Also acts as a medium for bacterial growth

Clinical features

Initially pitting then non-pitting oedema due to fibrosis

Skin ulceration

Pain

Lymphangiosarcoma may develop >10 years following the onset of lymphoedema and carries a poor prognosis – lymphangioma developing in a lymphoedematous arm following mastectomy = Stewart–Treves syndrome

Investigation of the patient with lymphoedema

Look for signs of venous hypertension and exclude DVT (Doppler/venogram)

Image the pelvic nodes for tumours (USS/CT/MRI) – CT shows a honeycomb appearance of subcutaneous tissues in contrast with normal subfascial tissues

Exclude hepatic, renal or cardiac causes

- serum albumin
- U and Es
- echocardiography

Lymphangiography

Differentiate from:

- lipoedema (lipodystrophy) – suitable for liposuction, often generally obese
- Klippel–Trenaunay syndrome – varicose veins, limb elongation, vascular malformations, limb oedema (some have lymphatic abnormalities)

Management of lymphoedema

Remove the precipitating cause if secondary

No form of treatment is curative

Surgery is rarely indicated (<10%)

Medical

- skin care – prevention of ulceration
- treatment of lymphangitis and cellulitis (common)
- dimethylcarbazine to kill *Wuchereria bancrofti*
- elevation
- foot pumps
- complex regional physiotherapy
- compression garments

Excisional surgery

- excision of all soft tissue down to fascia and SSG (Charles)
  - reserved for severe skin ulceration
  - poor aesthetic result
  - unstable grafts, keratotic overgrowths
- buried dermal flap (Thompson)
  - excision of subcutaneous tissue and burying of a dermal flap into the uninvolved muscle compartment

- creates a theoretical lymphatic communication allowing drainage of the skin via the deep compartment
- but few good results and rarely performed
- subcutaneous excision of lymphoedematous tissue preserving overlying skin flaps (Homans)
  - excess skin following reduction is excised
  - needs to be staged – medial side then lateral side
  - preserve vital structures – common peroneal nerve, sural nerve
  - good results and most commonly performed surgery

Physiological surgery

- microsurgical lymphovenous and lympholymphatic shunts
- pedicled omental or ileal flap
  - ileal segment on vascular pedicle
  - bivalved and mucosa stripped off to expose lymphatic-rich submucosa
  - contraindicated following radiotherapy due to possibility of established radiation-induced endarteritis of gut vessels

Use of a lymphatic bridge for head and neck lymphoedema

Withey. *Br J Plast Surg* 2001

Main cause is bilateral neck dissection and radiotherapy, particularly where lymphatic drainage is further compromised by repeated infections or tumour recurrence

- Late development of lymphoedema should raise the suspicion of recurrent tumour. Lymph from the facial and scalp skin drains first to the occiptal, auricular, parotid and facial nodes and then via valveless channels to the deeper cervical nodes
- Spiral muscle system maintains orthograde lymph flow. The deep cervical chain also drains lymph from the upper aerodigestive tract. The authors describe a case of severe head and neck lymphoedema ameliorated by the inset of a tubed deltopectoral flap to act as a lymphatic bridge. Similar pedicled flaps have been described in the management of lymphoedema at other sites including use of a pedicled groin flap to reduce contralateral lower limb oedema
- Tubed flaps should be designed to exploit the axial drainage pattern of the lymphatics

Tissue expansion

Neumann 1957 – expansion of postauricular skin for ear reconstruction
Radavan 1975 – silicone expander
Austed 1982 – histological evaluation
Aims:

- enables replacement of like with like – colour, texture, and hair-bearing quality
- uses local skin → good colour and texture match and is sensate
- donor site can be closed directly

Technique

Donor area must avoid scars
Multiple expanders reduce overall duration of expanders

Simple rotation or advancement flaps planned

Placement either through an incision which will be later excised or one remote from the scar/defect

Port can be internal or external

Initial expansion takes up dead space

Commence expansion after 1 week

Excision of the capsule makes the expanded flap thinner and more compliant

Histological changes

Epidermis

- thickens due to cellular hyperplasia
- loss of rete ridges
- increased mitoses in the basal layer

Dermis

- thins despite increased dermal collagen
- realignment of dermal collagen – fibrils straighten and become parallel
- rupture of elastin fibres
- appendages unaltered

Muscle

- sarcomeres thin and become compacted
- increased mitochondria

Adipose tissue

- adipose cells atrophy
- some permanent loss

Nerves – altered conductivity

Indications

Burn scar alopecia

- TE placed beneath the galea
- galeal scoring may aid expansion
- expansion over 6–8 weeks
- base rotation or advancement flaps on named artery – temporal, occipital
- care to orientate direction of hair growth
- can expand to double the size of the scalp without separating follicles unduly

Forehead expansion for nasal reconstruction

Burn scar excision of the face (including ear) and neck – TEs placed in the neck do not appear to cause vascular compromise

Large burn scars of the chest and abdomen – INTEGRA also useful in this situation

Extremity expansion, especially lower limb, associated with more complications

Expansion of myocutaneous pedicled and free flaps

- increases volume of tissue transported
- facilitates donor site closure

Complications

Migration – less with textured expanders

Extrusion

Infection

Rupture

Wound dehiscence

Choice of expander

Consider shape of defect, site of defect and type of flap to be used

Make the largest pocket possible and chose the expander base size to fill this pocket

Expand to the limits of patient tolerance

Check the available amount of expanded skin by subtraction of base size from the circumference of the expanded skin

Cyclic loading

Gibson. *BJS* 1965

Apply load to skin → stretches

Remove load → relaxes back

Apply excessive load → stretches without subsequent relaxation

Creep vs. stretch

Wilhelmi. *Ann Plast Surg* 1998

Dermal collagen is a mixture of types 1 and 3 collagen

Type 1 collagen synthesis decreases with ageing

Mechanical creep is the elongation of skin under a constant load over time

- collagen fibres stretch out and become parallel
- microfragmentation of elastin
- displacement of water
- occurs during intra-operative tissue expansion and skin suturing under tension

Biological creep is the generation of new tissue secondary to a persistent chronic stretching force – the type of creep seen in pregnancy and conventional TE

Stress–relaxation describes the tendency for the resistance of the skin to a stretching force to decrease when held at a given tension over time

- skin tight when expanded
- next visit skin no longer tight

Molecular basis for tissue expansion

Takei. *PRS* 1998

Mechanical stretch → activation of signal transduction pathways (via protein kinase C receptors) → increased DNA synthesis and cell proliferation – activation of transcription factors *c-fos*, *c-jun* → gene expression

PDGF has been shown to mediate in strain-induced cell growth

Changes in the binding properties of adhesion molecules to the extracellular matrix

Stretch-induced opening of ion channels including calcium → signal transduction and effects on the cytoskeleton (microfilament contraction)

Vascular supply of expanded skin

Increased vascularity and blood flow

Neo-angiogenesis due to expression of VEGF; Lantieri. *PRS* 1998

Radiotherapy effects on expanded skin

Goodman. *Plast Reconstr Surg* 2002

Study in rabbits to investigate effect of radiotherapy upon the skin overlying a tissue expander and upon the surrounding capsule

External beam radiotherapy administered 3 weeks after expander placement

- half of the expanded area treated, the other half acted as an internal control
- three treatment groups receiving 20 Gy, 25 Gy or 35 Gy in unfractionated doses

Animals euthanased at 2 months and histological assessment of skin and capsule undertaken

Results:

- dermal thickness and the surrounding capsule remained unchanged
- epidermal thickness increased to up to 130% in the highest radiation dose group

Molecular and physiologic influences on tissue expansion

De Filippo. *Plast Reconstr Surg* 2002

The mechanism of stretch induces molecular events in tissues that mediate in cell growth and regeneration (the stretch-induced signal transduction pathway) leading to:

- increased DNA synthesis and cellular proliferation
- up-regulation of growth factors such as EGF, PDGF and TGF-β
- increased cellular sensitivity to insulin

Mechanical strain modulates the extracellular matrix

- increased collagen synthesis

Changes in the cell membrane and cytoskeleton

- reduced cell–matrix adhesion due to deformational forces acting on the cell membrane and disruption of integrins
- actin cytoskeleton transmits mechanical forces intracellularly resulting in mitosis via interaction with protein kinases, second messengers and nuclear proteins
- conformational changes in membrane proteins allow for the influx of extracellular calcium through ion channels resulting in activation of signal transduction pathways such as phospholipase C (catalyses the activation of protein kinase C – potent signal tansducer)
- mechanical strain also shown to induce transcription of cellular proto-oncogenes such as *c-fos*, *c-myc* and *c-jun* while stretch-induced cell growth and proliferation preserves normal cellular morphology without evidence of malignant transformation

Biomechanical comparison between conventional and rapid skin expansion

Zeng. *Br J Plast Surg* 2003

Investigation of the biomechanical properties of rapidly expanded compared with conventionally expanded skin in a canine model

Rapid expansion regime

- expansion daily for 2 weeks

Conventional expansion regime

- expanded weekly for 6 weeks

Maintaining time after expansion

- 1 week, 2 weeks or 4 weeks

Results

- no difference in total area of skin expansion
- biomechanical properties of rapid and conventionally expanded skin are similar
  - stress–strain

- stress–relaxation
- tensile strength
- creep
- stretch–back ratio in both groups approach values of control skin after a maintaining time of 4 weeks

Conclusion

- rapid expansion can be undertaken to provide skin with similar biomechanical properties to conventionally expanded skin
- a 4-week maintaining time optimizes the stretch–back ratio

Tissue expansion in children

Tissue expansion in children – complications
Friedman. *PRS* 1996
9% overall complication rate in 82 patients
Internal (rather than remote) ports were associated with a higher complication rate (puncture)
Risk factors were burn scar surgery, soft tissue loss, age <7 years
?Lack of co-operation in the <7 years age group

Tissue expansion in children – complications
Gibstein. *Ann Plast Surg* 1997
Indications
- congenital naevus
- craniofacial anomalies
- aplasia cutis congenita
- myelomeningocoele

17% of 105 patients had complications (as above)
Traditionally accepted that there is a higher incidence of complications in children of ~20–40%

Calvarial deformity and remodelling following tissue expansion in a child
Calobrace. *Ann Plast Surg* 1997
Scalp expander → pressure → bone resorption and deformity: 'saucerization'
Case report of a 5-year-old boy undergoing scalp expansion for burn scar alopecia over 15 months
3 cm deep depression created in the calvarium
Bone lipping (deposition) at the margins
Reversible changes: fully remodelled by 6 months
Similar cases reported including full-thickness calvarium erosion
Burn scar is unyielding and so may transmit more pressure to the calvarium

Algorithm of hair restoration in children
Kolasiński. *Plast Reconstr Surg* 2003
Aetiology of hair loss in childhood
- congenital alopecia
- post-natal haematoma

- trauma including burns
- surgical scars
- irradiation for CNS neoplasms

Scalp skin in a child

- more pliable and responsive to expansion (but scars stretch more)
- less subcutaneous fat
- hair more sparse and widely separated

McCauley classification of hair loss

  I. single defect
- subtypes A–D depending upon size of defect (25% increments)

  II. segmental defects (2)

  III. multiple defects, multiple islands of intact scalp

  IV. total scalp loss

Treatment options

- excision with direct closure
- scalp flap reconstruction
- tissue expansion
  - cases of extensive hair loss (type IB,C,D, type II)
  - consider direction of hair growth when moving flap(s)
- hair transplantation
  - smaller areas of hair loss (type IA)
  - useful in cases of multifocal hair loss (type III below)
  - also useful for thinned hair after radiotherapy

Tissue expansion in the limbs

Tissue expansion in the lower limb

Manders. *PRS* 1987

Expanders at least as long as the defect to be closed

Placed **above** muscle fascia

Incisions perpendicular to the long axis of the expander are safest

Over-expand or expand as long as the patient tolerates it

Full advancement achieved by a back-cut in the **capsule**

High complication rate including 50% infection rate

Avoid expansion adjacent to open wounds at the knee

TE at or below the knee is much less successful than TE in the thigh

Use the other leg to guide the amount of extra skin generated

Tissue expansion in the lower limb

Vogelin. *BJPS* 1995

Vasculature in the leg is of the 'terminal' type with few axial vessels

Poorly formed subdermal plexus

TE placed above the deep fascia

Contraindications in the lower limb:

- extensive areas of scarring
- poor vascularity
- osteomyelitis

Incorporate a delay to the intended expanded flap (excluding incision of the capsule)

High local complication rate

Tissue expansion at limb and non-limb sites

Pandaya and Coleman. *Br J Plast Surg* 2002

Review of 113 expansion procedures in 88 patients

- 31 expansion procedures in limbs
  - performed under tourniquet where possible
- short incision for expander and port, radial to direction of expansion
- intra-operative expansion with saline and methylene blue
  - methylene blue useful at subsequent expansion to confirm correct needle placement in port
- non-limb expansion mainly for breast reconstruction
- limb expansion for post-traumatic scarring and other contour deformities

Complications: infection and exposure

- limb sites
  - overall complication rate 43%
  - more complications in the lower compared with upper limb
- non-limb sites
  - overall complication rate 27%
- exposed or infected expanders managed by hospitalization, antibiotics and dressings until healed and then further expansion was commenced
  - some expander complications were unresponsive to conservative management → expander removal after rapid expansion and judicious use of expanded tissue

Outcome

- successful outcome similar at limb and non-limb sites (83% and 86%)

Tissue expansion in the lower limb: complications in a cohort of 100 patients

Casanova. *Br J Plast Surg* 2001

Review of 103 expansion procedures (207 expanders) in the lower limb in 95 patients

- 54% remote internal valves
- 46% external valves

Complications

- sepsis, exposure, damage due to undermining
- complications recorded in 16 patients (15.5%)
  - expansion abandoned in 5 patients

Expander selection and placement

- avoid bony areas, joints, scars or irradiated skin
- place expanders in a longitudinal direction, multiple expanders preferable
- remote radial incisions
- atraumatic blunt dissection above fascia
- external ports:
  - risk of exposure of internal valves due to rigidity of port, thinness of overlying soft tissue and shearing forces associated with repetetive motion
  - prevent port failures (leakage)
  - but increased risk of infection
- use a plaster of Paris splint to immobilise joints in the post-operative period

Flaps

- advancement flaps preferred to transposition flaps

Self-filling osmotic tissue expander

Ronert. *Plast Reconstr Surg* 2004

Expander made from an osmotically active hydrogel

Manufactured to 10% of its final volume

Absorbs tissue fluid gradually to achieve final size over 6 to 8 weeks

Obviates the need for an inflation port, painful injections and regular clinic attendances for expansion

May be used for breast skin expansion prior to replacement with a silicone implant

- may be left *in situ* for up to 6 months before replacement
- requires healthy skin/muscle coverage
- unsuitable in previously irradiated areas

Also suited to other conventional tissue expansion indications, e.g. scar revision, alopecia, pre-expanded free or pedicled flaps

Results in 55 patients (75 expanders):

- visual analogue scores of pain showed discomfort abating after the early postoperative period
- wound dehiscence occurred in 4 patients and led to a modification to the expander with a silicone membrane to limit the rate of expansion

Lower limb trauma and reconstruction

Anatomy

Tibia bears 85% of the weight

Anterior compartment

- EHL
- EDL
- tibialis anterior
- peroneus tertius
- nerve – deep peroneal nerve
- artery – anterior tibial A
- main function – dorsiflexion

Lateral compartment

- PL
- PB
- nerve – superficial peroneal
- artery – peroneal A
- main function – eversion

Posterior compartments

- superficial
  - gastrocnemius
  - plantaris
  - soleus
- deep

- FHL
- FDL
- tibialis posterior
- nerve – tibial nerve
- artery – posterior tibial A
- main function – plantar flexion

Sensation
- lateral calf – sural N
- medial calf – saphenous N
- dorsum of foot – superficial peroneal N
- first web space – deep peroneal N
- sole of foot – medial and lateral plantar Ns from posterior tibial N

Sole of the foot

Layer 1
- abductor hallucis
- flexor digitorum brevis
- abductor digiti minimi

Layer 2
- flexor hallucis longus
- flexor digitorum longus
- lumbricals
- flexor accessorius

Layer 3
- flexor hallucis brevis
- adductor hallucis
- flexor digiti minimi brevis

Layer 4
- interosseii

Medial and lateral plantar nerves between layers 1 and 2

General considerations

'Debridement' described first by Pierre-Joseph Desault (1744–95) in the treatment of traumatic wounds

Sequential advances in lower limb trauma with the introduction of:
- debridement
- bone fixation
- antibiotics/asepsis
- vascular repair
- soft tissue coverage
- flaps of choice:
  - gracilis – long, thin defects, no need to turn
  - rectus – long, thin defects
  - latissimus – wide defects

Gustillo and Anderson compound tibial fracture classification

I – clean wound <1cm

II – wound 1–5 cm but no significant tissue disruption

IIIA – wound >5 cm but adequate soft tissue coverage with local tissues

IIIB – extensive soft tissue loss, contamination, periosteal stripping

IIIC – arterial injury requiring repair

Mangled extremity severity score (simplified)

Skeletal and soft tissue injury

- low/medium/high/very high energy
- multiple fractures
- contamination

Limb ischaemia

- pulseless but perfused
- pulseless, prolonged capillary refill
- devascularized

Shock

- no hypotension
- transient hypotension
- sustained hypotension

Age

- <30 years
- 30–50 years
- >50 years

Arnez and Tyler classification of degloving injuries

BJPS 1999

Type 1 – non-circumferential degloving

Type 2 – abrasion but no degloving

Type 3 – circumferential degloving

Type 4 – circumferential degloving plus avulsion between deep tissue planes

- intermuscular planes
- muscle–periosteum

Type 4 injuries require **serial conservative debridements** and delayed reconstruction – early radical debridement → functionless limb

General management

Adhere to ATLS principles of immediate management

Determining salvagability of the limb:

- is revascularization needed?
  - consider angiograms on-table for assessment of vascular status
  - is revascularization technically possible?
- is the soft tissue defect treatable with local flaps or free flaps?
- is there bone loss? Is this reconstructable?
- is there nerve injury?
  - does this preclude a functioning limb?
  - results of nerve repair and grafting in the lower limb are poor except in children

Reconstructive plan:

- reduce and stabilize the fracture (this alleviates vasospasm)
- restore perfusion by arterial reconstruction if necessary

- perfusion may be temporarily restored before fracture stabilization with the use of vascular shunts
- definitive vascular reconstruction before fracture stabilization can become disrupted during fracture manipulation/fixation
- fasciotomy (crush, reperfusion)
- debridement of all non-viable tissue and pulsed lavage under tourniquet – dark muscle, no contraction, no bleeding = dead
- soft tissue cover

Amputation

- BKA (6 cm below the tibial tuberosity) vastly superior to AKA in terms of rehabilitation
- may need to consider free flap salvage for a BKA stump – best suited tissue is a pedicled fillet of sole flap – best sensation – or a free sole flap with nerve repair

Fracture management in compound lower limb trauma

- IM nailing
  - reamed nails with proximal and distal locking
  - difficult in comminuted fractures
  - very stable → early mobilization
  - unreamed nails avoid disruption of the endosteal blood supply
- internal fixation
  - exacerbate periosteal stripping
  - infection risk
- external fixation
  - method of choice
  - Orthofix, Ilizarov frames
  - may get pin track infections
  - allows easy access for repeated debridement
  - site pins carefully – avoid compromising local flap options

Management of bone gaps

Non-vascularized bone graft

- small defect
- well-vascularized graft bed
- wait 6–12 weeks post-trauma before introducing non-vascularized bone graft into the defect

Vascularized bone graft

- complex reconstruction in the early post-trauma phase
- DCIA, free fibula
- large segmental defect >8 cm
- bone and soft tissue free flap cover required
- transferred fibula hypertrophies with use

Ilizarov techniques

- useful where the traumatic bone gap is 4–8 cm
- limb **shortening** followed by **distraction osteogenesis**
  - compensates for inadequate soft tissue for primary closure
  - also used as a limb lengthening technique in the established shorter limb
- limb **held to length** followed by **bone transport**
  - corticotomy to develop the mobile segment – preserving medullary and periosteal blood supply

- need adequate soft tissues or must be able to close the defect with a free flap
- avoids soft tissue contracture in the shortened limb
  - muscle atrophy
  - joint contracture and stiffness
  - disuse osteoporosis
- latent period of ~5 days following corticotomy before commencing distraction
- one-quarter turn QDS lengthens 1 mm/day
- bone must be healthy
- monitor rate of distraction by serial X-rays – avoid premature fusion or the appearance of lucency indicating that distraction is too fast
- at the required length leave the frame for ~2 months to allow for consolidation of the distracted segment
- complications
  - leg length discrepancies
  - refracture
  - pin track infections
    - minimize tension at the interface between pin and skin
    - recalcitrant infection may necessitate removal of the wire
  - incomplete docking/non-union requiring secondary bone grafting
- physiology of distraction histogenesis
  - tension–stress effect – tissues under tension respond by forming more tissue (regeneration)
  - distracted bone regenerates by intramembranous ossification orchestrated by the periosteum – osteoblastic differentiation of periosteal mesenchymal cells
  - hence not analogous to endochondral ossification, which occurs at a fracture site
  - in patients with bone dysplasia – fibrous dysplasia – new bone is also dysplastic hence cannot use this technique (but osteogenesis imperfecta **can** be so treated)

	Ilizarov	Free fibula
Time to full mobilization	18 months	18 months
Secondary fracture	Can nail	Cannot nail
Technique	Safe, quick	Difficult, slow, flap failure
Donor site	None	Morbidity fairly high

Soft tissue closure

Fracture/soft tissue defect	Flap options	Comments
Upper third	Proximally based FC flap	First described by Ponten
	Gastrocnemius muscle	Medial and/or lateral
	Free flap	
Middle third	Proximally/distally based	Perforators of peroneal A or posterior tibial A
	FC flap	
	Soleus muscle	
	Free flap	

Fracture/soft tissue defect	Flap options	Comments
Lower third	Distally based FC – can be islanded for greater arc of rotation to reach the ankle	Perforators of peroneal A or posterior tibial A
	Adipofascial turnover flap	Better donor defect than FC flaps in young female patients
	Sural artery island flap sacrifices the nerve and is small and unreliable	Based on a small artery and vein supplying the sural nerve
	Free flap	
Ankle/heel	Distally based islanded FC flaps as above	
	Medial plantar island flap	Based on a cutaneous branch of the medial plantar A, sensate with medial plantar
	Dorsalis pedis flap	FC flap based on DPA used as pedicled or free flap
	Free flap	

Healing by secondary intention (Paineau)
- no local flap option, patient unsuitable for free flap surgery
- drill cortex and keep moist to encourage granulation tissue formation, then SSG
- may take 3–4 months to heal

Primary closure	– Gustillo I and II
SSG	– Gustillo IIIA
FC flap	– Gustillo IIIA and B (but beware raising within a degloved area)
Free flap	– Gustillo IIIB
Cross-leg flap	– poor solution: immobilization (DVT, contracture) and need a well-vascularized recipient site

Radial artery forearm flap can be used as a flow-through flap for revascularization of the distal extremity

Distally based FC flaps based on posterior tibial A perforators.
- main perforators are 6 and 12 cm above the medial malleolus
- situated in the intermuscular septum between soleus and FHL
- venous drainage via VCs accompanying the perforating artery
- using the 12 cm perforator allows for a greater arc of rotation to reach the ankle

Timing of free tissue transfer
Advantages of early or emergency cover of the open fracture:
- less infection
- fewer operations

- shorter hospitalization time
- earlier mobilization
- lower treatment costs

Emergency free flap – at the time of first debridement, <24 h

Early – 24–72 h post-injury

Delayed ≥ 72

Recipient vessels:

- posterior tibial artery is usually well protected and is the best option for a recipient vessel (end–side)
- anterior tibial A is usually compromised by the trauma
- geniculate vessels in the popliteal fossa
- vein grafts to the SFA in the femoral canal
  - perform the proximal vein graft anastomoses before detaching the flap
  - leave the vein graft as a loop, then divide and anastomose to donor vessels

Chronic osteomyelitis

4.5% incidence in Gustillo III fractures

Risk minimized by thorough debridement

Investigations:

- plain X-rays
- bone scan
- wound swab/culture
- arteriography

Treatment:

- radical wound debridement (soft tissue and sequestrum)
- bone graft the bone defect (free or vascularized)
- rigidly immobilize
- microvascular transfer of muscle (brings its own good blood supply)
- antibiotics – local delivery systems/systemic for 2–6 weeks

BAPS/BOA working party report on open tibial fractures

BJPS 1997

Early cooperation between senior plastic and orthopaedic surgeons

About one-fifth of open tibial fractures occur in a multiply injured patient

Open tibial fractures occur in ~23/100 000 patients per year

Half of these fractures are Gustillo grades IIIA or B

~4% are Gustillo grade IV – these often proceed to amputation so rarely involve plastic surgery input

~70% of Gustillo grade IIIB injuries require flap cover (F/C, muscle, free flap)

Examine the wound once in casualty, polaroid photograph, dress and leave dressed until theatre

Fractures classified as high or low energy

High energy fractures

- have a poorer prognosis
- features in the history
  - RTA
  - fall from a height

- missile injuries
- clinical signs
  - large/multiple wounds
  - crush or burst lacerations
  - closed degloving
  - signs of nerve or vascular injury
- radiological signs
  - multiple bony fragments
  - more than one fractured bone in the same limb
  - widely spaced fragments
  - segmental injury

Open tibial fractures should be closed by a maximum of 5 days

- wound excision and fracture stabilization
  - diaphyseal open tibial fractures – IM nail
  - metaphyseal open tibial fractures – ex-fix or plate
  - negotiation of pin sites to avoid compromise of F/C flaps or free flap pedicle
- soft tissue reconstruction ideally as soon as possible – wounds closed within 72 h have highest success rate/lowest complication rate
- 6 litres normal saline pulsed lavage
- patient must be fit enough for reconstructive surgery

Immediate closure is not always required – delayed closure may enable serial debridements and compartment monitoring

Signs of compartment syndrome – see Chapter 5 – nerve injury

Gustillo grade IIIB fractures may be complicated by compartment syndrome – the skin wound does not necessarily adequately decompress the compartment and other compartments may also have increased pressures

Incidence of compartment syndrome in Gustillo grade IIIB injuries ∼6%

Fasciotomies should be placed anterior to the line of perforators both medially and laterally to preserve F/C flap options

- anterior and lateral (peroneal) compartments decompressed via a lateral incision
- both posterior compartments decompressed via a medial incision

Consider early amputation

- use of injury severity scores
- prolonged ischaemia
- nerve injury (insensate foot)
- multiple level injury
- avoids psychological trauma of late amputation

Degloved skin can be harvested as a SSG on the day of injury and stored

Colour and contractility of muscle as a predictor of viability may be unreliable

Islanded distally based flaps in the lower limb

Erdmann. *BJPS* 1997

FC flaps replace like with like in the lower limb

66 flaps based on perforators of the posterior tibial artery (medial)

Used preferentially in males and older females

Suitable for IIIB fractures but 20% of flaps in these patients were lost completely

Three-quarters of flaps closed lower-third defects

Also capable of filling Achilles/heel defects

Exploration of perforators rather than Doppler

Unsuitable where there has been vascular injury or degloving

Perforators emerge between soleus and FHL (NV bundle deep to soleus)

Sited at 6, 9 and 12 cm above the medial malleolus

Skin paddle between the long and short saphenous veins

Drained by VCs to the perforating arteries

Can rotate the skin paddle through 180°

Heavy smokers suffered more tip loss

Flaps raised on lateral perforators from the peroneal artery are less reliable because of the larger number of perforators: more must be divided to create the required arc of rotation

Midline approach to the posterior tibial artery

Godina. *PRS* 1991

Midline muscle splitting approach through gastrocnemius and soleus

Wide exposure of the posterior tibial artery

Facilitates end–side anastomosis, preserving blood supply to the foot

Avoids anastomosis at a site which is within the zone of trauma but is temptingly more superficial

Also offers decompression of the posterior compartments

Short saphenous vein and sural nerve, both lying in the midline, are retracted – can be harvested as grafts if necessary

Distal extent of incision stops at the Achilles tendon

After anastomosis the muscles are approximated but fascia is not closed to avoid compartment syndrome

Angiography before free flap reconstruction

Dublin. *Ann Plast Surg* 1996

23 patients with normal distal pulses → one case of abnormal angiogram

15 patients with abnormal distal pulses → all had abnormal angiograms

No need to perform angiography if distal pulses are intact

The fate of lower extremities with failed free flaps

Benacquista. *PRS* 1996, Discussion by Francel

Failure rate in trauma patients ~10% – mainly Gustillo IIIB and C

Failure rate in non-trauma patients ~7%

Commonest cause of failure was venous thrombosis – occurs later than arterial thrombosis by which time granulation tissue has formed beneath the flap allowing for SSG

Subgroup of patients with tibial fractures had a 35% amputation rate after a failed free flap

Timing of surgery did not affect rate of failure – no worse in those flaps performed on day 1 compared with later time points

- contrasts with Godina:
  - <72 h → <1% failure
  - >72 h → 12% failure

Overall ~80% of patients with a failed flap had their limb salvaged by other methods (SSG, local flap or a second free flap)

Seven patients had a second free flap – this failed in three but was successful in four

Vessel spasm, scarring and granulation tissue may make later reconstruction more difficult – may need vein grafts

High failure rate for acute free bone flaps – close the soft tissues first and leave bone reconstruction for later

Patients undergoing complex limb salvage, compared with primary amputation:

- take longer to full weight bearing
- less likely to return to work (salvage 25%, amputation 60%)

Lower limb salvage using parts from the contralateral amputated leg

Southern. *Injury* 1997

Two case reports

Large sections of skin harvested on septocutaneous perforators leading to the anterior and posterior tibial arteries and anastomosed to recipient vessels in the salvaged limb

Free flaps also help to maintain maximum length of an amputation stump

Vein, artery, nerve, split skin and bone grafts may all be harvested as spare parts

Comparison of bone transport and distraction-lengthening

Saleh. *J Bone Joint Surg* 1995

Bone transport more suited to **larger defects** in which shortening would be fairly dramatic and may have deleterious effects on soft tissues and joints

Hence distraction lengthening more suited to **smaller defects** and is generally simpler

Bone transport can also be followed by a period of distraction after docking

Bifocal lengthening is distraction occurring by the movement of two ends of the bone away from the central diaphyseal segment

Average time to union following bone transport was 16 months, 10 months for lengthening (but smaller defects)

After distraction, some patients also needed bone graft to aid consolidation

Union at the docking site was occasionally problematic after bone transport (leading edge may be relatively avascular or obstructed by soft tissues)

Other complications mainly related to pin track infections

Bone transport involves the wires cutting through soft tissues – may need skin releases under LA

Cross leg free flaps

Chen. *J Trauma* 1997

Performed when a free flap is required but there are no suitable recipient vessels and vein grafts are inappropriate

Cross leg pedicle flaps may also fail to provide the right volume or tissue type

In young patients only

Salvage manoeuvre

Latissimus dorsi, rectus abdominis, DCIA and parascapular free cross leg flaps have all been reported

Eight flaps in this series, average period of cross-leg fixation 24 days although muscle flaps require ~4 weeks at least

One of eight flaps failed

Cross clamp the pedicle to determine when it is safe to divide it – when the flap can tolerate the pedicle clamped for 1 h

Flap relies upon neovascularization for its blood supply

No significant joint stiffness

Reconstruction of the lower extremity after ablative resection for cancer

Walton. *Surg Oncol Clinics N Am* 1997

Commonest malignancy of the lower limb is skin cancer (SCC, MM)

One-third of all sarcomas arise in the lower limb

- malignant fibrous histiocytoma and liposarcoma are the commonest
- sarcomas require compartmental resection of composite tissues
- external beam radiotherapy or brachytherapy offer some benefit postoperation
- prerequisites for reconstruction
- patient accepting of multiple operations and lengthy hospitalizations
- surgical margins must be free of tumour
- must be able to expect reasonable function to avoid amputation
  - pain-free ambulation with a sensate foot
    - intact posterior tibial nerve
    - stable knee with good extension
    - good limb length

Consideration of the defect

- what tissues are missing?
- what is the functional significance of this?
- soft tissue defects closed using local or distant flaps as for traumatic defects
- bone defects require free fibula or DCIA vascularized bone flap or a distraction technique
- nerve reconstruction using autologous nerve graft only an option in children or young adults

Reconstruction in children

- epiphyses open → potential for growth
- resection of a growth plate → progressive limb length discrepancy over time – epiphyses at lower end of femur and proximal tibia (i.e. around the knee) are responsible for ~70% of limb growth and are common sites for lower limb sarcoma
- need to transfer vascularized bone with a growth plate but none really available – hence consider distraction-lengthening or bone transport

Lower extremity microsurgical reconstruction

Heller and Levin. *Plast Reconstr Surg* 2001

General principles covered in this tutorial:

- consider the defect and choose flap to address size of defect, contour, length of pedicle required, etc.
- nerve injury does not preclude salvage if distal enough
- advanced age not a contraindication to free flap salvage
- complex injuries with nerve damage may rehabilitate faster with an amputation
- initial treatment focuses upon thorough wound debridement and bone stabilization

- consider angiography for extensive wounds, especially if recipient vessels are potentially compromised
- anastomoses outwith the zone of injury preferable
- aim for soft tissue closure by day 5–7
- principles of microsurgical reconstruction applied to patients with osteomyelitis and extremity soft tissue and bone sarcoma
- free tissue transfer in diabetics (large vessels unaffected) facilitates radical debridement of chronic wounds where a useful limb can be salvaged
- bone gaps less than 6 cm managed predominantly by Ilizarov techniques; greater than 6 cm may necessitate vascularised bone grafts (fibula, iliac crest)
- compromised flaps demand immediate exploration for salvage
- failed free flaps should be debrided and consideration given to a second free flap

Long-term behaviour of the free vascularized fibula following reconstruction of large bony defects

Falder. *Br J Plast Surg* 2003

Retrospective review of 32 free fibula flaps

- Age range 8–61 years
- Mean length of bone gap 12 cm
- Mean length of harvested fibula 18 cm
- Three double-barrelled flaps
- Five osteocutaneous flaps, remainder all bone flaps
- femur (13) and tibia (8) formed largest group
- most indications either trauma (14) or tumour (13)
- trend towards Ilizarov bone fixation

Flap survival

- 29/32 flaps survived

Flap hypertrophy was assessed radiographically

- flap hypertrophy due to mechanical loading and periosteal vascularity
- hypertrophy was equivalent in patients treated for trauma and tumour
- greater hypertrophy in the lower limb group (more loading)
- median hypertrophy 71% (range 0–316%)
- age not a significant factor

Bone union

- 74% bone union achieved
- median time to union 4.75 months

Stress fracture

- Six stress fractures (21%)
- Four required plating and bone grafting
- Double barrelled flaps less likely to suffer stress fracture
- Triangular cross-sectional shape is resistant to angular and rotational forces

Ipsilateral free fibula transfer for reconstruction of a segmental femoral shaft defect

Erdmann. *Br J Plast Surg* 2002

The authors describe a technique for transferring a free fibula flap to a bone defect in the ipsilateral femur

The flap is raised and inset in to the bone defect, temporarily clamping the peroneal vessels after division in the lower leg

A sphenous vein graft is then harvested from the same leg

An interpositional vein graft loop is tunnelled between the flap pedicle and the site of detachment in the lower leg – the peroneal vessels thereby become the donor vessels

This avoids the requirement to identify and dissect donor vessels at the site of flap inset

Limb salvage using a free gracilis flap

Redett. *Plast Reconstr Surg* 2000

Series of 50 patients requiring gracilis free flap reconstruction of acute (22 patients) and chronic (28) lower limb soft tissue defects

Indications:

- Gustillo IIIb (48 patients)
  - Acute 20 wounds
  - Chronic 28 wounds
    - Osteomyelitis or deep soft tissue infection
- Gustillo IIIc (two patients, both acute wounds)

Outcome

- 19/22 successful limb salvage in acute trauma setting
  - 3 flap losses (2 in IIIc injuries)
- 26/28 flap survival in chronic wound setting
- donor site complications in 5/50 patients
  - infection, haematoma, seroma
- flap loss greater in smokers and IIIc injuries

Free flap reconstruction of chronic traumatic lower leg wounds

Gonzalez. *Plast Reconstr Surg* 2002

38 patients reviewed over an 11-year period

- open lower leg wounds, mean duration 40 months
- 23 patients had established osteomyelitis
  - localized 15 patients
  - diffuse in 8 patients
- 36 patients underwent pre-operative angiography
  - abnormal in 13 patients
- free flaps (38 primary reconstructions, 4 repeat flaps):
  - latissimus dorsi (27)
  - rectus abdominis (11)
  - gracilis (3)
  - lateral arm (1)
  - average of 2.3 debridements before flap reconstruction
- Outcome
  - eight flap losses
    - three due to infection
    - four patients had a repeat free flap (all survived)
    - two patients underwent amputation
    - five patients had normal angiograms, in three patients angiography was abnormal

- six patients had chronic osteomyelitis (diffuse in three)
- successful reconstruction finally achieved in 33 patients

Diffuse chronic osteomyelitis and an abnormal angiogram increased risk of flap failure

Use of vein grafts recommended to ensure anastomoses are performed outside of the zone of trauma or vicinity of the chronic wound

Classification of osteomyelitis

Cierny and Mader. *Orthopaedics* 1984

1. Superficial
2. Localised
3. Diffuse
4. Medullary

> **Self-assessment: A 50-year-old self-employed farmer has been knocked over by a car. He has a compound fracture of his right tibia. Describe how you would assess this patient and his injuries and formulate a management plan**

First priority is the airway with C-spine control

Continue with a primary survey, treating life-threatening injuries, and then a secondary survey

Once the patient is stable, take a history and examine the limb

Senior plastic surgery and orthopaedic input required jointly (BAPS/BOA working party report)

History (beyond AMPLE):

- time and mechanism of injury – high energy vs. low energy
- previous health
  - drugs
  - allergies
  - PMSH including diabetes
  - social history – married, smoker, alcohol
  - systems review
  - tetanus status

Examination

- concomitant injuries identified during primary and secondary surveys
- degree of soft tissue injury/loss
- degree of bone injury/loss
- vascularity of the limb
- sensation in the limb
- assessment for compartment syndrome

Investigations

- AP and lateral X-rays
- angiography if pulseless following fracture reduction

From the history, examination and investigations the following are determined:

- Gustillo and Anderson grade of injury
  - I – <1 cm wound
  - II – 1–5 cm wound
  - IIIA – >5 cm wound, closes with local tissues

- IIIB – extensive periosteal stripping or contamination
- IIIC – vascular injury
- Mangled extremity severity score
  - degree of injury
  - duration of ischaemia
  - shock
  - patient age
- Arnez and Tyler degloving type
  - non-circumferential degloving
  - abrasion
  - circumferential degloving superficial plane
  - circumferential degloving deep plane
- salvagability of the limb
  - bone and soft tissue injuries are reconstructable
  - circulation is intact or can be restored
  - limb remains sensate (children → can graft)
- suitability for salvage
  - concomitant life-threatening injury
  - needs and wishes of the patient – earlier return to work if amputated (e.g. self-employed farmer)

Management of the bone
- no bone loss – reduction and stabilization, external fixator versus unreamed IM nail
- bone defect <4 cm, options – autologous bone graft >6 weeks
- defect 4–8 cm, options – shorten limb and distract later
- defect 8–12 cm
  - hold out to length and bone transport – problems include docking non-union requiring bone graft
  - hold out to length with external fixator and reconstruct secondarily with vascularized bone flap (preferred flap – free fibula)
- defect >12 cm – hold out to length with external fixator and reconstruct secondarily with vascularized bone flap (free fibula)

Management of the soft tissues – preferred options
- upper third – medial gastrocnemius and SSG
- middle third – fasciocutaneous flap – medial perforators
- lower third – free flap

Examples of the author's preferred free flaps
- big defect – latissimus dorsi muscle flap and SSG (in lateral position to avoid turning)
- medium defect – rectus and SSG
- smaller defect – gracilis and SSG
- sole of foot – free lateral arm flap (sensate – lateral cutaneous nerve of the arm)

Preferred anastomoses
- end–side posterior tibial vessels

Preferred timing of surgery: within 72 h of injury

Diabetic Foot

Sensory neuropathy → loss of protective sensation

Motor neuropathy → derangement of joints → pressure sores over metatarsal heads

Autonomic neuropathy → dry, cracked skin → infection
Peripheral vascular disease → tissue hypoxia → infection
Decreased cellular and humeral immunity → infection

Prevention
Effective glycaemic control
Chiropody/diabetic foot care regimes

Management
Wound debridement including bone where necessary (osteomyelitis)
Systemic antibiotics
Hyperbaric oxygen
Revascularization if the ulcer is predominantly ischaemic
Amputation/arthrodesis:
- amputation of non-viable toes
- amputation at level of TMT joints – Lisfranc
- amputation at level of talonavicular joint – Chopart
- amputation just above the ankle joint – Symes
- MTP joint arthrodesis for dorsal ulceration as a result of motor imbalance

Soft tissue closure:
- trial of dressings to allow healing by secondary intention
- granulation tissue may accept a SSG
- consider local flap options first, e.g. medial plantar flap or distally based FC flaps to heel defects
- free flaps to larger defects – dorsum of foot – FC free flap, e.g. lateral arm
  - heel/ankle
    - FC or muscle plus SSG
      - muscle flaps less bulky than myocutaneous flaps
- **SSG just as stable**

Pressure sores

Pure pressure sores begin with tissue necrosis deep near the bony prominence leading to a cone-shaped area of tissue breakdown with its apex at the skin surface
Worsening this situation is the soft tissue damage caused by moisture, infection, shear forces, etc. (see below)
~10% of patients in acute care facilities develop pressure sores (mainly sacral)

Risk assessment
Daily assessment in every patient
Waterlow score
- body mass index
- age/sex
- continence
- mobility
- nutrition
- skin changes

- adverse wound healing factors
- neurological deficit
- surgical intervention(s)
- drugs (steroids, cytotoxics, etc.)

Pathogenesis

Stages

- hyperaemia
- ischaemia
- necrosis
- ulceration (ultimately Marjolin's)

Unrelieved pressure → ischaemic necrosis

- tissue P > perfusion pressure
- muscle more susceptible than skin
- proportional to pressure and duration

Altered sensory perception

- incontinence and exposure to moisture
- friction and shear force – shear forces can lead to subcutaneous degloving
- infection → deepening of the sore

Grading of pressure sores

1. Erythema
2. Blistering
3. Subcutaneous muscle breakdown
4. Bone/joint involvement

But this does not reflect the underlying extent of the sore

Position of the patient

Supine patient → sacral and heel sores

Sitting → ischial sores

Lying on one side → trochanteric sores

Management

General

Optimize nutrition

Correct anaemia

Prevention and treatment of infection

Catheterize to avoid exposure to moisture if incontinent

Relieve pressure by regular turning and a suitable bed

- effective pressure relief for 5 min every 2 h
- relief of spasm – baclofen
- treatment of contracture – Botox, tenotomy, **amputation**

Dressings

Sloughy – saline soaks or betadine soaks

Deep cavity – betadine sorbsan

Ulcers – intrasite gel and/or hioxyl (if sloughy)

Topical rhPDGF and FGF – experimental use only

Surgery

'Oncological' debridement of the sore (including osteomyelitis)

Excision of bony prominences

Wound closure with healthy tissues

Direct closure if no tension but in general avoid leaving the suture line in the area of pressure

Maintain future flap options

TE brings in healthy **sensate** tissue and is a fairly well tolerated but prolonged treatment

Free flaps a last resort for large defects or where local options have been exhausted

- recipient vessel – superior gluteal A
  - curvilinear buttock incision
  - reflect gluteus maximus
  - vessel diameter ~5 mm
- free flaps include latissimus dorsi myocutaneous flap

Ischial pressure sores

Commonest sores in paraplegics – sitting in wheelchairs

The most difficult sore to treat

Posterior thigh FC flap (medially or laterally based)

- based upon the descending branch of inferior gluteal A
- rotation
- transposition + SSG

TFL – sensate (but distal third unreliable and may not reach)

Gracilis (but flimsy flap)

Hamstring V–Y advancement – based upon the descending branch of inferior gluteal A

Pedicled VRAM flaps can be used for recalcitrant/recurrent sores of the ischium and trochanter; Kierney. *PRS* 1999

Trochanteric sores

TFL

Lateral thigh FC flap

- posteriorly or anteriorly based
- first lateral perforator of the profundis femoris A

Rectus femoris

Sacral sores

Buttock rotation flap(s)

- can be re-raised and advanced further if sore recurs
- straightforward and reliable

V–Y gluteus maximus myocutaneous flap – but burns bridges – cannot be re-raised

S-GAP flap pedicled on a perforator of the superior gluteal A (below)

Gluteus maximus muscle flap

- upper half of the muscle supplied by the superior gluteal A, lower half by the inferior gluteal A
- exposure of the muscle using a buttock rotation flap incision
- detach insertion on the femur and reflect muscle as a turn-over flap into the sacral defect

- needs SSG
- can be used to close lower lumbar defects

Gluteus maximus rotation flap

- as for buttock rotation flap but raised in the plane between gluteus maximus and medius
- origin of the muscle is divided off the gluteal surface of the ilium and the edge of the sacrum to allow rotation into the defect
- arc of rotation may be limited by the superior gluteal vessels – these can be divided and the flap will survive on the inferior gluteal vessels

Complications

Haematoma

Infection

Dehiscence

Recurrence

Beds

Clinitron – optical beads fluidized by warm air

Mediscus

- low air loss
- cells which inflate and deflate independently
- GORTEX material → evaporative fluid loss to keep patient dry

Electronic mattresses

Pegasus – alternating pressure system

Nimbus – dynamic floatation system

Closure of lumbosacral defects using perforator-based flaps

Masakazu. *PRS* 1998

Use of the S-GAP flap pedicled upon its dominant perforating vessel

Lumbar perforators may also be used to distally base a skin paddle for closure of large defects

Pre-operative assessment and postoperative rehabilitation of patients with pressure sores

Kierney. *PRS* 1999

High rate of recurrence (40–60%) may be reduced by optimizing rehabilitative care (25% in this study)

Skin care optimized pre-operation (general management – above)

2–3-week period of immobilization on a clinitron bed, during which time patients receive physiotherapy

Then a graduated 7–10-day sitting programme finally achieving three periods of sitting per day, each lasting 4 h – pressure-relieving manoeuvres every 15 min while sitting

Patient education

Long-term outcome of pressure sores – sites and flaps

Yamamoto. *PRS* 1997

FC flaps – posterior and lateral thigh (ischial sores) and buttock rotation and S-GAP flap (sacral sores)

Muscle flaps – TFL, rectus abdominis and gracilis (ischial) and gluteus maximus (sacral)

Concepts in sore management:

- ischial sores → large dead spaces → more likely to need muscle flaps
- sacral → smaller dead space → FC flap

but:

- **fasciocutaneous flaps → less recurrence than myocutaneous flaps**
  - muscle flaps provide good early cover
  - but muscle becomes atrophic
  - and muscle is more susceptible to ischaemia
  - all pressure points in the body are naturally covered by skin-fascia not muscle

Conclusion:

- muscle flaps are inadequate for the surgical management of pressure sores in the long-term
- ischial sores → slightly higher recurrence than sacral sores

Gluteal V–Y flap

Ohjimi. *PRS* 1996

Conventional gluteus maximus V–Y requires mobilization of the insertion ± origin of the muscle which sacrifices function in the ambulant patient

This method raises a V–Y skin paddle but the medial portion is elevated in a FC plane

This alone provides the mobility required to reach the midline with the muscle advanced as a result

> **Self-assessment: Discuss the management of a patient with an ischial pressure sore**

History: how did the sore develop?

- duration of history
- current dressings – improving or worsening?
- cause of unrelieved pressure?
  - paraplegia?
  - poor bed mattress at home?
  - poor chair cushion?
  - insensate area?
- cause of macerating forces?
  - urinary incontinence?
  - faecal incontinence?
- difficulty in turning?
  - help at home?
  - upper body weakness?
- poor nutrition?
  - average calorie intake
  - weight gain/loss
  - smoking
  - drinking
- adverse drug factors?
  - steroids (MS)
  - immunosuppressants
- adverse medial conditions?

- diabetes
- general fitness for surgery

Examination of the sore and the patient

- general body habitus – poor nutrition?
- presence of a urinary catheter
- posture – **contractures**?
- sore itself:
  - position of sore
  - size of sore
  - grade of sore
  - clean vs. infected
  - bony sequestrum
  - scars – local flaps may already have been used

Investigations

- bloods – albumin, FBC, ESR, U and Es, glucose
- wound swabs
- X-ray to identify bony sequestra

Planning and treatment within the context of a multidisciplinary team environment

Nursing staff → Waterlow grade and turning, dressings, care of other pressure areas

Community nurse → provision of a mattress at home

Physiotherapist → treatment of contractures, mobilization, passive joint movement

Occupational therapist → provision of gel cushions

Dietician → dietary assessment and optimize nutrition

Treatment options

- dressings until healed
- VAC pump ± surgery
- surgery
  - oncological principles
  - debridement of bony sequestra and spikes
  - vascularized tissue cover
    - individual flap options
    - do not burn bridges
    - no pressure for at least 2 weeks post-operation
    - use of drains and antibiotics

Discharge only after home assessment and mattress in place

Ischial pressure sores: a rationale for flap selection

Foster. *Br J Plast Surg* 1997

A review of the management of 139 ischial pressure sores in 114 patients

Ischial sores most difficult pressure sore to treat

Most commonly used flap for reconstruction

- inferior gluteus maximus island flap
  - also had highest success rate
  - first reported by Mathes and Nahai, 1979
  - Modified by Scheflan (*PRS* 1981) and Stevenson (*PRS* 1987)
  - A trunk-based flap that allows for ischial reconstruction while avoiding tension generated by hip flexion

Other flaps used:

- gluteal thigh flap
- hamstring V–Y
- TFL
- Gracilis

Mean time to healing 38 days

Complications in 37%

- Wound edge dehiscence
- Partial flap necrosis
  - Gracilis (3/16)
  - TFL (5/12)
    - Distal part of flap too unreliable for coverage of the ischial area
    - Delay to the tip of the flap increases viability
    - Can also consider expansion prior to transfer
  - V–Y hamstring (2/12)
- Wound infection

Predictors of poor outcome

- Large sore size
- Previous flap history
- Adverse wound healing factors
  - Elderly
  - Smokers
  - Diabetes
  - Local or systemic infection
  - Immunosuppression
  - Poor nutritional state

Management of pressure sores by constant tension approximation

Schessel. *Br J Plast Surg* 2001

The authors describe their management of chronic pressure sores by:

- wound excision
- partial suture
- dressing
- constant low grade tension Proxiderm device
  - acts on subcutaneous tissues
  - principle of internal tissue expansion

Contraindications

- inflamed wound
- deep cavity
- excessive wound discharge
- persistent faecal contamination of wound

Sores treated:

- sacral/ischial (15/23 healed)
- trochanteric (10/12 healed)
- heel (13/14 healed)

Time to healing measured in days (range 5–42)

Avoids major surgery in a debilitated patient

Reconstruction of paediatric pressure sores

Singh. *Plast Reconstr Surg* 2002

Surgical management of 25 sores in 19 patients at the Children's Hospital of Philadelphia reviewed

Pressure sore risk factors in this series included:

- spina bifida
- cord injury
- cord tumour

Sores treated:

- ischial
- sacral
- trochanteric
- iliac crest

Myocutaneous flap reconstruction:

- gluteal flap
- posterior thigh flap
- total leg flap

Recurrence at mean follow-up of 5.3 years in 15 patients

- 5% at the same site
- 20% at another site

Necrotizing fasciitis

Mixed anaerobe and Group A streptococcal infection – group A *Streptococcus* carried in nose/throat of 15% of the population

Mortality rate up to 53%

Risk factors

IDDM

NSAID (most correlation)

Varicella zoster virus infections

Pathogenesis – production of

Pyrogenic toxins

Haemolysins

Hyaluronidase

Streptokinase

Clinical features

No obvious entry portal

Local swelling, redness, intense pain

Very rapid spread subcutaneously

Systemic toxicity

- apathy

- confusion
- septic shock
- elderly may be unable to mount a pyrexia

Dusky hue, areas of purple necrosis

Management

Clindamycin (also stops the production of toxins) and imipenem

Radical surgical debridement

ITU supportive therapy

- ventilation/oxygenation
- inotropic support where necessary
- dialysis

Necrotizing fasciitis of the face and neck

Sepulveda. *PRS* 1998

Dissemination of infection through tissue planes causing thrombosis of blood vessels

Violaceous skin changes and haemorrhagic bullae

Fascial necrosis more extensive than overlying skin changes

Crepitus and anaesthetic zones

Mixture of *Streptococcus, Staphylococcus*, Gram-negative bacilli and anaerobes

May follow pharyngeal or tonsillar abscesses

Extensive debridement, systemic antibiotics, hyperbaric oxygen

Vital structures in the head and neck makes radical debridement difficult

More commonly affects abdominal and thoracic walls and perineum (Fournier's)

Gas gangrene

Similar onset, sick patient

Surgical emphysema (crepitus)

Bloody blisters: aspirate → *Clostridium (C) welchi* (Gram-negative bacilli)

Aggressive surgical approach

Some evidence to support role of hyperbaric oxygen

High mortality

Necrotizing fasciitis of the breast

Shah. *Br J Plast Surg* 2001

The authors present a case of necrotising fasciitis affecting the breast necessitating expedient surgical debridement amounting to mastectomy

Diagnosis based upon clinical features with a high index of suspicion

Crepitus due to gas forming organisms diagnosed by aspiration Gram stain microscopy:

- Gram +ve cocci – peptostreptococci
- Gram +ve rods – clostridia
- Grame –ve rods – coliforms

Delayed reconstruction indicated several months after the acute episode

Vacuum-assisted closure

First described by Argenta. *Ann Plast Surg* 1997, Banwell. *J Wound Care* 1999

Aims to convert a wound into one that may be healed by a lesser surgical procedure than before

125 mm Hg subatmospheric pressure – **higher pressures →collapse of vessels and decreased blood flow**

Removes chronic oedema from tissues

- facilitates oxygen delivery
- wound fluid also inhibits fibroblast and keratinocyte activity and contains matrix metallo-proteins responsible for collagen breakdown
- analogy with hypoperfusion in the zone of stasis in Jackson's burn wound model

Encourages formation of granulation tissue

Increases local blood flow – **sucking blood through vessels?**

Decreases bacterial colonization – clinical infection at 10^5 organisms g^{-1} tissue

Encourages wound contraction – **analogous to tissue expansion relying upon creep**

World-wide licence belongs to KCI (Kinetic Concepts, Inc.)

Evacuation tube within a polyurethane foam dressing tailored to fit the wound precisely

Airtight seal created by overlying occlusive dressing

Vacuum pump connected via a canister for collection of wound 'effluent'

All non-viable material should be debrided from the wound before vacuum therapy either surgically or using debriding dressings

Dressings are changed every 48 h (at which point the wound is cleaned with copious irrigation before application of a new foam dressing)

Fungating tumour is the only contraindication to therapy – increased blood flow may → increased growth

Can be used in the community

Technique may be used to secure SSG at continuous subatmospheric pressures of 50–75 mm Hg for 4 days

If used on the abdomen, separate abdominal viscera from Marlex mesh using omentum then apply VAC device

Pressure sores (stages III and IV) and chronic, subacute and acute wounds – intermittent therapy (5 min on/2 min off) used for all chronic wounds after the first 48 h – **cyclical loading phenomenon?**

- included wounds with exposed orthopaedic metalwork and exposed bone
- large volumes of exudate may be removed – up to 4 litres/24 h – so monitor fluids and electrolyte balance
- acute wounds respond more rapidly than chronic wounds

Venous ulcers

- need lower pressures ~50 mm Hg
- continuous rather than intermittent
- cultured keratinocytes or SSG applied to granulating tissue

Complications

- pressure necrosis of adjacent skin if the patient lies on the vacuum tube
- pain – mainly related to venous ulcers → turn down the suction

- over-granulation → ingrowth into sponge and traumatic dressing changes with bleeding
- late infection is rare and due to inadequate debridement

Topical negative pressure (TNP) for treating chronic wounds

Evans. *Br J Plast Surg* 2001

TNP removes interstitial fluid and exerts a mechanical deformational forces upon the extracellular matrix and upon cells

Animal studies have demonstrated increased local blood flow, accelerated granulation tissue formation and a decrease in bacterial count

Systematic review of studies entered on the Cochrane Wounds Group Specialist Trials register evaluating TNP in the management of patients with chronic wounds:

Only 2 randomised controlled trials published and examined in detail:

- Joseph *et al. Wounds* 2000
  - Significant reduction in wound volume at 6 weeks in favour of TNP
- McCallon *et al. Adv Wound Care* 2001
  - Decreased time to healing in favour of TNP

Both studies provide weak evidence in support of TNP compared with saline gauze dressings as both are open to criticism over potential selection and observer bias

Conclusion: little current evidence base to support TNP and more randomized controlled trials are required

VAC in the management of exposed abdominal mesh

Vooght. *Plast Reconstr Surg* 2003

Four patients treated by VAC for abdominal wall dehiscence after hernia surgery exposing prosthetic mesh

wound debridement undertaken prior to application of the VAC

Three/four patients avoided mesh removal

- One patient failed to heal but was receiving chemotherapy

mean time to healing with VAC 24 days

Two patients needed a split skin graft

VAC in the management of sternal dehiscence

Harlan. *Plast Reconstr Surg* 2001

VAC well established in the management of sternal dehiscence

- stabilizes the wound improving the mechanics of ventilation
- removes exudate and bacterial contamination
- reduces the size of the defect in preparation for flap reconstruction
  - superiorly pedicled VRAM
  - pectoralis major flap

But sponge adherence to the epicardium, great vessels or bypass grafts remains a hazard

- authors describe use of a silicone sheet sutured to the underside of the sponge to prevent adherence

VAC in the management of lower extremity wounds with exposed bone

De Franzo. *Plast Reconstr Surg* 2001

Continuous negative pressure (minus 125 mm Hg) used in the management of 75 patients with open wounds on the lower limb exposing bone or orthopaedic metalwork

VAC therapy preceded by wound debridement, often serial, until necrotic tissue was eliminated

- wounds inspected and dressings changed every 48 hours

Rapid decrease in limb oedema within 3–5 days

Successful wound closure in 71/75 patients

- delayed primary closure in 12 patients
- split skin graft in 58 patients
- local musculocutaneous or fasciocutaneous flap in 5 patients

Wounds remain stable at up to 6 years follow-up

Index